The Therapist's Use of Self
in Family Therapy

The Therapist's Use of Self in Family Therapy

Daniel A. Bochner, Ph.D.

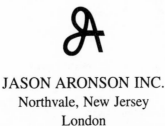

JASON ARONSON INC.
Northvale, New Jersey
London

This book was set in 11 point Times by Pageworks of Old Saybrook, CT and printed and bound by Book-mart Press, Inc. of North Bergen, NJ.

Library of Congress Cataloging-in-Publication Data

Bochner, Daniel.
    The therapist's use of self in family therapy/ by Daniel Bochner.
        p. cm.
    Includes bibliographical references and index.
    ISBN 0-7657-0248-7
    1. Family psychotherapy.   2. Countertransference (Psychology).
    RC488.5 .B635 2000
    616.89'156—dc21   99-055415

Printed in the United States of America on acid–free paper. For information and catalog write to Jason Aronson Inc., 230 Livingston Street, Northvale, NJ 07647-1726, or visit our website: www.aronson.com

For Mary Jo, Henry, Owen,
and my family of origin

Contents

Preface

The process involved in this study has been therapeutic. I have been caught within the general scheme of it for some time now. The divisions within the field of family therapy had always bothered me, and what began as frustration and simply wondering why there would be so much conflict, over time became a desire to integrate theories and knowledge so that those divisions would not be necessary. On a personal level I recognize all of this as connected to my childhood desires to solve conflicts within my family and within myself, which probably resulted in my choice of career as well. And it reminds me that sometimes our own conflicts are also our strengths. I have tried to be understood here. I have thought about my reader and I have considered what tactic to take in presenting the material within. I am afraid that the lengths I went to in detailing many perspectives will bore some readers, but I like the fact that those perspectives can be found here. I have struggled with the clarity of my writing at the same time that I have struggled with the clarity of my ideas. At times my own feelings of being overwhelmed have been projected into my readers because I reacted to those feelings by going into more explanatory detail, and by providing a grand scope, which made me feel satisfied with my completeness rather than overwhelmed. I only hope that my efforts will be valued for their therapeutic potential, and that the bulk of information and the difficulty of some of the material will not be overwhelming for the reader, as they once were for me.

This book comes at a time when there is a wide proliferation of new ideas on how to treat patients. My colleagues are trying to figure out ways to treat patients more quickly but just as meaningfully as has been done in long-term psychotherapy models. Although this book is about family therapy, most of the ideas for integrating analytic and systems models came from analytic theory. Analytic theory, of course, provides the most prominent viewpoint for doing long-term psychotherapy. For this reason it becomes important to say that these newer models presume an understanding of analytic theory that has never been adequately presented in any one context. Rather, for most practitioners, the study of analytic theory must come together over time in some cohesive, personal fashion. One of the most important attributes of this book is that my own personal integration of analytic theory is presented in a cohesive manner within these pages. This integration, which is most systematically presented in Chapter 6, but is used as the viewpoint throughout the book, is perhaps the only integration of its kind. While all practitioners using analytic theory must come to their own integration, this particular integration is the only one I am familiar with that is fully compatible with systems theories and developmental research, and which fits an experiential way of working. I present it to you, in this nascent form, with the suggestion that it holds great potential as a unifying theory.

The totalistic view of countertransference as defined by Winnicott (1949) and described by Kernberg (1976) was the initial inspiration for this project. In doing family therapy I had often wondered about the therapist's part in the therapeutic system. Family therapy is, of course, a very emotional situation, and I have not been immune to strong emotions in its practice. Plainly stated, the totalistic view of countertransference naturally leads to understanding the therapist as part of the therapeutic system. The task from there, however, was to explain how countertransference makes the therapist a part of the system, how the therapist's part in the system is systematic, and how those particular points are helpful. I believe this task has been accomplished in this integration. The totalistic view of countertransference, a concept unknown to most family therapy practitioners, allows for integration in a field where so many unnecessary walls exist between different understandings of the subject. We know, however, that if we are describing the same subject, the subject of humanity and mental health, there must be vast similarity in what is being said. Sometimes it seems that it is merely language getting in the way.

In concluding this preface, I would like to offer my grand vision for the book which places family therapy in a general psychotherapy context. When reviewing the development of the therapist's use of the self in family therapy, it is impossible to ignore the overall effect of family therapy's growth away from analytic thinking. In its own development, it seems family therapy needed to differentiate from its parent. In that differentiation many new paths were followed and much new ground was broken. In the meantime, however, the analytic parent became a wise old grandparent, learning new approaches inconceivable in its early adulthood. By ignoring this parent now, family therapy has much to lose. Fortunately, some of family therapy's children are returning to their analytic grandparent. Sometimes the grandparent's teachings are taken as gospel. At other times the children are confident enough to retain their own knowledge and continue to learn from the grandparent's teachings. This study is an addition to that integrationist approach. It is hoped that the broad use of the word countertransference, discussed here as the use of the self, will help to integrate analytic and systems thinking without the fear that either one must overcome the other. Thus, this study aims for a healthier family therapy family in which every generation plays a part.

Acknowledgments

I would like to acknowledge several people who provided emotional sustenance and/or help during the life of this project. My family has been a great inspiration. My wife, Mary Jo, is always there to continue the work, and my sons, Henry and Owen, are living proof that the work is worthwhile. The members of my family, in their interaction with me, provide daily instruction on core concepts. I thank my parents, Sheldon and Sandra or Mom and Dad, for fostering my two most prized therapeutic attributes, kindness, and the desire for understanding. I thank my four brothers for insuring in me a healthy amount of self-doubt, yet confidence in interpersonal conflict. I would also like to thank my closest adviser in this project, Stephen J. Schultz, for showing me a path and guiding my journey. I thank several friends who read my work and gave instructive feedback, including Dr. David Goldberg, Dr. Cliff Weller, and Dr. Mark Lessard. Finally, I would like to thank whatever power it is that motivates me and allows me to gain new insights. It is truly wonderful to feel that life is a wonder.

1

Introduction

The concept of countertransference has evolved in the psychoanalytic literature and now holds great potential for integrating clinical approaches. Its importance has been elevated from an obstacle to be avoided (Freud 1910) to a tool that is often very useful in understanding the patient (Heimann 1950, Kernberg 1965, Little 1951, Racker 1953, 1957, Sandler 1976, Winnicott 1949). The therapist's use of the self—the use of countertransference—refers to the therapist's emotional reactions. These emotional reactions become a tool when they are recognized as being related to certain characteristics of the client or client-family as well as of the therapist, instead of reflecting the therapist's idiosyncrasies alone. In the family therapy literature this broader understanding of countertransference has been neglected. Only a few family therapists have considered it (Ackerman 1959, Framo 1965, Luepnitz 1988, Nichols 1987, Scharff 1991, Scharff and Scharff 1987, Shapiro 1981, Skynner 1981, Slipp 1984, 1988). By applying this broader view of countertransference to family therapy more extensively than has been done in the past, this study hopes to shed new light on the therapist's role.

From a perspective that includes this broader view of countertransference, the therapist must be viewed as within a therapist–family system. And from within the therapist–family system, I will argue that if all the therapist's emotional reactions are considered to be representative of his part in that system, the use of the self—or the use of countertransference, is unavoidable. I will also argue that, although many therapists do use countertransference intentionally, they do not use it as effectively or as widely as is warranted, given its value. This study aims to demonstrate this new perspective for family therapy by integrating systems approaches and psychoanalytic thinking. From this perspective, which will be referred to as the *relational systems perspective*, the use of countertransference always occurs, whether the therapist intends its use or not. However, intentionally using countertransference, with an understanding of the relational systems perspective, is practicable and especially powerful. It is hoped that the views advanced here will help family therapists intervene at intrapsychic as well as interpersonal and systemic levels. The recognition that countertransference is always involved in therapy can enhance any therapist's ability to intentionally implement an effective use of self.

In this opening chapter I will introduce several key contentions that will lead to a better understanding of how countertransference is used—and can be better used—in family therapy. What has been called the "totalistic" definition of countertransference (Kernberg 1965) has been associated with the use of this response as a tool in psychotherapy, and will be differentiated from the classical view of countertransference as exclusively problematic. A brief discussion of the lack of discourse about countertransference in family therapy, and some of the reasons for its absence, will lead to several arguments in support of the position that the totalistic definition of countertransference is essential to a full understanding of the family therapy paradigm. I will show how the application of the totalistic definition unavoidably leads to the conclusion that countertransference is used at least unintentionally by all therapists. And I will argue that acceptance of the unintentional use of countertransference is especially necessary in family therapy, where the therapist's activity makes her personality an integral part of the treatment situation. From the relational systems perspective, unintentional uses of countertransference are a regular part of the therapeutic process. The therapist can acknowledge her unintentional use of countertransference as well as intentionally use countertransference reactions to enhance the treatment approach.

THE CLASSICAL AND TOTALISTIC DEFINITIONS

In the family therapy literature most articles on countertransference have been written by a minority of authors who accept psychodynamic principles (Ackerman 1959, Carr 1989, Framo 1965, McElroy and McElroy 1991, Nichols 1987, Pittman 1985, Pollak and Levy 1989, Reynolds and Levitan 1990, Scharff 1991, Scharff and Scharff 1987, Shapiro 1981, Shay 1992, Skynner 1981, Slipp 1984, 1988, Springer 1991, Stierlin 1977, Wallerstein 1990). Even in those papers where psychodynamic principles are accepted, often the definition of countertransference employed is limited to a focus on its problematic aspects (Carr 1989, Halperin 1991, McElroy and McElroy 1991, Pittman 1985, Pollak and Levy 1989, Reynolds and Levitan 1990, Shay 1992, Stierlin 1977). But limiting the definition of countertransference in this way obscures its potential importance to family therapy.

The limited view of countertransference is typically referred to as the "classical" definition derived from the work of Freud (1910). In Sandler's (1976) words, according to Freud "countertransference is 'an obstruction to the freedom of the analyst's understanding of the patient'" (p. 43). In this view, countertransference feelings need to be analyzed out of the analyst as a precondition for doing analysis.

A broader definition of countertransference has since become common in the psychoanalytic literature. It has been called *totalistic countertransference* by Kernberg (1965), who included in it "the total emotional reaction of the psychoanalyst to the patient" (p. 38). The idea that countertransference could be a source of information was first discussed by Winnicott in 1949. Beginning in 1950 other psychoanalytic authors suggested that countertransference could even be useful as well as informative (Heimann 1950, Little 1951, Racker 1953, 1957, Sandler 1976). Kernberg's term "totalistic countertransference" summarized what these authors had been discussing. Winnicott's definition of countertransference, although he advocated it before Kernberg called it "totalistic countertransference," in my view continues to be the most useful definition yet conceived.

Winnicott (1949) differentiated three parts of countertransference. He saw it as consisting of (1) emotional reactions that occur due to the therapist's unresolved conflicts, (2) unconscious aspects of the therapist's personality that help him be therapeutic, and (3) emotions that occur as objective reactions to the personality or behavior of the patient. The information gained in the objective reactions, spelled out in the third part of his definition, was Winnicott's primary focus. Other contributors to the literature on the totalistic notion of countertransference also emphasized objective reactions and elaborated on the best ways to use them (Heimann 1950, Little 1951, Racker 1953, 1957). It is important to note, however, that in the first part of Winnicott's totalistic definition, the Freudian view of countertransference is clearly included. It is the second part of Winnicott's definition, which includes aspects of the therapist's personality that, although unconscious, help him do therapeutic work, that addresses a part of therapy that is seldom even recognized but is nonetheless essential. Using this totalistic definition, countertransference can be viewed as informative, useful, and unique to every therapist, as well as problematic. Which view is correct for a particular therapy at a particular time depends on what has evoked the countertransference response, and the way the response is handled by the therapist.

Only a smattering of articles in the family therapy literature adopt a similar definition (Ackerman 1959, Framo 1965, Luepnitz 1988, Nichols 1987, Scharff 1991, Scharff and Scharff 1987, Shapiro 1981, Skynner 1981, Slipp 1984, 1988). However, using the totalistic definition, it appears that various schools of thought within the field of family therapy have many different ways of describing what might be considered countertransference phenomena. Within these schools, the use of countertransference as I am viewing it is often implicit in the way the work is described, rather than being explicitly called "using countertransference." In fact, based on the totalistic definition (especially the second part of Winnicott's definition), it is possible to say that countertransference is *always* used in *any* therapy. The therapist uses countertransference whenever his emotional reaction is involved in the therapeutic process. The therapist cannot avoid having emotional reactions to patients, and those emotional reactions are inevitably related to the interventions the therapist uses and the way the therapist acts.

THE ABSENCE OF "COUNTERTRANSFERENCE" IN FAMILY THERAPY

Perhaps the timing of family therapy's emergence is a primary factor in understanding why the current psychoanalytic understanding of countertransference has not been thoroughly explored in family therapy. Family therapy began around 1950. In that year Nathan Ackerman published his paper "Family Diagnosis: An Approach to the Preschool Child" (Ackerman and Sobel 1950). In 1954 Gregory Bateson's Project for the Study of Schizophrenia received a grant for studying the communication of schizophrenics; he was soon joined by Don Jackson. Also in 1954, Murray Bowen was seeing family members of schizophrenics at the National Institute of Mental Health (NIMH) as part of his research on interaction in schizophrenic families. Headed by Lyman Wynne, another branch of family researchers at the NIMH was working with schizophrenic families and in 1958 Wynne and associates published the now famous paper "Pseudomutuality in the Family Relations of Schizophrenics."

Many of family therapy's founders, including Jackson, Theodore Lidz, Salvador Minuchin, Virginia Satir, Carl Whitaker, and Wynne, received training in psychoanalytic methods before branching off into family therapy. However, as indicated above, the notion of totalistic countertransference was only beginning to be articulated within the psychoanalytic literature around 1949. Thus, at the moment when psychoanalytic therapists were just beginning to discuss the totalistic definition of countertransference, family therapy was already breaking away from the individual therapy model. As a result of this breaking away, much of the psychoanalytic theory that had been developed in treating the individual was discarded by family therapists.

Since the totalistic view of countertransference has become so widespread within contemporary analytic theory and practice, one might expect that family therapists who maintained a psychodynamic approach would have introduced it within the family therapy literature long ago. However, although there have always been psychodynamic therapists within the family therapy movement, only recently has a totalistic understanding of countertransference been widely advocated by them. Such a view has emerged within the work of psychodynamic family therapists beginning in 1981 (Box et al. 1981, Luepnitz 1988, Nichols 1987, Scharff 1991, Scharff and Scharff 1987, Shapiro 1981, Skynner 1981, Slipp 1984, 1988). But currently, while psychodynamic family therapists are finally embracing the totalistic definition of countertransference, very few other therapists within the family therapy movement are doing so.

The time during which family therapy developed is clearly one major factor in understanding why family therapists have not often considered a totalistic approach to the use of countertransference. Two other factors contribute as well. One of these is that using countertransference intentionally may appear to require analyses of multiple countertransferences to parts of a family as well as to the family as a whole, resulting in extreme complexity. The high level of therapist activity typically involved in family therapy might further complicate dealing with this complexity.

A second and alternative explanation is equally compelling. Perhaps family therapy is, in fact, discussing the use of countertransference, but is using other words to describe it. As structural and strategic methods for family therapy have gained preeminence, there appears to have been not only a lack of knowledge about psychodynamic thinking, but also a desire to leave psychodynamic concepts behind. This desire is clearly evident in articles like the popular one by Madanes and Haley, "Dimensions of Family Therapy" (1977). It has its theoretical underpinnings in the erroneous assumption that psychoanalytic theory is based exclusively on the linear thinking that is apparent in Freud's (1905) libido theory (Watzlawick et al. 1967). Regardless of its origin, however, it seems that the desire to leave psychodynamic thinking behind might be a factor making it unlikely that family therapy would refer to certain phenomena as "countertransference." Instead, family therapy is more likely to discuss similar phenomena with a new language. Thus the two issues that must be addressed here are (1) the complexity of using countertransference in the family therapy situation, and (2) the identification of other concepts in family therapy that seem related to the use of countertransference.

It is my view that the therapist's use of countertransference or use of self is, in general, very much a part of doing family therapy, in spite of the complexities involved. This is true even if other terms are at times used in describing it. Also, although these other terms for the use of countertransference can be identified in many schools of family therapy, I will demonstrate that countertransference is used to some extent in every school, even when the literature of a school has nothing in it that would suggest this use. The therapist's emotions are always part of the work, even though some schools of family therapy simply do not consider how they come into play when working with families.

THE INTENTIONAL AND UNINTENTIONAL
USES OF COUNTERTRANSFERENCE

That countertransference is used to some extent in every therapy is a consequence of the very inclusiveness of the totalistic definition. In considering countertransference as a part of every therapy, it is helpful to divide its use into two categories: the intentional use of countertransference and its unintentional use. The intentional use of countertransference is what most therapists using the totalistic definition discuss. With the conscious effort to self-reflect on one's emotions and their meaning in relation to a client or client-family, the intentional use of countertransference can lead to empathic interventions as well as to the feeling in the client or client-family that the therapist is able to handle the problems addressed in the therapy. But, as is indicated by the second part of Winnicott's countertransference definition, whether or not a therapist is aware of countertransference reactions, the interventions she formulates and uses are derived to some extent from countertransference feelings. The therapist at least partially responds to clients in a way that is based on her unique personality before it is possible for her to reflect on her perceptions or interaction. Thus even when the therapist is unaware of using her emotions, the way she reacts to a family's behavior has some effect on that family. To the extent that the therapist's feedback to a family, verbal or otherwise, is the result of her own emotional experience of the family, this feedback has been determined by countertransference, even if the therapist is unaware of such feelings.

The countertransference aspect of the therapist's response is useful only to the extent that it has contributed to a *therapeutic* stance. To the extent that that feedback is incongruent with therapeutic goals, the therapist's emotional reaction, or countertransference, will interfere with treatment. Moreover, it is important to clarify, in describing the unintentional use of countertransference, that it is possible for the therapist's expression of positive feelings to be destructive for the client and for the expression of negative feelings to be salutary. What is most important in the unintentional use of countertransference is that the therapist act in a way that is beneficial to the client. For example, sympathizing with a patient who is dangerously regressing might lead to further regression. Confronting that same patient might be very helpful in stopping the regression.

Using the countertransference response to move toward positive outcomes, but unintentionally, means the therapist must rely heavily on her tendency to think and act in ways that benefit the client without becoming completely aware of her internal motivation for thinking or acting in those beneficial ways. Thus another factor that will be addressed here is the difficult subject of the psychological functioning, or level of mental health, of the therapist. Although relying on the unintentional use of countertransference leaves room for destructive acts of the therapist, to the extent that the therapist's acts are constructive, such use can also be valuable.

Because family therapists are inevitably affected by countertransference in the totalistic sense (sometimes using it unintentionally), it would be beneficial for them to become aware of its value, and to use it intentionally to enhance family treatment. It seems most family therapists would agree that countertransference reactions are at times provoked when sitting with families. For example, systemic therapists (Palazzoli et al. 1978) discuss the avoidance of "suction" into the family. They attempt to avoid the acting out of countertransference feelings that can occur if one loses one's objectivity. Avoiding such acting out apparently requires a great deal of effort. But if one is faced with experiencing these feelings, why not intentionally use them as opposed to only avoiding the acting out associated with them? Even though a therapist can successfully use countertransference without doing so intentionally, making that use of countertransference intentional will improve the family therapist's ability to treat families.

There are many benefits to using countertransference intentionally. It is most commonly considered important for the therapist when it leads to empathic interventions in situations where such empathy is not common, and in handling emotions that are difficult to tolerate, an ability that, in itself, can be beneficial to a client or client-family. What is perhaps more intriguing to some family therapists is that the intentional use of countertransference brings with it, as is obviously necessary given concepts like "suction," partial control over the harmful acting out, or loss of objectivity, that sometimes results from countertransference reactions. Most important, however, if the therapist chooses to use countertransference intentionally, she can track the emotions of the family by experiencing them, and then formulate powerful interventions that incorporate both interpersonal and intrapsychic dimensions of the family's life.

By considering both the intentional and unintentional uses of countertransference within a totalistic view, it becomes evident that all therapists use countertransference. Because, at a minimum, the unintentional use of countertransference is evident in the work of all therapists, the integration of various family therapy concepts under the heading "countertransference" could prove fruitful for family therapists from many different schools of thought. And since the unintentional use of countertransference is a part of every therapist's approach, it is possible that every therapist can also use countertransference intentionally. That is, if the therapist is able to understand the emotional interaction that occurs between herself and family members, then that understanding can be put to use in formulating interventions. Using countertransference intentionally could prove fruitful even for therapists who maintain strategic, structural, experiential, or narrative approaches. The dynamics that are revealed can be universally related to any perspective on therapy.

THE TRANSFERENCE–COUNTERTRANSFERENCE SYSTEM AND FAMILY THERAPY

With an understanding of the intentional and unintentional uses of countertransference it becomes possible to envision a family therapy that integrates psychodynamic and systems perspectives. It is undeniable that in family therapy a particular kind of system is formed that includes both the therapist and the family. Some psychoanalytic family therapists have already described family systems as being constructed of a mass of projections and introjections (Bowen 1978, Scharff and Scharff 1987, Slipp 1980, 1984, 1988, Zinner and Shapiro 1972). Samuel Slipp (1984) has even described family systems as being made up of transference and countertransference manifestations. Essential to these perspectives is the fact that family members communicate expectations and mold one another's behavior through a mechanism of communication called *projective identification* (Scharff and Scharff 1987, Slipp 1980, 1984, 1988, Zinner and Shapiro 1972).

Projective identification, loosely defined, is an interpersonal and intrapsychic phenomenon in which a person, the projector, uncomfortable with certain emotions, behaves in a way that creates one-half of a dynamic between himself and another, thus evoking in that other a similar uncomfortable experience, and thereby allowing that experience to reside in the other while not being fully experienced by the projector. The therapist–family system also operates via projective identification. Just as transference and countertransference communicated through projective identification are essential in understanding family dynamics, they are also essential in understanding the therapist–family system. Families and therapists communicate expectations both consciously and unconsciously and mold each other's behavior through those expectations. By recognizing themselves as part of a system with families, therapists will be able to make better use of their own personalities as well as the deeply ingrained psychodynamics within families and their individual members.

Any of the therapies developed for working with families could benefit from access to interventions that address both interpersonal and intrapsychic dynamics at the same time. A very powerful way to gain access to such interventions is through an understanding of how the therapist's experience comes to reflect the singular way his personality interacts with the personalities, both aggregate and individual, of the family members with whom he works. From the relational systems perspective, the only possible obstacle to using countertransference effectively is that its intentional use requires in the therapist a well-ingrained and integrated knowledge of an interpersonal/intrapsychic theory that allows the therapist to recognize the process that has led to his emotional experience. Object relations theory will be used within this study because no other has been as well developed. The relational perspective within object relations theory (including intersubjective, two-person, and social constructivist views) will be emphasized because its interactive focus parallels the activity level of family therapy. Finally, the relational systems model will be offered as an integration of analytic and systems theories that fully accounts for the relationship between intrapsychic action and interpersonal interaction.

THIS STUDY

In summary, in this study I will argue that countertransference can and should be intentionally used in family therapy. In developing the relational systems perspective, it will be shown that countertransference is always used in therapy, whether intentionally or unintentionally. From this perspective, because the therapist's personal influence (and tendency to be influenced) must be accepted as an undeniable part of doing therapy that cannot be eliminated by inaction, it will be further argued that it is the therapist's responsibility to gain an understanding of that mutual influence. From within the therapist–family system, the therapist must self-reflect on her own contribution to the therapeutic interaction as well as on the contributions of the family or family members. The unintentional use of countertransference will always be present in every therapy and, when possible, the intentional, self-reflective use of countertransference should be considered an important tool in assessing and formulating interventions.

This study is organized into the following seven chapters. The first chapter is this introduction, where I have outlined my main premise. In the second chapter, I will discuss how the totalistic understanding of countertransference can already be found in the family therapy literature; I will also show that it has not been used to its full potential in any family therapy model. In Chapter 3, psychoanalytic perspectives related to the use of countertransference will be presented that demonstrate the movement within the analytic literature toward viewing the therapeutic situation as a transference–countertransference system. The fourth chapter is concerned with the analytic literature that pertains to aspects of using countertransference that make it therapeutic, with special emphasis on the therapist's empathy, personality, activity level, and boundaries. Chapter 5 is a foray into the small subsection of analytic family and group therapy literature that focuses on the connection between intrapsychic and family or group dynamics. In the sixth chapter, I will present the relational systems model, which integrates systems and analytic thinking in developing an intrapsychic model that is compatible with systems thinking. Finally, in Chapter 7 the application of the relational systems model will be shown to facilitate the understanding of countertransference and its use within the family therapy situation.

2

The Use of Self in
Family Therapy

THE EARLY WORK OF FAMILY THERAPY PIONEERS

Family therapy has taken several disparate courses since its inception. With
the advent of systems theory models in explaining family interaction, and
the experiential approach to treating families, a methodology emerged re-
putedly so different from psychodynamic methods and theories that, by
the 1970s, almost all psychodynamic thinking had become anathema to
the family therapy movement. However, even though psychodynamic theory
was discarded by most family therapists, many pioneers of the family
therapy movement had some psychoanalytic background. The fact that so
many family therapists did have that background suggests that a use of
countertransference would not be so foreign to many of them. In fact, there
is a solid foundation for connecting the use of countertransference, or the
use of self, to the primary impetus for the family therapy movement. Interaction between people, and the attempt at salutary intervention in that
interaction, is the focus of family therapy, just as it is in the use of countertransference. Several of family therapy's leaders have considered the
therapist a part of that interaction, and thus interpersonally integral to the
intervention.

In early family therapy, works published by clinical theorists from the
psychodynamic, experiential, and systems camps, clearly discuss the is-

sue of using countertransference, even though, in the case of the experiential and systems camps, the issue was less emphasized or entirely forgotten later. In the early work of Ackerman, Whitaker, and Jackson, the therapist's countertransference was considered an essential aspect of therapy. It should be no surprise that the work of Ackerman (1959), as representative of these psychodynamic family therapists, integrated uses of transference and countertransference. What is more surprising is that the foundation of Whitaker's (Neill and Kniskern 1982) early work involved a use of countertransference similar to that found in the work of those analytic therapists who have contributed to the psychoanalytic literature on the use of countertransference. Most surprising among these early works, perhaps, is that of Jackson (1956), conceivably the greatest influence in the systems therapy movement, who ardently believed that the use of countertransference was integral to the therapeutic process. I will begin with the work of Ackerman.

Nathan Ackerman

In 1966 Ackerman published *Treating the Troubled Family*, in which he included his 1959 paper on transference and countertransference. In his book, Ackerman distinguished the model Freud used with individuals from the view he was using with families. Of the Freudian model, Ackerman said that the "blank screen" requires that the therapist not fulfill the part of a real person. Therefore, the Freudian model does not provide the "architecture for a true social experience" (p. 101). "What happens the moment we join, conceptually, transference to countertransference?" Ackerman asked. He explained that intrapsychic and interpersonal phenomena mix together in a two or more person community where a circular interchange of emotions occurs between family and therapist. The transference and countertransference of a therapy become a testing of the real against the unreal. The family members and the therapist perceive each other based on their personal backgrounds, and the therapist attempts to judge his perception against reality in formulating interventions.

In discussing what to do with countertransference feelings that do occur, Ackerman (1966) stated, "The real issue is not whether the analyst has or shows emotions, but rather, which emotions are right and which wrong for the healing of the given patient" (p. 104). Generally, within this circular interchange of emotions, withholding of emotion is not helpful. Ackerman wrote, "The withholding of emotion on the [therapist's] part, therefore, the hiding of the [therapist's] real self, is no answer to the dangers of emotional contamination" (p. 105). He then asked rhetorically, "Is there a risk in the analyst's use of his own sense of self, and in the injection into the process of certain selected emotions?" and went on to answer, "Certainly there is. But nothing ventured, nothing gained. Risk is inherent in omission as well as commission" (p. 104). In these statements, Ackerman made it clear that in his view countertransference is used because it is an integral part of an interpersonal dynamic. When the therapist believes his emotional experience might help the client or family, that experience is offered.

Ackerman (1966) also discussed how the therapist accesses deeper involvement with a family, clearly indicating a use of countertransference.

> To achieve access in depth, the therapist uses as an instrument his own being, his own emotions as he experiences them. The emotions stirred in a therapist facing a family group are diagnostic, provided that the therapist can correctly read his own emotions. The thesis is a simple one. The emotions aroused in a therapist as he confronts a troubled family offer specific clues to the shared currents of feeling among the family members. That part of the therapist's own depth experience that pertains to his family feeling is especially relevant. He must be able to distinguish clearly which of his inner responses are his own private emotions toward family and which others are specifically induced by the unspoken, conflict-ridden feelings of the family sitting before him. [p. 110]

In this statement Ackerman made it unmistakable that he used his personality in a way consistent with psychoanalytic theory, yet in a way far more active and spontaneous than is typically associated with psychoanalytic work. He adjusted the knowledge he gained from psychoanalytic training to fit a therapy of interaction.

Carl Whitaker

The emphasis on spontaneity found in Ackerman's work is also essential in the work of Whitaker, but with Whitaker there is far less emphasis on self-reflection. His early work with schizophrenics and delinquent adolescents was the foundation of his philosophy of psychotherapy. It was in connection with his work with schizophrenics that Whitaker postulated that an interpersonal cure could take place if the therapist was willing to undergo a mutual regression with the patient. According to Neill and Kniskern (1982), two authors who chronicled and integrated Whitaker's work,

> [Whitaker's] strategy consisted in the therapist's replacing the mother as the symbiotic partner in the schizophrenic dyad. The therapist himself had to experientially replace her. He himself had to experience the "agony and ecstasy" of that mutually double-binding relationship. The difference was that the therapist was comfortable with the regression in himself. It was this very regression in herself that the biological mother feared and had defended against projectively, and which stabilized the schizophrenic dyad. Thus the therapist imposed a therapeutic double-bind in lieu of the pathologic one. [p. 16]

Although Whitaker believed the genetic antecedents to schizophrenia were to be found in the early experiences of the patient, he did not believe that the uncovering and working through of that experience were the curative factors in therapy. Rather, Whitaker (1946) guessed that it was the reworking within a relationship that would be curative. He did not believe that the therapist's knowledge of the patient's past or knowledge of forces within the patient's personality were important, but he emphasized the therapist's understanding of how to help an individual mature.

Whitaker's work thus differed from traditional psychoanalytic methods in that understanding the genetic cause of a patient's current malady was not emphasized. He did not consider this understanding important for either the therapist or the patient. At the same time, his work bore great similarity to the work that was concurrently being developed by the psychoanalytic theorists from the object relations school. Although object relations therapists do attempt to explore historical data, and employ a great deal more restraint in their approach than Whitaker, their emphasis too is on the interpersonal process of the therapeutic relationship. In their book, Neill and Kniskern (1982) compare Whitaker's work to an object relations approach. Central to this comparison is the use of countertransference via the processing of projective identifications.

> The therapist forces in himself an epigenetic series of complementary projective identifications we call "therapist." In this state, he experiences, by projective identification, the patient as his own (the therapist's) adolescent self. The patient internalizes this projection and becomes (i.e., experiences himself as) an adolescent. In this adolescent ego state, the patient then experiences (i.e., projectively identifies) the therapist as a sibling. The therapist, in response, begins to experience himself as a parent and projectively identifies the patient as his own child-self. The projection of the therapist's child-self onto the patient activates the patient's own child-self representation or imago, which is altered by the therapist's projection of his child-self. The most primitive pairing is that of the patient's child-self state and the therapist's "primordial parent state." In this process of exchanging projections, or partial counteridentifications in the language of ego psychology, the patient's self-images are repaired or polished, becoming more acceptable and more accessible to him, less likely to be split. [pp. 28–29]

It is evident in this excerpt that countertransference is being used. The therapist allows his own experience to match the patient's in the mutual regression. Further, it is the more mature development of the therapist that is expected to be beneficial to the client who did not have a relationship with an equally well-developed person as a child. Thus, although there is an intentional use of countertransference within Whitaker's work, it does not require self-reflection. Rather it is the therapist's willingness to take part in a natural process of experiencing a relationship at a very deep level that constitutes this use of countertransference. However, the emphasis on the therapist's better ability to cope with intense affects and impulses is an essential aspect to the therapy, and one that brings the therapist's psychological health into the picture. The process is very active, including handholding, arm wrestling, and even mutual face-slapping with schizophrenic patients (Neill and Kniskern 1982). The process includes whatever is activated in the therapist at the time of therapy.

Whitaker did not focus on understanding but emphasized the curative power of experience within a relationship. That same emphasis on process, including a natural use of countertransference without much self-reflection, has been evident in Whitaker's work throughout his career. However, self-reflection is not absent in Whitaker's therapy. According to Neill and Kniskern the use of a co-therapist allowed for self-reflection. With such teamwork in family therapy, "the therapists gained power in their ability to reflect and comment on both their own and the family's feelings and activities" (p. 17). Co-therapists would observe the process of a session and, with comment, pull each other away from enmeshment or taking sides, so that they could each observe their own process within the therapy.

Don Jackson

It is a surprise, given his place within the pantheon of family therapy, that among my grouping of Ackerman, Whitaker, and Jackson, it is Jackson who was most specific about the use of countertransference in his early work. In 1956, two years before co-founding the Mental Research Institute, Jackson published a paper called "Countertransference and Psychotherapy." Although this paper did not specifically address the issue of countertransference in family therapy, the interactive view espoused in it seems to indicate the way that Jackson might have thought about families if he had continued to advocate a psychoanalytic framework. In that paper Jackson described two views on the handling of countertransference: "I think the extreme right position would be held by those analysts who feel countertransference is a rather specific reaction on the therapist's part to unconscious aspects of the patient, and that the therapist needs to resolve the threat to on-going therapy by becoming aware of the conflict and suppressing any manifestations on his part that tend to erupt into action" (p. 235).

This definition closely resembles the classical stance. That is, the therapist must be aware of his own unresolved conflicts which, when evoked during a therapy, should be understood and controlled. Jackson in fact described his second view as such: "The extreme left position, which is the one I hold, states that countertransference is a too limited concept that does not do justice to the fact that the whole way of life of the therapist is very much in the room" (p. 235).

Jackson was making a statement here that is similar to what many psychoanalytic authors have written about the effect of the therapist's countertransference on the client (Atwood and Stolorow 1984, Balint and Balint 1939, Little 1951, Ogden 1994a,b, Searles 1958). Jackson believed that the client's perception of the therapist's personality and behavior is, in reality, not only a part of the client's transference but is often a reaction to who the therapist really is or what the therapist is really feeling. Jackson stated that this second view is especially important because the therapist's personality is much more a part of psychotherapy, which is somewhat interactive, than it is a part of psychoanalysis, which is much less interactive. If this second view is more important in psychotherapy than in psychoanalysis, then it seems that it would certainly be even more important in family therapy where the therapist's activity and interaction are so common.

Later in that paper, rejecting the stance of the first description above, Jackson (1956) advocated that therapists be more interactive with clients. He wrote, "it would seem that much of the 'good' therapist's energy may be spent on suppressing his reactions, and thus limiting his available self to the patient" (p. 236). With this logic, the more interaction between the mentally healthy therapist and the client, whether it be verbal or nonverbal, the better the treatment.

In discussing his view of countertransference, Jackson felt the need to find a different word for the complex interaction that takes place between therapist and client. If there were such a word, Jackson suggested, then the term "countertransference" could be retained to indicate those aspects of the interaction that do require management. Although he pointed out that the term countertransference might best be left to the problematic aspects of the therapist's reaction, the lack of a better term brought Jackson to discuss the positive aspects as well. Also, by acknowledging that some aspects of countertransference require management, Jackson seemed to be indicating that some use of intentional self-restraint and self-reflection would be necessary when working so freely with one's personality. Nevertheless, the primary argument in the 1956 paper remains that maximum access to the therapist's personality, without too much intentional self-restraint, is the most therapeutic way for the therapist to embody his goal in working with the client.

The crux of Jackson's point was that, although countertransference reactions can be problematic, if all the therapist's reactions are included within the concept, then the therapist's personality, its development and its use, must be as healthy as possible. Countertransference reactions should be monitored, but equally important, the therapist must enrich his own personality as much as possible so that maximal contact with the client will be enriching for that client.

In this paper Jackson discussed many aspects of countertransference that are important in applying the concept to family therapy but have not often been discussed in the family therapy literature. He combined two issues, the activity level of the therapist and the maximal contact of the therapist's personality with the client. When the content of this paper is applied to the family therapy context, it would seem to be Jackson's view that if a therapist is "good," simply maximizing his contact with a family will be beneficial.

But Jackson later renounced all positive thought about the concept of countertransference. In 1961, his association with the Mental Research Institute then well on its way, he wrote a paper with John Weakland on the theory and technique of family therapy. In that paper the authors suggested that transference and countertransference have very little meaning for family therapy.

> Many analysts have had strong doubts about the idea of family therapy, which are often put on transference and countertransference grounds. Thus the terms "transference and countertransference" are troublesome unless it is kept in mind that they refer strictly to aspects of a very special situation—psychoanalysis. We have no doubt that our therapists have feelings about the family members and vice versa; on the other hand, no clarity is achieved if we label such states of mind transference and countertransference.

From this excerpt it is clear that the authors believe that both countertransference and transference have little use in family therapy. But it is also clear that they are not referring to the totalistic definition, even though Jackson had emphasized what appeared to be a totalistic view in his earlier psychoanalytic work. Nevertheless, in the next several paragraphs of their paper, if one views their work from within the scope of the totalistic definition, these authors seem to describe a way of using countertransference. In their description of the lack of importance of countertransference these authors use the following example: "If [the therapist] finds himself irritated by the mother's quietly nagging, martyred tone, he may turn to the father and ask what he experienced in himself during the time when the wife was speaking" (p. 33).

Although this statement is meant to show how the therapist is not affected by the problems caused by countertransference, it also demonstrates how the work of the authors suggests working with countertransference. The therapist notices a feeling developing within himself and then uses that feeling to both better understand the family interaction, and keep the family interaction moving toward better communication. Although Jackson and Weakland put forth the point of view that "countertransference" has no place in family therapy, if the totalistic definition is applied in evaluating their methods, it can be seen that they do believe in a use of countertransference. That belief, however, is not described as a use of countertransference.

This paper is a good example of how systems theorists completely disavowed psychoanalytic concepts even though some of those concepts may have retained utility. It is interesting that the authors' negative comments about countertransference here contradict Jackson's (1956) descriptions only in that they say the concept (evidently referring to its classical definition) has no usefulness in family therapy. Perhaps their denunciation of the concept of countertransference, despite their own inadvertent demonstration of its utility (if one thinks of it in the totalistic sense), was an early example of family therapy's tendency to reject psychoanalytic thinking of all kinds.

The Early Family Therapy Movement

In family systems methods developed later, the therapist's self was plucked out of the system, and emotions he experienced were not considered important. For example, Jay Haley (1976) is known for going so far as to discourage therapists in training from self-reflecting when a therapy appears to be awry. In place of insight, method and action became paramount. Haley encourages therapists in training to find a strategy that will work. Intentionally using countertransference, however, is not an acceptable strategy since it requires self-reflection.

The common current running through the three examples above (the early work of Ackerman, Whitaker, and Jackson) is the emphasis on the interpersonal relationship in therapy, including a use of countertransference. Ackerman (1966) used his personality spontaneously, stating that the psychoanalytic method in which the analyst was to be a "mirror" to the patient did not allow for a "true social experience" in which perception or transference could be tested against reality by way of examining the therapist's countertransference. Whitaker's emphasis (Neill and Kniskern 1982) on reparenting the patient by being comfortable with regressive tendencies that the original parent defended against, and his belief that with such a relationship the genetic antecedents did not require uncovering, relied on an intense degree of freedom in the use of countertransference. Jackson's desire to declare that the therapist's personality is integral and beneficial to therapeutic relationships demonstrates the degree to which he believed the therapist's interpersonal experience of the therapeutic dyad was vital to treatment.

These perspectives can also be seen as forerunners to the family therapy movement as a whole. Like Ackerman, those therapists who wanted to maintain the psychoanalytic framework further developed psychoanalytic concepts as they pertain to families. It could also be said that Ackerman's desire to modify psychoanalytic technique as necessitated by the family therapy context influenced some integrationist authors to do the same. Like Whitaker, therapists who focused on the interpersonal emotional experience of families continued to develop methods for using the self of the therapist as a way to connect to that emotional experience. The early paper by Jackson may best be seen as a forerunner to systems methods in that it expressed a certain frustration with the one-sidedness of the psychoanalytic paradigm most common at that time. Jackson perceived the psychoanalytic paradigm as not acknowledging the presence of the real person of the therapist. But his paper with Weakland demonstrates that, instead of developing the use of his presence as a therapist, his understanding of the complicated nature of human interaction motivated him to develop methods of working with the complicated interaction between family members, without further consideration of the emotions of the therapist. This change might be seen as the result of Jackson's respect for the complicated nature of family interaction, which required a great deal of exploration in itself, rather than a disavowal of the therapist's importance.

Despite the different directions taken in the family therapy movement, these early reports demonstrate that the use of countertransference in family therapy is perhaps not as uncommon an idea as would be guessed from contemporary mainstream literature. It has a history in several of the major branches of the family therapy movement. The movement of family therapy away from psychoanalytic ideas even makes sense. The experiential movement could be a sensible outgrowth of the desire to maintain the deep understanding of psychoanalytic thought at the interactional level without the geometrically multiplied complications that would be involved in the analysis of every person and subgroup within a family. Likewise, it can be speculated that systems theory was a sensible place for Jackson to turn, given the complication that results when families are explained by analytic epistemology. It is important to note, however, that in the diaspora of family therapy the reasons for turning away from psychoanalytic thinking would seem not to apply to the use of countertransference. The use of countertransference, a concept that directly focuses on interactional process, could not only continue to be a good fit within all these methods, but would also be especially appropriate, given the emphasis of these methods on interactional dynamics.

THE SELF-REFLECTION VERSUS ACTION CONTINUUM

Since the concept of countertransference is not often discussed in family therapy, and yet the totalistic perspective suggests that its use is ubiquitous, it will be helpful to identify a unifying construct that can help indicate the extent to which countertransference is used in any particular school of thought. Such a construct is the self-reflection versus action continuum. It has been argued (e.g., Madanes and Haley 1977) that therapeutic approaches can be ordered along a continuum depending upon their emphasis on *insight versus action* as the curative factor. I propose that a parallel continuum exists that can be used to describe a therapist's use of *self-reflection versus action* with respect to countertransference reactions. This self-reflection versus action continuum is especially useful for delineating the current state of the intentional use of countertransference in family therapy because self-reflection is always a part of that use.

Four primary views on the use of countertransference, or the use of self in family therapy can be differentiated along this self-reflection versus action continuum. These four views, ranging from the psychoanalytic/object relations view to the self-reflection as unimportant view (see Table 1–1), are used here primarily to capture the extent to which self-reflection is used by the therapist in various therapies. But the four views also have implications with respect to the unintentional use of countertransference and the extent to which different therapists perceive themselves as part of the therapist-family system. Proponents of these four views may be grouped as seen in Table 1–1.

The Psychoanalytic/Object Relations View.   On one end of the continuum are some psychoanalytic authors who consider countertransference to be an essential tool in doing family therapy. All of the contemporary therapists in this category make object relations theory a primary focus of their work, and the totalistic definition of countertransference is now universally accepted among them. They can be differentiated in that regard from classically oriented psychoanalytic family therapists, who limit their view of countertransference to the classical definition. Therapists at this end of the continuum emphasize self-reflection in therapy, viewing the action of the therapist, when not the product of self-reflection, as acting out. With these methods, if the therapist has adequately "metabolized" (Langs 1976b) her countertransference reaction and can interpret it for the client-family, then essential insights can be gained. Among these authors are the object relations family therapists (Scharff 1991, Scharff and Scharff 1987, Slipp 1984, 1988), the analytic family therapists (Box et al. 1981), and Ackerman (1959, 1966), whose work was not apparently influenced by object relations thinking but was nevertheless consistent with such an approach.

The Integrationist View.   Next on the continuum, closer to the psychoanalytic/object relations authors than to those who view self-reflection as unimportant, are some experiential and eclectic therapists who integrate various forms of therapy (Aponte and Winter 1987, Nichols 1987, Shapiro 1981, Skynner 1976, 1981). These therapists advocate an understanding of the therapist's feelings that can lead the therapist in new directions. These

The Psychoanalytic/Object Relations View
   The classical view in psychoanalytic family therapy
      Lyman Wynne
      Murray Bowen
      Ivan Boszormenyi-Nagy
      Helm Stierlin
   The totalistic view in psychoanalytic family therapy
      Sally Box, Beta Copley, Jeanne Magagna, and Errica Moustaki
      Samuel Slipp
      Jill and David Scharff
      James Framo
      Nathan Ackerman
  The Integrationist View
      Robin Skynner
      Michael Nichols
      Rodney Shapiro
      Harry J. Aponte
  The Experiential View
      Virginia Satir
      Shirley Luthman
      Carl Whitaker
      Walter Kempler
  The Unimportant View
      Don Jackson
      Salvador Minuchin
      Paul Watzlawick, Janet Helmick Beavin, and Don Jackson
      Jay Haley
      Mara Selvini Palazzoli, Luigi Boscolo,
      Gianfranco Cecchin, and Giuliana Prata
      Narrative and solution-oriented therapists

Table 1–1. The self-reflection versus action continuum. Therapists are presented in order from the greatest use of self-reflection to the least.

integrationist approaches are differentiated from the psychoanalytic/object relations schools in that the blending of approaches results in less emphasis on self-reflection in their work. It can also be shown that they are more consistently likely than psychoanalytic/object relations therapists to recognize that countertransference difficulties are common even among experienced therapists. They are differentiated from the next group on the continuum, experiential therapists, in that the theory they apply includes some self-reflection. The integrationist therapists show the greatest potential for a full use of countertransference as both its intentional and its unintentional use can be applied within an integrated theory.

The Experiential View. Further along the continuum, among the experiential family therapists, some suggest either a very natural, empathic "use of self" (Luthman 1974, Satir and Baldwin 1983) or the open expression of countertransference reactions (Kempler 1965, 1968, Whitaker et al. 1965, Whitaker and Keith 1981). These therapists use a very active approach in dealing with their emotional reactions, with the hope that a genuine relationship between family and therapist will have a salutary effect. This emphasis on "genuineness" or "authenticity" is motivated by the belief that the therapist's personality is the primary therapeutic tool. These therapists can thus be said to use countertransference both intentionally and unintentionally. The belief that the therapist's personality is the primary therapeutic tool and, as a part of that belief, the desire to allow the therapist's emotional reactions into the therapeutic process, constitutes an intentional use of countertransference. The desire to do so without much self-reflection constitutes an unintentional use of countertransference. Self-reflection is typically a part of some applied theory of development and/or interpersonal process that is de-emphasized in experiential approaches.

The Unimportant View. On the other end of the continuum are those authors who advocate the use of systems, strategic or solution-oriented methods, and who seem to suggest, through their lack of discussion of the topic, that countertransference responses are for the most part unimportant. These authors emphasize action in therapy to such an extent that they do not recognize a use of countertransference in their literature. It is difficult to describe these therapists as being opposed to a use of the self in therapy since they do not discuss concepts like countertransference in their work. Authors who seem to represent this position include Beavin, Epston, Fisch, Haley, Jackson, Madanes, Selvini-Palazzoli, de Shazer, Watzlawick, and White. More than any other group of authors, those that I categorize within the "unimportant" view would be unlikely to recognize their use of countertransference reactions. Yet their emphasis on action without self-reflection suggests that they are more likely than the other groups discussed to use countertransference unintentionally.

Thus, the more a particular therapy views self-reflection of the therapist as positive, the more likely that therapy is to recognize the intentional use of countertransference. The more a particular therapy views the activity of the therapist as positive, the less likely that therapy is to recognize the intentional use of countertransference. The unintentional use of countertransference has not been elucidated in the literature within any of these schools, yet each view suggests certain implications in that regard as well. The unintentional use of countertransference is probably most likely to be recognized by therapists who fall toward the center of the continuum since these therapists do not deny either the importance of countertransference or that some countertransference reactions go unrecognized.

In the following review of countertransference in family therapy, the therapists presented are in order from the greatest use of self-reflection to the least, or from the least emphasis on activity to the most, within the four categorical views that have been outlined. In focusing on the way countertransference is used in family therapy given the totalistic definition (rather than on how it has or has not been described), I will sort out the impact of the classical versus totalistic definitions, and the intentional versus unintentional use of countertransference, while uncovering the extent of its use within each of the four perspectives.

THE PSYCHOANALYTIC/OBJECT RELATIONS VIEW

The Classical View in Psychoanalytic Family Therapy

The psychoanalytic/object relations view, as placed on the self-reflection versus action continuum, captures the most self-reflective, and therefore most intentional, use of countertransference. Many contemporary object relations family therapists epitomize this stance (Scharff 1991, Scharff and Scharff 1987, Skynner 1981, Slipp 1984, 1988), and Ackerman (1966), discussed above, certainly held a totalistic view of countertransference. But not all psychoanalytic family therapists have advocated this view. In fact, the classical definition has been the only one considered in the work of several of family therapy's earlier psychoanalytic therapists. Perhaps the work of classically oriented therapists does not belong at this end of the continuum. On the other hand, all of these therapists seem to be very self-reflective, and in spite of the fact that they did not discuss totalistic countertransference, it can be speculated that they used countertransference without emphasizing that use enough to explicitly describe it. I will present these authors at the beginning of this section because their work is used by systems therapists (Madanes and Haley 1977) to represent the "antiquated" insight-oriented approach to family work that is considered to be the opposite of their own view. As such, these therapists would fall on the insight end of the insight versus action continuum, and are perhaps characterized by a lack of activity. Their work also helps to provide a context for the psychoanalytic/object relations family therapy which developed later.

Lyman Wynne

A group including Lyman Wynne wrote a paper called "On the Nature and Sources of the Psychiatrist's Experience with the Family of the Schizophrenic" (Schaffer et al. 1962) that indicated some of the many difficulties that may arise for the family therapist working with schizophrenic families. In this paper the authors referred to issues of countertransference as "counter-resistance." The next excerpt demonstrates that these authors viewed counter-resistance as something that could create a stumbling block in treatment, especially with reference to the fragmented nature of schizophrenic families. "[I]f the therapist analyzes the counter-resistance, then something of the experience of fragmentation is revealed, and he is thus able, however tentatively and indirectly, to grasp such previously neglected components of the culture and structure of the family group" (p. 40).

The description given here, although seemingly indicative of a totalistic use of countertransference, refers primarily to the necessity for the therapist to grasp the nature of the family without getting caught up in countertransference reactions. But these authors were also describing, to some extent, how the therapist's experience of fragmentation, however slight compared to the family's experience, can be helpful to her work. It is interesting that the perspective given in this paper is so close to an intentional use of countertransference and yet the authors did not choose to take that path in their discussion. Although these authors describe the general difficulty a therapist might experience with families, and even point out by example how that difficulty might be turned into an asset, they do not suggest that these experiences are useful to the family or the therapist in any routine way. They focus only on the necessity for the therapist to be aware of her denial and resistances that could result in failure to understand the family.

Wynne (1965) described the problems that arise due to countertransference in more detail in a later paper. Here he stated that fully developed transference–countertransference interactions do not usually occur in family therapy because there are not several sessions per week for long periods of time to intensify the work. He did not make it clear whether he was referring to countertransference in the totalistic or classical sense in that statement. However, Wynne did use this paper as a vehicle for listing the many difficulties that can be encountered when working with families, which suggests that his meaning was classical. Where countertransference difficulties were acknowledged, Wynne wrote very little about how such problems could be avoided beyond the suggestion that the therapist must constantly analyze her own emotions to prevent them from affecting the therapy. He generally seemed to support the Freudian notion that a therapist must resolve her own issues before dealing with similar issues in family therapy.

These two papers, although focused on the extensive countertransference difficulties that can arise in family therapy, can be interpreted to suggest that, if harnessed, countertransference experiences could be very helpful. The self-analysis used by Wynne to avoid countertransference problems seemed to broaden his understanding of the families with whom he worked. Although he did not suggest an intentional use of countertransference, the analysis of his own countertransference reactions demonstrates the extent to which self-reflection was a part of his work. For example, in the first example given above, such self-analysis results in the ability to grasp certain components of the family's experience that would not have otherwise been uncovered. Perhaps it is best to say that Wynne's intentional self-reflection is beneficial to treatment even though the effort is not primarily motivated by the desire for a deeper understanding of the family.

Murray Bowen

Bowen, despite an extensive background in psychoanalytic training and the compatibility of his work with psychoanalytic theory, is often associated with systems theory. Many of the concepts he used to describe family therapy continued to be used and integrated into systems theory. Yet Bowen never compared his own work with the cybernetic systems and games theory that became so prominent in family therapy. His work is presented here because of his association with psychoanalytic thinking as well as his historic significance to family therapy, beginning in the mid-1950s. Bowen did not specifically write anything extensive about countertransference. Yet several of his techniques seem designed to avoid countertransference difficulties.

Bowen's work (1978) included a way of avoiding the "undifferentiated ego mass" of a family in two ways, both of which seem specifically related to the negative aspects of countertransference. First of all, by acting as coach to the family or the couple, Bowen maintained an atmosphere that was much less charged than that experienced by families at home. Because family members had to explain their emotional process rather than experience it fully, the total power of that emotional process did not enter the room. Secondly, it could be said that a primary aspect of Bowen's work as a therapist was to remain "detriangled" and thus unaffected by countertransference. When Bowen got the feeling that he was being pulled by a family, he avoided the full impact by detriangling. He stated: "I attempt to back out emotionally to the point where I can watch the ebb and flow of the emotional process while always 'thinking process,' and without getting caught in the flow" (p. 250). His ability to avoid countertransference reactions, or the pull of the "emotional system," was very important to his work. According to Bowen, "A basic principle in this theoretical-therapeutic system is that the emotional problem between two people will resolve automatically if they remain in contact with a third person who can remain free of the emotional field between them, while actively relating to each" (p. 251). Although Bowen did not attempt to use the information that came from being emotionally pulled, the effort put forth in avoiding countertransference that can be seen in his work seems to constitute a very specific way of dealing with its negative aspects.

With regard to the unintentional use of countertransference, I suspect that it was extremely important to Bowen's work. By "thinking process," he could remain "free of the emotional field." Thinking about process must have included an understanding of what family members were doing to him, or wanting from him, and his reaction was to put the ball back in the court of his clients. I would assume that Bowen accomplished this tactic quite naturally, with a quick or instinctive reference to his knowledge of triangles, and that the ability to do so was related to his unique personality and to what he might have called his high level of "self differentiation" (Bowen 1972).

Ivan Boszormenyi-Nagy

Boszormenyi-Nagy represents an analytic stance that on the surface appears to leave little room for an intentional use of countertransference. He does, however, discuss how the family therapist avoids countertransference difficulties. He (Boszormenyi-Nagy and Krasner 1986, 1987) believes the therapist's safeguard against countertransference reactions is maintaining multidirected partiality. "Multidirected partiality is the therapeutic attitude that protects the therapist from becoming unilaterally attached to one person via countertransference, or from turning into a fragmented referee who gets caught between the conflicting goals and aspirations of competing family members" (1986, p. 52).

Boszormenyi-Nagy (Boszormenyi-Nagy and Krasner 1987) also describes multidirected partiality as "a process of consecutive siding with now one and now the other relating partner in order to help family members state their respective terms with some confidence that opposing views can be heard and tolerated" (p. 221). In this same discussion he directly associates this process with avoiding countertransference dangers. He states that "consecutive siding with relating partners is a protection against the dangers of countertransference reactions" (p. 221).

Although Boszormenyi-Nagy (Boszormenyi-Nagy and Krasner 1987) does not appear to believe in a use of countertransference, he does write about how a therapist can channel strong feelings elicited in him into action. He believes that "the best use of affect is its investment in a courageous and forceful exploration of options for reworking deep-rooted patterns of unfairness" (p. 311). Here he is referring to the therapist's strong feelings of inequity in the family, and not to feelings transferred to the therapist through projective identification. Perhaps it could be said, however, that he is experiencing the inequity of the family through their projections. But because Boszormenyi-Nagy is so highly focused on the issue of fairness, it is difficult to differentiate whether the feelings he describes emanate from projections or from his own adept sensitivity.

Even though he does not believe in using countertransference, it is interesting that some of the processes recognized by Boszormenyi-Nagy, which are considered by many authors to be essential in using countertransference, are not harnessed for use within his model for therapy. In one of his papers (Boszormenyi-Nagy and Framo 1987) he describes a process by which a hospital staff becomes, through transference and countertransference, like the family of a schizophrenic patient. Perhaps, despite this description of very powerful countertransference reactions in a hospital staff, Boszormenyi-Nagy's own multidirected partiality protects him from the same reactions affecting his own practice of therapy.

It can be speculated that Boszormenyi-Nagy's sense of fairness, of right and wrong, and his desire for family members to discover these values within themselves, is very much related to who he is as a person. These values also speak to the issue of the therapist's mental health in that balancing many emotionally laden viewpoints without becoming stuck on any one side, coupled with the ability to make decisions based on one's own beliefs, is the sine qua non of a mentally healthy person. Perhaps his unintentional use of countertransference is very central to his approach. The following excerpt, in referring to empathy, is very suggestive of an unintentional use of countertransference that fits perfectly with multidirected partiality:

> Empathy is an aspect of partiality, that is a therapist's openness to imagining the feeling mode of each family member as he or she proceeds to describe personal perspectives and conflicted interests. The therapist's own natural feelings and reactions towards particular family members are reined in by his efforts to be partial. One family member may evoke resentment in him, another may evoke contempt . . . At the very least a therapist has to find room in his feelings to imagine how the offending person has himself suffered as a childhood victim. [Boszormenyi-Nagy and Krasner 1986, p. 302]

In his use of empathy, Boszormenyi-Nagy apparently uses countertransference to the extent that he struggles to understand each member of a family.

I would argue that Boszormenyi-Nagy intentionally uses countertransference as he perceives the anguish of family members and identifies with family members' feelings of unfairness. I wonder how his countertransference might be piqued by a person who is treated extremely unfairly but believes she deserves such treatment. It is certainly conceivable that some persons like this do not experience themselves as victimized but do, via projective identification, bring about sympathy in the observer (often becoming constant help refusers) as well as poor treatment from others. Perhaps given such a situation Boszormenyi-Nagy would naturally have multidirected partiality at work and would become sympathetic with this person and then move his sympathies to another family member, thus making the complementarity of the situation come to light. In my view this sequence might require a quasi-intentional use of countertransference, and if such behavior just comes naturally to Boszormenyi-Nagy, it certainly involves at least an unintentional use of countertransference. It is likely that the absence of consideration of a use of countertransference in his work is mostly due to the limitations of the classical definition. It is also possible that his style of work is so natural to him that it does not require such meta-level explanation.

Helm Stierlin

Stierlin (1977) defined countertransference as "any deviation from a therapeutic position of involved impartiality" (p. 311). Involved impartiality is the therapist's ability to maintain fairness in approaching the family under conditions of increasing involvement with each member. Involved impartiality (almost the opposite of Boszormenyi-Nagy's multidirected partiality) emphasizes the avoidance of taking sides with various members of the family. Stierlin's model seems to suggest the psychoanalytic concept of neutrality. It is interesting that Stierlin, although suggesting a classically analytic stance of neutrality for the family therapist, seems to advocate the possibility of using countertransference. The definition of countertransference as a deviation from involved impartiality does not, at first, seem to fit with the idea that countertransference, being a response to the transferences of the family, can provide information for the therapist. Perhaps Stierlin's involved impartiality suggests that countertransference thoughts may occur but countertransference actions should be avoided (countertransference "thoughts" and "positions" or actions were differentiated by Racker in 1957), which would allow countertransference to be informative as long as the therapist did not act upon the associated feelings.

Although most of Stierlin's statements on countertransference emphasize the problems it can cause, there does seem to be some suggestion in his writing about when countertransference can be useful. Toward the beginning of a therapy Stierlin believes that countertransference is typically only of the problematic kind. He writes about problematic countertransference developing as a result of the therapist's reaction to family myths. As therapy progresses, however, helpful kinds of countertransference may develop as a reaction to transferences, collectively referred to by Stierlin as "family myths," from various family members.

Family myths are described in detail by Ferreira (1963), who maintained that the family myth is to the relationship what the defense is to the individual. Stierlin's view of family myths is that they "fulfill the major function of providing a shared formulation which makes some sense out of the family members' involvement with, and their rights and obligations toward, one another . . . They provide cognitive, relational, and ethical meaning and are therefore affectively charged" (p. 307). These myths distort as well as disguise the family's transference–countertransference dynamics both within the family and to outsiders. To the extent that these myths can be "sold" to the therapist, they invite typical countertransference responses. The countertransference here is seen as an unwitting reaction to, as well as acceptance of, the family's collaborative and distorted script of the family drama. As such, it will prove a stumbling block to the therapy, attributable to a blind spot in the family therapist's perceptiveness and objectivity.

According to Stierlin, in family therapy, "while he tries to gain each member's trust, the therapist explores and thereby punctures the family myths" (p. 310). The therapist punctures these myths while maintaining his "involved impartiality" (p. 311). If the therapist is maintaining this impartiality, he is not buying the family myths, but challenging them. This impartiality also leads family members to trust the therapist because the challenges are made in a fair way.

A different kind of countertransference reaction can occur when myths are challenged and trust develops. With views in part similar to Wynne's

(1965) that transference–countertransference dynamics do not fully develop in family therapy, Stierlin (1977) contends that the family group, before trust with the therapist develops, holds its transferences and counter-transferences within the family system where they originated. He believes this happens because "it is family transactions which give rise to those relational patterns which later, inappropriately and repetitively, are transferred to non-family contexts" (p. 307). As the therapist develops trust with family members, however, transferences are loosened between them and become free to be projected onto the therapist. He explains the phenomenon:

> To the extent that trust develops, transferences are pried loose from within the family and the therapist becomes their likely recipient. Once this happens, classical views and formulations as to the development of transference–countertransference reactions become more applicable. We observe how parents increasingly relate to the therapist as they related to their own parents, while their children bring to bear on him those relational patterns which originated in their parent relationships. [pp. 310–311]

It is when this trust develops that a therapist might use countertransference reactions to better understand the family and its members. Although Stierlin seems to use countertransference toward positive ends, it is important to note that he does see it as stemming from problems. He writes, "the therapist's 'countertransference' might be a response to taxing treatment challenges and then serve primarily as a source of information about the family or some member, or it might primarily reflect certain defenses, personality traits, growth lacunae, or blind spots in himself which interfere with his therapeutic task and require corrective action" (p. 312).

In this statement Stierlin seems to define countertransference in a classical sense, even though he is willing to go one step beyond the classical definition. That is, even when countertransference poses a problem (when it is "a response to taxing treatment challenges"), it can be used to benefit the treatment. Even if the therapist ends up using countertransference feelings to better understand the family, they are first noticed as a problem for the therapist.

The Totalistic View in Psychoanalytic Family Therapy

The split in the field of psychoanalytic family therapy between therapists who advocate the totalistic or the classical definitions of countertransference complicates what I refer to as the psychoanalytic/object relations view. The therapists discussed above all limited their discussion of countertransference to the classical definition. But the totalistic definition that had been developing in the psychoanalytic literature, especially in the object relations school, was not completely unknown in family therapy. Ackerman (1966) certainly employed a totalistic understanding of countertransference even though he did not use object relations explanations. Views similar to Ackerman's did not reappear in family therapy until object relations thinking was applied to family interaction. The first major influence in applying object relations to family therapy came from Henry V. Dicks (1967), who authored a study that discussed the importance of projective identification in marital couples. Although Dicks did not discuss the use of countertransference in any depth, his followers soon applied such thinking to families. Like Dicks, several authors in the United States, most notably Edward R. Shapiro, Roger L. Shapiro, and John Zinner, were applying object relations theory to the inner workings of families without discussing the therapist as part of that object relations system. But countertransference was soon to become a powerful tool in some therapists' work.

In 1981 a group of psychoanalytic family therapists from the Tavistock Clinic (Box et al.) published a book called *Psychotherapy with Families: An Analytic Approach*, in which countertransference was used extensively. Also influenced by British object relations thinking, but integrating systems theory (therefore part of the section on the integrationist view below), Robin Skynner's work was just beginning to receive notice around the late 1970s. By the late 1980s the work of Jill Savege Scharff and David Scharff, and also the work of Samuel Slipp, began gathering notice. These therapists use countertransference quite deliberately, making it a central element within their method. Object relations thinking brought a totalistic understanding of countertransference to these therapists' work. Although it had been developing since the 1940s, the intentional use of countertransference did not appear in the family literature until introduced by these therapists in the late 1970s and early 1980s.

Sally Box, Beta Copley, Jeanne Magagna, and Errica Moustaki

At the time of its publication, *Psychotherapy with Families* represented the most comprehensive psychoanalytic approach yet conceived within the family therapy movement. Box and colleagues (1981) based much of their work on the psychoanalytic group theory of Wilfred Bion. It is clear that in Bion's (1959a,b) work, the use of countertransference is extremely important. Likewise, examples of using countertransference are found throughout the book by Box and colleagues.

Box and colleagues (Box et al. 1981) stated that when the family comes into treatment, the projections they have been carrying can be experienced by the therapist. It is through countertransference, they wrote, that the therapist knows what requires containing in the family. "The therapists in their interaction with the family by means of their countertransference experience attempt to take the projective identifications into themselves, find space for and try to understand the nature of the elements disowned by the family and thereby provide some containment. They also need to remember that this may be a communication that the family does not know how to make in any other way" (p. 166).

Owing to the complex nature of working with families, Box and colleagues (1981) employed co-therapists in their work. Their viewpoint was that although each therapist reacts differently to the family, the co-therapy team members also react to each other. They believed the processing of countertransference occurred both within the session and between sessions. Naturally, this processing would occur with both therapists together as well as apart. In general, these authors believe countertransference helps them understand and analyze a family. They use their countertransference experiences both to understand what aspects of the family require containment, and in formulating interpretations.

One seemingly significant omission in the work of Box and colleagues (1981) is that no mention is made of acting out, or any other form of the classical view of countertransference. It is interesting that among those family therapists who advocate working with countertransference, this same omission is common. But when the therapist's acting out is deliberately not acknowledged within a therapeutic method, an unintentional use of countertransference would also most likely be denied. If the classical form of countertransference supposedly does not affect the therapist, then is one to assume that such a therapist has perfect control over all his emotions? Such control seems unlikely. Does containment require perfect control, or just relative control? The potentially important unintentional use of countertransference is precluded from discussion by these therapists due to what seems to be an assumption that perfect control is possible.

Samuel Slipp

Slipp described a use of countertransference in his object relations approach to family therapy (1984, 1988). Slipp (1988), in what he refers to as the "middle phase" of family therapy, advocates that a therapist concentrate on the interpersonal realm of interaction. In an earlier stage he works more systemically but still with an object relations formulation. While concentrating on this interpersonal realm in the middle phase, he contends that the therapist's concentration on his own countertransference reactions, both to the family as a whole and to each individual within the family, is of utmost importance. If the therapist can distinguish certain thoughts or feelings that are not typical of his own manner, then he might postulate that these thoughts and feelings are the result of projective identification—the same mechanism that evokes certain feelings of family members within the family. (In fact, throughout his writing Slipp often refers to the effects of projective identification within the family as countertransference reactions.) If the therapist is affected by projective identification, Slipp (1988) says, he "needs to contain these feelings, understand where they are coming from, and then weave them into an interpretation of the projective identification that is [then] presented to the family" (p. 196).

The interpretation of projective identification is considered by Slipp to be the most important task of the interpersonally oriented "middle phase" of treatment. Slipp (1988) sums up his use of countertransference in this excerpt:

If the objective countertransference can be contained, and not ignored or acted out by the therapist, then the therapist can think through what the transference is that the member is using in the here-and-now interaction. This is termed metabolizing the countertransference. Thus the therapist can experience how that person felt he or she was treated by the parents as a child. If the objective countertransference is interpreted in an empathic manner, and tied to a genetic reconstruction that links the present interaction with a past relationship, the net result usually is an increase in the depth of empathic understanding and a furthering of the therapeutic alliance. [p. 196]

Slipp proposes using countertransference almost exactly as it would be used in working with an individual. It is interesting that he does not indicate that the activity level the therapist uses in doing family therapy requires any changes in technique. Yet his model does seem to be quite interactive.

It is also interesting to note that Slipp does acknowledge the classical view of countertransference within his totalistic view, yet is no more likely than Box and colleagues (Box et al. 1981) to acknowledge an unintentional use of countertransference. In Slipp's case this oversight is likely due to his particular view of projective identification rather than the belief that a therapist can completely overcome countertransference difficulties. His view of projective identification is confusing because he postulates that it requires a certain kind of closeness between the projector and the recipient, and at the same time he discusses it as though the recipient is only a passive receptacle. That is, Slipp (1988) views the projector in projective identification as having sole responsibility for the effect of the projection even though the recipient must share a certain amount of intimacy with the projector. He believes there is a clear distinction between an objective countertransference response and a subjective countertransference response. And once he has distinguished his response to be objective, he uses it as a tool. The problem with such a formulation, however, is that there is no room for the possibility that a countertransference response is both subjective and objective, that it is meaningful and can be useful even though it is not purely the result of projective identification from the patient.

Many individual therapists writing on the phenomenon of projective identification have postulated that the recipient of a projective identification is a participant in the interaction (Bion 1959b, Malin and Grotstein 1966, Ogden 1994a,b, Sandler 1976). Such a view of projective identification can accommodate the relational systems perspective and the unintentional use of countertransference, in which the therapist unknowingly influences the family in a preconscious way, as well as the self-reflective, intentional use of countertransference. But Slipp sees countertransference reactions as either subjective or objective without considering the fact that they may be a mixture of the two. While he might determine that his reaction is more of one and less of the other, he instead chooses to believe that he is able to determine the issue absolutely one way or the other. It appears that a black-and-white decision must always be achieved. His view leaves no room for the middle ground where the therapist might arrive at an intervention that communicates his responsibility in taking on the projection as part of the process.

The outcome is that, because he does not acknowledge that his reactions to projective identification are uniquely his reactions, Slipp's view of projective identification limits the extent to which he might find his own personality dynamics of use in therapy. Slipp does not consider his own sensitivity, and actions related to that sensitivity, to be an integral part in understanding projective identification even though he believes that intimacy is required for the transmission of projective identification. Thus it is difficult to consider his view of countertransference as within the perspective that views the therapist as part of the therapist–family system. Within the therapist–family system the therapist has an effect on the family and its members, just as they have an effect on him, and countertransference interventions must be offered within that context, tempered by an understanding that there is no purely objective countertransference.

Jill and David Scharff

The Scharffs use a straightforward psychoanalytic approach with object relations theory as the base. Jill Scharff's book, *Foundations of Object Relations Family Therapy* (1991), points to their major influences within the psychoanalytic family therapy movement, and includes papers published throughout the time expanse of family therapy. The work of Zinner and Shapiro (1972, 1974) is especially important to their approach but, as stated earlier, these authors only apply object relations thinking to family dynamics without considering the therapist's part in the therapist–family system. Scharff and Scharff (1989) have outlined their view of using countertransference, one that goes well beyond the work of other authors. They see countertransference as the cornerstone of their work. David Scharff (Scharff 1991) describes transference and countertransference in object relations family therapy this way: "They offer the living bridge between therapist and family through which the family's shared unconscious assumptions, mutual projective identifications, pained relationships, and deficits in providing holding to one another can be experienced, understood, and fed back to the family in modified form" (p. 422). In this paper by David Scharff, and a joint paper that appears as a chapter in a book by both these therapists (1987), several ways in which the use of countertransference in family work differs from its use in work with individuals are described. These authors differentiate two kinds of countertransference that correspond to two kinds of transference, the "focused" and the "contextual" countertransference.

"Focused" countertransference refers to those feelings experienced by the therapist that relate to projective identification coming from one member of the family. When a therapy is dominated by this kind of countertransference, the family is likely to be substituting individual experience for shared experience. This might happen when the identified patient is using projective identification. Here is an example given by David Scharff (1991): "If we find ourselves feeling bullied by an angry adolescent, it is likely that the family feels bullied by him and that the members' shared feeling that they cannot provide holding to his anxiety is being expressed to us in the parents' collusion to make his bullying the prominent message" (pp. 424–425). In this situation the Scharffs would use the experience of feeling bullied to speak to the family's shared difficulty, without focusing only on the bullying adolescent, because their work is aimed at understanding why the family needs to speak through the bullying adolescent.

"Contextual" countertransference refers to the therapist's feelings in relation to the family's need to be held or to feel safe. It is the contextual countertransference that organizes the therapist's work in that the overall field is too complex to organize from the multiple transferences of individual family members. "The organizing responses are more apt to come out of the therapist's feeling of the confusion that the family as a whole is conveying, or from the fantasy that emerges spontaneously as the therapist listens to the family and to the subgroups or individuals who are speaking. The ability to understand and then to organize this understanding grows out of a capacity for 'negative capability'" (Scharff and Scharff 1987, p. 223).

By "negative capability" the Scharffs (1987) refer to the capacity to tolerate "not knowing," "being in uncertainties, mysteries, doubts," and similar states, "without any irritable reaching after fact and reason" (p. 210). It is by allowing for uncertainty that countertransference feelings are allowed to take root in these therapists. Negative capability allows these therapists to communicate with the family at a deep level where reason and knowledge do not always explain complex emotions, and where immediate action interferes with complete understanding.

Related to the use of countertransference and negative capability is the concept Jill Scharff (1992) refers to as a "use of self." Scharff states:

My self is what I have to offer. I am both myself and the person the patients need me to be. Because I am there, they can experience and remodel their own selves in individual, couple, or family therapy. In each modality I aim at gaining access to the experience that has shaped their psychic structures. Metabolizing my own experience of the expression of their internal structures, I arrive at understanding, which I communicate in the form of interpretations that ultimately have the explanatory power to modify intrapsychic and interpersonal dynamics. The therapist's self is the therapeutic instrument. She becomes a necessary object of use to the patient. How she is used determines her understanding of the patient's psychodynamics. How she is used in contrast to her own concept of herself yields the material for her interpretations. In the gap between what she is and how the patient perceives her and needs her to be lies therapeutic leverage, room for interpretation of the burden of fantasy upon reality. At the same time the therapist may come to perceive aspects of herself hidden from her until brought to light by the patient's fantasy. Each patient calls forth our higher reach. As they improve, our patients succeed in making us better, too. [p. 12]

This one excerpt points out several important aspects of the use of countertransference. Scharff recognizes the value of allowing her total self to be with the client or client-family at the same time as she recognizes the influence of their projections within her. Her interventions are aimed at both intrapsychic and interpersonal change. Scharff even recognizes that there may be aspects of herself of which she is not yet aware. The main difference between the Scharffs' approach (assuming that Jill Scharff speaks for herself and her husband in the excerpt above) and what I suggest, is that they seem to lack a full appreciation of the unintentional use of countertransference. There appears to be room for such a concept, but meaningful explanation is not offered. The Scharffs would appear to believe that their personalities do not unintentionally influence client-families in the same way that client-families attempt to influence them. They appear to believe that they become aware of almost everything, at least eventually. There is no discussion within their work about the therapeutic intangibles of the therapist's personality.

David Scharff (1991) recommends several techniques in relation to countertransference experiences. Some of these techniques are very similar to those suggested in the writing of object relations individual therapists, but a few are designed specifically for family work. Among these techniques are:

- *Reflecting and Digesting.* This technique is a direct analog to the "containing" and "processing" (originally from Bion [1959a,b]) that individual object relations therapists assume is essential in therapy with relatively regressed patients. It also includes self-reflection as the path to understanding how and why the family is affecting the therapist in a particular way.
- *Supporting and Advising.* This technique is basically educational. Supporting and advising are considered useful when the family seems to be simply in need of understanding or information. At times the Scharffs choose not to support or advise, because the family's need for these functions might be part of a projective identification. When the family's need does seem connected to some projective identification the Scharffs would examine the deficits in the family's shared "holding" (originally from Winnicott [1960a]) capacity, which would lead to the family coming up with its own solutions.
- *Feedback and Interpretation.* This technique includes clarifying, mirroring, and confronting the family. In ways similar to those found in individual technique, the Scharffs use clarifying comments until

they are reasonably sure about the accuracy of an interpretation.

- *Working in the Here and Now.*   This technique involves the therapist's understanding of the family's communication within the room as being reflective of transference and countertransference occurrences. The immediacy of these events allows for powerfully emotional interventions.
- *Working Through.*   In the ending phases of their work with a family the Scharffs believe that, with repeated interpretation and confrontation of projective identification, the family works through its conflicts.

In general, it appears that the object relations model given by the Scharffs is very much like individual therapy within the object relations school. However, their addition of the contextual and focused countertransference concepts offers additional explanatory power for the use of countertransference, specifically as used in family therapy. An especially intriguing aspect of their work is their view that a family's inability to contain certain aspects of its functioning can result in contextual countertransference, which then may be harnessed by the therapist to inform interventions. Where other therapists might describe the analysis of countertransference with so many individuals and subgroups as impossible, the Scharffs maintain that a generalized feeling occurs in the therapist that can be extremely valuable and useful.

It is important to add that the Scharffs (D. and J. S. Scharff 1987) do see some problems for the therapist who attempts to use countertransference as part of her work. However, the Scharffs limit their discussion of this issue to the training of therapists, as if the experienced therapist has no countertransference reactions left unchecked. They believe that novice therapists must overcome countertransference difficulties as they progress toward being object relations family therapists. Among these difficulties are "distancing," "unempathic interpretation," "taking sides and reversal," "reverting to the dyad," and "simplification." All of these manifestations of countertransference are considered to be acting out, which occurs as a result of the inability to handle the anxiety of doing analytic family work. The therapist may "distance" due to fear of becoming too emotionally involved with the family. "Unempathic interpretation" results from a particular kind of distancing where the therapist hopes to solve problems quickly and be rid of the family. "Taking sides and reversal" occur when the therapist is uncomfortable with being left out; by taking sides the therapist becomes part of a subgroup and projects his or her own discomfort into the group, which often results in someone else being left out. "Reverting to the dyad" refers to focusing one's work on individuals within the family rather than viewing the family as a whole. "Simplification" allows the therapist to work with a family without addressing depth issues.

These descriptions of forms of defending against the anxiety inherent in doing family therapy are very interesting, especially in reference to acting out. But the Scharffs stop short of explaining why or how these anxieties may develop within the therapist. Their solutions for overcoming these anxieties are similar to those of many other therapists: to begin with smaller family groups, like couples, and to see families as part of a co-therapy team. These solutions are probably very important training tools. Yet the idea that difficulties of this kind can be completely overcome with training seems an oversimplification. By attributing these problems to therapists in training, and not including them in their own work with countertransference, the Scharffs seem to be suggesting that these difficulties are not part of the work for the experienced object relations family therapist.

Furthermore, as I suggested in reference to the work of Box and colleagues (1981), by not attributing any unchecked countertransference reactions to the experienced therapist, the Scharffs preclude the possibility that the therapist's unique personality influences a transference–countertransference exchange. Jill Scharff comes close when she states that the reality of who she is is checked against the fantasy of the patient, and that she may even discover something in herself of which she was not aware when doing therapy, but in general the Scharffs do not acknowledge that they may have an unintentional influence on their patients.

James Framo

Framo uses the classical definition of countertransference, yet his approach to family therapy seems to acknowledge both its useful and problematic aspects. His writing focuses on technique, and is largely atheoretical, but object relations influences are often referenced in it. Framo's (1965) perspective on countertransference generally comes from his belief that, although a therapist must have his or her own therapy in order to become aware of blind spots, countertransference is unavoidable and ubiquitous when working with families. With the classical view as the focus of his direct investigation of countertransference, Framo discusses the use of a co-therapist and consultation with a team as the primary ways to avoid countertransference pitfalls.

While the classical definition of countertransference is most often associated with cautions on the avoidance of countertransference, Framo's (1968) forthright depiction of his own thoughts during therapy sessions in the paper "My Families, My Family" is suggestive of both its intentional and unintentional uses. In that paper, Framo not only presents statements of family participants but also parenthetically presents the thoughts that occurred to him at the time those statements were made. As a result both Framo's personal experiences and the effect that the family has on him are shown. Unfortunately, since he does not present any ongoing therapy in this paper, it is impossible to discern the overall effect of his having these thoughts during sessions. He states his thoughts and feelings in such a way that it is clear that the therapy was to some extent influenced by that experience, but since the influence is never demonstrated through ongoing discourse, one cannot be sure how important a factor his personality becomes. However, it is apparent that there is some effect that could be called an unintentional use of countertransference.

Although Framo's association with object relations theorists may be suggestive of an intentional use of countertransference, the extent to which he believes such a use is helpful in family therapy is difficult to discern because he does not discuss any theory related to it. His writing does, however, suggest that self-reflection is used in his method. From his descriptions one would be led to believe that his work with countertransference fits within a totalistic definition. Nevertheless, given his comments, it is difficult to place Framo's approach on the self-reflection versus action continuum. Because he appears to emphasize both action and self-reflection in the therapist, his approach might well fit toward the action side of the psychoanalytic/object relations view.

Nathan Ackerman

Although I have already discussed Ackerman's (1959, 1966) approach to using countertransference, I would like to place his work on the self-reflection versus action continuum. Ackerman's extensive use of his personality, joined with his self-reflective, intentional use of countertransference, is indicative of a spontaneous yet analytic approach. He was aware of an unintentional use of countertransference and even referred to the reciprocal processes involved in transference and countertransference in a way that seems similar to what some would call a transference–countertransference system. He states, "Just as soon as we view [transference and countertransference] as reciprocal processes, the head and tail of a single phenomenological entity, we have, in effect, executed a shift from a theoretical model of analysis as a "one person" process to a two-or-more-person phenomenon. . . . The relationship now involves a circular interchange of emotion" (Ackerman 1966, pp. 102–103).

Ackerman realized that within this circular interchange the therapist could not be completely cognizant of every aspect of his countertransference reaction. Thus he advocated the use of the therapist's self, believing that the emotional influence of the therapist could not be completely eliminated, but the therapist's willingness to show himself could be helpful. Both self-reflection and spontaneity, both the intentional and unintentional uses of countertransference, were thus essential to his approach. Ackerman's work seems to indicate that he viewed himself as part of the therapist–family system. The self-reflection he advocated clearly places his work on the self-reflection, or psychoanalytic, side of the self-reflection versus action continuum.

Summary and Conclusions

The psychoanalytic/object relations position on the self-reflection versus action continuum includes leaders in the family therapy movement who have defined countertransference both classically and totalistically. But all these theorists share the view that the therapist's self-reflection is a central component in effective therapy. The analytic authors presented at the beginning of this subgrouping are the therapists who advocate a use of countertransference the least. My placement of these therapists at the far end of the self-reflection side may seem contradictory in light of my insistence that this continuum is reflective of a greater intentional use of countertransference where self-reflection is more emphasized. But perhaps where self-reflection is overemphasized, the appropriate level of action required for using countertransference cannot occur. These therapists do, however, seem to use countertransference, even if they do not emphasize its use. It might be said that their use of countertransference is limited due to their extreme focus on insight. Their emphasis on insight and self-reflection, as opposed to action, positions them at the extreme of the continuum.

As one moves along the continuum within the psychoanalytic/object relations view, the more action is combined with self-reflection, the greater the extent to which countertransference seems to be used. Even though a few therapists, like Box and colleagues, Slipp, and Scharff and Scharff, use the totalistic definition of countertransference, their work is not necessarily reflective of the greatest use of countertransference. If the unintentional use of countertransference is considered as a complement to the intentional, then therapists who recognize the unintentional use of countertransference may well use countertransference more often, and more effectively, than do modern analytic therapists. There are therapists like Ackerman or Skynner (who will be presented in the next section) who can be clearly shown to use countertransference unintentionally as well as intentionally. And whereas Box and colleagues, Slipp, and Scharff and Scharff seem to limit their unintentional use of countertransference by not acknowledging it, therapists like Ackerman and Skynner embrace the idea that their own unique but integrated personalities are part of their therapy.

THE INTEGRATIONIST VIEW

In this section four therapists who integrate theoretical viewpoints in their use of countertransference will be presented. A primary difference between the views held by these therapists and those of Ackerman, and thus one differentiating the integrationist position from the psychoanalytic/object relations position, is the level at which interpersonal theory is used as a frame of reference for the therapeutic approach. The therapists in this section recognize the importance of theory, but it appears that as action becomes a greater part of their approach theory is less emphasized. The presentation of views in this section ranges from an integration of theory by Skynner that is very self-reflective but also experiential, to a mostly experiential but sometimes self-reflective integration by Harry J. Aponte and Joan E. Winter. These two approaches seem to reflect the most effective use of countertransference among the integrationist therapists. Both approaches recognize intentional and unintentional uses of countertransference. The middle two therapists here, Michael Nichols and Rodney Shapiro, use countertransference in what seems to be a much less effective way. Nichols and Shapiro both recognize only the intentional use of countertransference, and, by failing to comprehensively apply the theory of such a use, appear to lose much of its benefit.

Robin Skynner

Skynner (1981) presented a way of working with countertransference that bears a resemblance to the suggestions of both Jackson and Ackerman, as discussed above. His method appears to be somewhat experiential in nature, thus suggesting similarities with the work of therapists like Whitaker as well. Yet Skynner (1981) describes his own approach, calling it "group analytic," as using object relations thinking as a "particularly powerful source of understanding" (p. 40), and he integrates systems theory to great benefit (1976). Skynner's work is an excellent example of how a psychoanalytic/object relations formulation is helpful in understanding therapy of any kind, whether it resembles a classical analytic approach or an experiential approach. His psychotherapeutic perspective also appears to posit object relations theory as a systems theory.

On first meeting with a family, Skynner (1981) describes his experience as including vague feelings of unknown origin that increasingly seem to be information about the family. Soon these vague feelings become associated with an increasing sense of conflict. At first they are a "vague discomfort" but gradually they "crystallize" into an impulse toward some action that is felt to be "somehow inappropriate and better kept concealed"

(p. 60). Finally, "there is the conviction that the response aroused is perhaps exactly what the therapist needs to put into the family system, since one realizes on reflecting on the interview that it is exactly what has been missing throughout it—some emotional attitude conspicuous by its absence—and that one is feeling inhibited because one is resonating to the family's taboos on expressing this particular aspect of human nature" (p. 60).

The "resonating to the family's taboos" described here sounds similar to Stierlin's (1977) idea that being taken in by family myths can cause countertransference difficulty. But, instead of limiting this experience, Skynner allows himself to become a part of the family's system and thus experience the family myths. He is then able to use his countertransference reactions. He states that this is not a logical, step-by-step process. Rather, what occurs is a sudden flash of insight with a coming together of all the other experiential fragments into a meaningful whole.

In further discussing his work, Skynner distinguishes between the insight that can be gained through verbal interpretation and the change that occurs when the therapist acts on his understanding of the family dynamic. Although he suggests that insightful families can benefit from interpretation, he believes that the most powerful intervention is when the therapist allows himself to enact the "scapegoat" role. Skynner (1981) states about interventions at a later stage of treatment: "It is as if the family members have been fleeing from a monster and finally find refuge in the safety of the therapist's room only to discover, as they begin to feel secure and to trust him, that he turns into the monster himself!" (p. 61).

In this method, the trust that is built up with the family is essential in enabling them to tolerate the therapy experience. Skynner (1980), with confidence that he can tolerate the family members' experience, allows his own experience, molded by the influence of intrapsychic and interpersonal patterns, to inform him of what the family's experience is. He sums up the strength of his method by indicating that becoming part of the therapist–family system allows him to address and contain defenses and resistances as well as denied or repressed emotions. He states (1981): "By absorbing the projective system of a disturbed family, the therapist suffers from their dilemma himself first, but the solution, if found, is inevitably tailored to that particular family's exact defensive structure" (p. 61).

Skynner does not refer to countertransference in his work, but his use of the terms "containment" and "projection" clearly indicates how he uses his countertransference. As in Ackerman's work, it seems that a transference–countertransference system starts to develop and that it is Skynner's ability to recognize that system through self-reflection that is the crux of his final interventions.

In his description of "absorbing the projective system" of the family, Skynner is also describing how he works with projective identification. Just as he does not discuss the use of countertransference, he does not generally use the term "projective identification." However, in his book *Systems of Family and Marital Psychotherapy* (1976), he does discuss the influence of the family's projections on the therapist and states that this term has been used to describe such phenomena. In discussing transference, Skynner (1976) states that there is a complicating aspect, often neglected, which leads to naive and limited techniques: "This complicating aspect is that the projected model can actually affect the internal experience and behavior of the therapist himself in such a way that he is manipulated into enacting the behavior pattern predicted by the model and so verifying its correctness once again" (p. 77).

He goes on to say, "The prime necessity is for the therapist to receive the projection without being taken over by it and acting it out, so that he can maintain his own identity and respond in a way which is related to the expectations inherent in the model projected, but which is different and, hopefully (if the therapist is more mature or healthy than the person on whom the original model was based), a more accurate and effective guide to dealing with the world" (p. 79).

By "without being taken over by it" Skynner is obviously not referring to lack of action but rather is emphasizing that the action taken be related to the therapist's intact identity. Skynner emphasizes that the action must come from the therapist's center. He explains that the action the therapist chooses may be most effective if it embodies the more mature way that the therapist, with his identity intact, would react to the emotions created in him.

The eye of the storm in a family interview is the still center, reached by allowing oneself to move willingly into the middle of the emotional cyclone, through the region of greatest turbulence and danger to one's own stability, into the "I" where one is most truly oneself and, since it is one's own center and point of balance, the point where one is most free and most in control of oneself. If one can reach this point, probably any response one makes will be valuable, whether interpretation, action, or simply waiting in order to allow others to interpret or act instead. . . . [Skynner 1976, p. 81]

Thus Skynner advocates an unintentional use of countertransference, one that relies on the therapist's intact and well-developed identity. The therapist's behavioral response is the outcome of feeling the pull toward confirming the family's transferential perspective commingled with the therapist's unique personality. The therapeutic quality of that behavior is dependent on the stability of the therapist's personality. Although a minor part of the first excerpt above, even Skynner's reference to detecting feelings in himself that are not entirely his "alone" is suggestive of his knowledge that the feelings he does experience are a combination of his own personality dynamics and those being projected by the family. If the therapist is effective in maintaining his emotional balance, the action that is born of that combination might just be exactly what is most needed in the intervention.

More than any other therapist thus far presented, Skynner's work is reflective of a transference–countertransference, relational systems perspective. In his work it seems likely that the interactive nature of the therapist's role relies heavily on what I have referred to as an unintentional use of countertransference. In becoming "the monster," it appears that Skynner may risk some nontherapeutic action. However, after the therapist has been with a family for some time, his ongoing experience allows for recognition of an overall pattern within the projective system that is, when noticed by the therapist through self-reflection, processed more fully, metabolized, and then given back to the family for reinternalization at a verbal level. Thus both an unintentional and an intentional use of countertransference are involved in his approach.

Although I believe that Skynner's approach nears the ideal in integrating object relations, systems, and experiential thinking, his reluctance to discuss the concept of projective identification in either the family's effect on him or his effect on the family leaves some room for clarification on the theory behind the therapeutic process he describes. The concept of projective identification is essential to the relational systems perspective. It could be guessed from his (1976) overview of systems theory, however, that Skynner understands the family as an open system and allows himself, in the role of therapist, to be an open system in experiencing and affecting the family. Such a view, a view that would value the therapist–family system construct highly, seems to reflect the way he works. Skynner does not, however, discuss his role as a therapist in these terms.

Michael Nichols

Nichols (1987) draws from psychodynamic models in enhancing his systems approach. Nichols defines countertransference in a totalistic way but seems to emphasize the classical aspects. He starts with the premise that therapists cannot avoid induction into a family. "They can try, but it won't work. The important factor is not the therapist's ability to avoid the family's pull or avoid the temptation to react emotionally to them, but rather the ability to recognize when he or she is trapped and immersed in the system, and to work his or her way out" (p. 278).

Nichols takes the position that avoiding negative aspects of countertransference is best achieved by approaching families "without needing anything from them" (p. 284). He describes this attitude as a kind of neutrality in which the therapist does not need a family to like him, does not need them to get better, and does not need them to act in any particular ways. According to Nichols, "The neutral therapist eschews determining how families should behave in favor of helping them discover what is right for them" (p. 280).

Nichols differentiates two specific types of countertransference both of which he describes as potential problems. The first kind of countertransference is "the therapist's own personal and idiosyncratic response, stemming from unresolved conflict and constituting a potential undesirable bias, which client families should not be burdened with" (p. 282). According to Nichols this kind of countertransference will not cause difficulty if the therapist maintains neutrality.

The second kind of countertransference is "the therapist's natural and valid reaction to important messages, unconsciously transmitted by family members" (p. 282). This second type can lead to the use of countertransference. However, Nichols cautions that if therapeutic neutrality is lost when influenced by this second type of reaction, even though it might constitute a communication from the family, then its hold on the therapist comprises a potential undesirable bias similar to that found with the first type of countertransference reaction. The therapist must not act according to the countertransference felt but must self-reflect in order to make use of it. Nichols writes: "When the therapist is at an appropriate distance and maintains neutrality, his or her response to the family's behavior should be trial action— that is, thought— rather than impulsive reaction" (p. 280).

When this thought is imposed on the first type of countertransference response, the therapist prevents herself from bringing her own conflicts into the therapy. When this thought is imposed on the second type of countertransference response, the therapist learns something about the family that can be used to further treatment. When any countertransference feelings are not scrutinized by self-reflection, then impulsive reaction is likely to result. In that event, according to Nichols, a family could be unfairly burdened by the therapist's actions anytime a countertransference reaction occurs without the maintenance of neutrality freeing the therapist's mind for scrutiny of those feelings. Nichols presents his general approach in saying, "When feelings do get stirred up, the first thing to do is to notice them. Try to be neutral, but face what you do feel. A phobic attitude toward your feelings leads only to denial. Countertransference can be useful if you begin to understand it, what it says about the family, about you and about the therapeutic relationship" (p. 284).

Nichols's work is a clear demonstration of his view that the therapist's self must be used within a therapy. Perhaps his use of self is a good compromise between the introspection necessary within analytic methods and the activity of the therapist necessary in family systems therapy. But this "use of self" is far different from what experiential therapists mean by the phrase. Experientially speaking, the use-of-self approach (Aponte and Winter 1987, Satir 1987) would certainly not emphasize neutrality.

In general, Nichols's approach sounds very similar to that of the object relations therapists. However, he not only advocates interventions based primarily on interpretation, like those of the object relations school, but also structural and strategic interventions. Nichols believes in an integrative approach that relies on what has been discovered from systems theory as well as what has been learned in psychoanalytic therapy. His work is especially interesting in that it is an integrative approach that seems to come primarily from the systems view. Most of the authors who discuss countertransference as a useful part of their work seem to find the origins of their techniques within psychoanalytic theory.

But Nichols only applies the most rudimentary aspects of the theory behind the use of countertransference, thus limiting its usefulness. Also, he does not elaborate on the extent to which he becomes a part of the therapist–family system. He acknowledges that countertransference reactions are sometimes left over from the therapist's unresolved conflicts and sometimes are the result of projections from the family or its members. He even suggests that the therapist's feelings can be informative about the therapeutic *relationship*, which suggests that he is aware of unintentional aspects of countertransference (at least up to the point where they should be analyzed for meaning). The missing ingredient in Nichols's work is in the area of a more comprehensive theoretical explanation for what happens in family therapy. The depth of understanding that can be provided by applying psychoanalytic/object relations thinking to the therapist's countertransference reactions is reduced when it is not applied in a comprehensive way to the therapist and the family. Nichols never addresses the processes involved in transmission of countertransference phenomena, specifically projective identification, projection, and introjection.

One step that can make Nichols's integration of theory more meaningful is to conceive of the therapist as part of the therapist–family system. As has been the case among many of the other therapists I have presented, Nichols never addresses the effect of the therapist's unique personality on the family, thus eliminating the relational systems perspective. Although Nichols's work is in my view the best attempt to date at integrating object relations thinking into systems thinking (as opposed to integrating systems thinking into object relations thinking, which has been best accomplished thus far by Skynner), the therapeutic system cannot be complete without the therapist.

Rodney Shapiro

Shapiro is known for integrating systems and psychodynamic thinking. His (1981) article, cited here, represents that viewpoint. However, perhaps because of the need to make his thought palatable to a mainstream family therapy audience, his ideas are presented in what seems to be an overly simplistic way. The idea of viewing countertransference as anything but

problematic would have been a long stretch for the average family therapist at the time this paper was published. Shapiro introduced a clearly
totalistic view of countertransference into the family therapy mainstream
by having his paper published in a widely read book edited by Alan Gurman
called *Questions and Answers in the Practice of Family Therapy* (1981).
(Skynner's 1981 article, also published by Gurman in 1981, did not discuss the totalistic view of countertransference but simply presented an
approach in which the totalistic view was obvious.) Much as Nichols did,
in work that would be published later, Shapiro attempted to integrate a use
of countertransference into family systems thinking. In his article, Shapiro
discusses countertransference as both problematic and useful.

Shapiro (1981) succinctly states that "Strong feelings in the therapist
may be a normative experience in successfully engaging with a family. It
is to the therapist's advantage to regard his/her reactions to the family as
valuable data that can help the progress of treatment. The task for the
therapist is to distinguish what is being conveyed by the family or individual members, from feelings that he/she may be inappropriately attributing to the family" (pp. 196–197). Shapiro believes countertransference
can be beneficial. But there is surprisingly little explanation in his paper
as to why countertransference can be beneficial.

In explaining how the therapist might discern what has been "conveyed"
by the family from his own inappropriate attributions, Shapiro goes on to
say that "the criterion for what is said by the therapist should be the therapeutic needs of the family and not the personal needs of the therapist" (p.
199). But, like Nichols, Shapiro does not discuss how countertransference
feelings are conveyed. His main point is that "a more productive approach
[to countertransference] is to explore the possibility that such reactions
reflect the feelings of the family" (p. 199). Perhaps Shapiro felt this idea
would be so new to family therapists that it would be better to keep it simple.
But if it is a true reflection of his work, then the absence of theory involved in it indicates a fairly superficial rendering of the use of countertransference.

While it is clear that Shapiro would advocate self-reflection in his use
of countertransference, thus conveying the meaning that an intentional
use of countertransference is an aspect of his therapy, the unintentional
use of countertransference goes for the most part unrecognized. Again, in
a way that resembles Nichols's work, this oversight seems to be connected
to a failure to fully include the therapist in the therapist–family system.

The theory Shapiro applies to the family system is seemingly not well developed, nor is it applied to the therapist. That the therapist's emotions might be reflective of emotions in the family is a fact he does present well. However, without an explanation for what motivated the family or its members to create those emotions in the therapist, or even how, behaviorally, those emotions can be created in the therapist, the options for intervention would seem to be severely limited. Some readers may even feel that Shapiro is asking them to believe in some mystical or extrasensory phenomenon. Nevertheless, although it is a relatively superficial attempt, Shapiro's integration of a use of countertransference into his systems therapy was the first widely known straightforward attempt to do so.

Harry J. Aponte

Aponte, who is best known for furthering the development of structural family therapy (Aponte and VanDeusen 1981), has discussed the therapist's use of self (Aponte and Winter 1987). His integrationist stance can best be seen in his references to experiential therapists like Satir and Whitaker. Aponte's "use of self," a term he borrows from Satir (Satir and Baldwin 1983), clearly includes both intentional and unintentional uses of countertransference. However, Aponte's integrationist stance is very different from that of Nichols or Shapiro owing to its experiential influences. The unintentional use of countertransference is much more important in his approach.

Among the four "fundamental therapeutic skills" Aponte (Aponte and Winter 1987) identifies as essential in the well-trained family therapist are the therapist's "internal skills, or the personal integration of the therapist's own experiences and self in order to become a useful therapeutic instrument" (p. 86). One great element of contrast between Aponte and the other therapists presented so far is that for him this personal integration is considered essential; this is the case because for him the therapist is inevitably part of a system with the family: "It is inevitable that both patient and therapist will bring into the therapeutic relationship each person's real and psychological linkages with their respective lives which bear all the scars of their past along with the wounds inflicted by their current lives" (p. 92).

Similar views will be seen in the work of Satir and Minuchin presented below. But Aponte (Aponte and Winter 1987) goes one step further in this next statement: "Successful clinicians learn to be aware of what material they currently bring into the therapeutic process, both strengths and problems, and how to employ these resources for the client's growth and change" (p. 94). Here, Aponte seems to be suggesting that even the problems or idiosyncrasies of the therapist can be useful if the therapist is aware of them and keeps them in check. This statement is truly reflective of the relational systems perspective.

Aponte emphasizes the fact that the therapist responds to the family in a natural way as it fits him into their patterns, and them into his, thus suggesting an unintentional use of countertransference. He also emphasizes that the therapist self-reflects on his experience of this process. In self-reflection the therapist uses the knowledge he gains to inform his treatment approach. Thus the unintentional and intentional uses of countertransference are both clearly a part of his work. But Aponte falls short in describing how emotional exchanges take place in family therapy.

Perhaps the general structural model is supposed to clarify this issue; however, structural therapy never developed a comprehensive theoretical model for understanding the transmission of emotions. Even the boundary concept falls short of making clear why boundaries are crossed. Structural theory is primarily clinically based, and change is the emphasis of the therapy. By contrast, an intrapsychic and interpersonal theory of human behavior, like object relations theory, is more helpful in obtaining a clearer understanding of the actual connection between family members and the therapist, rather than vaguely stating that it exists. The better understanding a therapist can have of that kind of theoretical system, the more likely the therapist is to understand how to intervene in the process by which the family members and therapist exchange emotions. Such focus is not evident in Aponte's writing.

Summary and Conclusions

On the self-reflection versus action continuum, the integrationist view is comprised of four therapists from disparate backgrounds. Skynner's central approach is most informed by psychoanalytic and object relations theory, Nichols's by systems theory, Shapiro's by psychodynamic theory, and Aponte's by structural systems theory. Yet all these therapists attempt to weave into their work what I call a use of countertransference or use of the self. So all these therapists make self-reflection a part of their work. With regard to the continuum, perhaps the most interesting factor revealed in reviewing the work of these therapists is that, even though self-reflection is absolutely essential in the intentional use of countertransference, the most intensive use of self-reflection may not always reflect the most intensive use of countertransference. In Skynner's work we see a great amount of self-reflection as well as freedom to act on the experiential aspects of doing therapy. Both the intentional and the unintentional uses of countertransference are emphasized, so that the use of countertransference is integral to his work. In the work of both Nichols and Shapiro, the use of self-reflection appears to be less emphasized than in the work of Skynner yet more emphasized than in the work of Aponte. Both Nichols and Shapiro fail to recognize the therapist's unintentional use of countertransference, a situation that further limits their use of countertransference. In Aponte's work, although self-reflection is used, it is de-emphasized. The unintentional use of countertransference becomes prominent with his "use of self." Since both the intentional and the unintentional uses of countertransference do find a place in his work, however, Aponte generally uses countertransference more than either Nichols or Shapiro. It seems the acknowledgment of the experiential aspects of therapy, as seen in the work of both Skynner and Aponte, is essential to a full use of countertransference within the integrationist view. But the experiential and unintentional use of countertransference may be of greatest benefit when complemented by the self-reflective and intentional.

THE EXPERIENTIAL VIEW

The experiential view has had a very strong following in family therapy. In this section are included two therapists, Virginia Satir and Carl Whitaker, who in many ways tower above the field in their renown and expertise. Examining the use of countertransference among these therapists is especially interesting when their work is viewed from a perspective of the unintentional use of countertransference complementing the intentional use. The views of experiential authors are central to the topic explored here since the desire for authenticity and the "use of self" which they describe bear a great resemblance to the unintentional use of countertransference. In the previous section, movement toward a very effective unintentional use of countertransference could be seen in the work of Aponte, who cited Satir's influence on much of what he referred to as the "use of self." In this section the unintentional use of countertransference reaches full bloom. First, in Satir's work we see no reference to the word "countertransference" and yet find an elegant use of both its intentional and unintentional aspects. Toward the end of the section the work of Whitaker will be presented. Whitaker defines countertransference in the classical tradition and does not use it intentionally, but the unintentional use he makes of it can be demonstrated to be an important part of his work. Perhaps one way of organizing this section would be to separate two central views. Satir's work, and that of Shirley Luthman that follows it on the continuum, could be described as a "use of self" view in which the therapist intentionally uses her personality to benefit treatment. Whitaker's work, and that of Walter Kempler that follows it on the continuum, could be described as an open-expression view in which the therapist's personality is integral to what occurs in the therapy, but self-reflection is subordinated to authenticity (which seems to translate into the full and relatively uncontrolled expression of the therapist's experience). Thus, what is clearly shown in the experiential school of family therapy is a progression along the self-reflection versus action continuum, from an emphasis on self-reflection in being with client-families, to an emphasis on genuineness in reacting to client-families. Both positions place at least de facto importance on the view that the therapist becomes part of the therapist–family system.

Virginia Satir

Satir is well known for her association with the Mental Research Institute, along with Jackson and Haley. But unlike Jackson and Haley, who emphasized systems models and approaches, Satir became much more humanistic in her view of therapy. She also had a great deal of psychoanalytic understanding that seemed to affect her work. Even though Satir's work had so many different influences, her approach was generally thought of as experiential; she emphasized experiencing as well as communication between family members. Many therapists now hold her in high regard for her "use of self" (Aponte and Winter 1987) and for her dedication to maintaining an empathic and nurturing environment in family therapy (Luepnitz 1988).

Perhaps one reason that Satir is not considered a major contributor to family therapy theory is that some of the techniques she used so naturally and elegantly did not fit well with the systems thinking of the time. But in viewing the contributions she was able to make toward the use of countertransference in family therapy, it seems her work may be more important than the work of most of her contemporaries. Satir's use of self included a way of working with empathy as well as countertransference. It could be said that she was in the business of healing via nurturance. She took a nurturing attitude toward the families with whom she worked. She also attempted to teach family members to have more nurturing attitudes toward one another. Although Satir did not state that she was "using countertransference," this next statement clearly demonstrates what I would consider its very natural and empathic use.

> The therapist's ability to check on his own internal manifestations is one of the most important therapeutic tools he has. If his internal experience of an interview is different from all other data he is observing and he is fairly sure his reaction is not related to something going on in his personal life, then the most effective way to proceed is on the basis of that internal data. It takes time for the therapist to become aware and be able to trust his internal manifestations, but when he does, he will always have another way to proceed in a therapy situation when he feels stuck. [Satir and Baldwin 1983, p. 233]

In this excerpt it appears that using countertransference is simply a natural part of using one's self. Perhaps one of Satir's most noteworthy abilities was to simply integrate nurturance, including a natural use of countertransference, into her therapy. Her use of countertransference as shown in this excerpt, although intentional, appears to have been naturally integrated into her methods. It seems as though she was able to use countertransference well both intentionally and unintentionally.

Satir's approach is generally atheoretical. Yet it would not be true to say that she was unaware of an unintentional use of countertransference.

Despite her lack of explanation of her methods in theoretical terms, Satir made great use of the unintentional use of countertransference. By being nurturing and extremely empathic, she reparented whole families. She was a role model and an expert in emotional communication. Her therapy is more marked by a positive but unintentional use of countertransference than by its intentional use, although the evidence of her using counter-transference intentionally as well, as in the excerpt above, demonstrates a balanced approach.

Satir also indirectly described her method as allowing her to make her-self a part of the therapist–family system. Aponte and Winter (1987), in quoting Satir and Baldwin (1983, p. 191) on Satir's method, wrote: "This theoretical framework incorporates the total life experience of both family and the therapist, conscious and unconscious, real and fantasized. A sys-tems approach holds that 'every part is related to the other parts in a way that a change in one brings about a change in all others. Indeed, everyone and everything impacts and is impacted by every other person, event and thing'" (pp. 91–92).

For Satir, as with Aponte and Winter, the inclusion of the therapist as part of the therapist–family system makes the therapist's mental health important to a therapeutic outcome. In this next statement Satir and Baldwin (1983) describe several essentials of Satir's stance, including her view of the therapist's mental health, and what I would call the unintentional use of countertransference in the form of nurturance:

Using oneself as a therapist is an awesome task. To be equal to that task one needs to continue to develop one's humanness and matu-rity. We are dealing with people's lives. In my mind, learning to be a therapist is not like learning to be a plumber. Plumbers can usually settle for techniques. Therapists need to do more. You don't have to love a pipe to fix it. Whatever techniques, philosophy or school of family therapy we belong to, whatever we actually do with others has to be funneled through ourselves as people. [p. 227]

Satir emphasized the person of the therapist no matter what kind of therapy is practiced.

It is clear that from Satir's perspective the therapist is part of the thera-pist–family system, and also that she understood the interpersonal processes of that system extremely well. She valued a high degree of personal development in the therapist, as marked by her desire to develop her "humanness and maturity." Therefore it is clear that Satir made use of both unintentional and intentional uses of countertransference. But as in the case of Aponte and Winter, evidence of her theoretical understanding of the therapeutic process is lacking. Although I have a strong suspicion that Satir simply subordinated theoretical language to the simpler language of what she thought was most important in therapy, no clear concepts are presented as a guide to the use of self she described. By not conceptualizing in terms of theory, and by relying exclusively on the natural mental health and creativity of the therapist, it is likely that she missed many therapeutic opportunities. An understanding of how certain dynamic concepts work, for example that of projective identification, clearly offers an opening to many additional possibilities for intervention in interpersonal and intrapsychic process.

Shirley Luthman

Luthman's (1974) approach is very similar to Satir's. She adds to Satir's viewpoint, however, in her descriptions of ways to approach some of the negative aspects of countertransference (although, like Satir, Luthman never uses the word countertransference). Luthman believes the most important things a therapist can do to avoid negative feelings related to a therapy are to be aware of those feelings and to take care of one's own needs outside the therapy. Like Whitaker and his associates, presented below, Luthman believes that negative feelings are inevitable. But because she uses herself spontaneously within a therapy, most feelings experienced by the therapist using her model do not cause countertransference difficulties. This is not to say that Luthman encourages acting on negative feelings. Rather, within her model for therapy, negative feelings experienced by the therapist are channeled toward benefiting the family by seeking to find their source and encouraging expression from that source. For example, if a therapist can come to an understanding of the anger she is experiencing as having its source in a conflict between a mother and child, it is the therapist's responsibility to find a way to bring out expression of that conflict between the mother and child, rather than through her own expression of the feeling. This might be the logical next step to what Satir (Satir and Baldwin 1983) said was "another way to proceed" when strong emotions are experienced in the therapist. Thus Luthman's views seem very similar to those discussed more indirectly by Satir. Her language indicates both an intentional and an unintentional use of countertransference as well as a conceptualization of the therapist as within the therapist–family system. However, in Luthman's work, as in Satir's, a theoretical system through which to understand her approach is lacking.

Carl Whitaker

Earlier in this chapter, I described the use of countertransference in the background of several of family therapy's pioneers, including Whitaker. Before becoming a family therapist, Whitaker (1946, 1947) wrote of his strong belief in the curative powers of a therapeutic relationship in which the availability of the therapist's personality was of central importance. As a family therapist, Whitaker, along with two of his closest cohorts, wrote a seminal piece on countertransference in family therapy that aimed at highlighting the problematic aspects of the concept. Even though this paper focused on problematic aspects of countertransference, it is evident throughout the paper that Whitaker's ideas about how the therapeutic relationship cures had not changed much since his early work. Whitaker continued to emphasize what I would call an unintentional use of countertransference with relatively little self-reflection.

In this paper, entitled "Countertransference in the Family Treatment of Schizophrenia" (Whitaker et al. 1965), the authors extensively describe their ideas about countertransference. Although the paper focuses on families with schizophrenic members, its contents are generally applicable to Whitaker's approach. As Whitaker and his associates view it, the therapist does not maintain a neutral stance, as is advocated by some psychoanalytic family therapists. Rather, the therapist must become intimately and emotionally involved in order to have an effect. These authors believe the therapist must become part of the therapist–family system. However, they also assert that countertransference is primarily a problematic occurrence within a therapy. As Whitaker and his associates (1965) wrote, "we must warn that countertransference is non-therapeutic but the depth of involvement which it evidences is necessary in the successful treatment of any psychotic patient" (p. 325). Thus they attempt to avoid countertransference even though they aim to become involved in depth with their clients.

Whitaker and associates (1965) employ an unintentional use of countertransference from within the therapist–family system, but hope to avoid problems associated with the therapist's becoming too close to the family system. They make a small attempt to use countertransference intentionally, but only indirectly and as a consequence of relying on a co-therapist to guard against too intimate a relationship between the other co-therapist and the family. Since they take the position that countertransference is generally nontherapeutic, their methods for avoiding the associated problems are an integral part of this discussion.

In clarifying how Whitaker and associates (1965) generally view countertransference issues, the following statement, which exemplifies the complicated processes involved in the work of a therapist using their model, is helpful:

> The family is intact and he is enacting only a functional role. His normal warmth in relating to an individual suddenly becomes a countertransference vector. His affect must be attached to the family unit, yet he may not belong to it. He must help the family to break up their group loyalty, to develop new subgroups, and gradually to sense their right to "belong" yet not lose their identity in the group . . . Through all this process he must be "in," yet not "of," the family and its subgroups. He must be available to each person of the family, yet belong to none; he must belong to himself. [p. 335]

I begin with this excerpt not only because it expresses the complications involved in the work of these therapists, but more specifically because it reflects the desire to be both a part of the therapist–family system and out of the family system at the same time. Whitaker clearly values the experience of being "in" the therapist–family system and this is precisely why he wrote an article (Whitaker et al. 1965) about the perils of countertransference. The problem seems to be that once he gets "in" the system, he may become "of" the system. If, through countertransference difficulty, he becomes "of" the system, he is no longer effective.

Whitaker and associates (1965) believe that two main problem areas arise in countertransference reactions, with both areas having the potential to cause difficulty in maintaining the therapeutic separateness necessary for therapeutic effectiveness. They state that "to maintain his separateness throughout the therapeutic process, the therapist must avoid not only the countertransference problem of overinvolvement but also the countertransference problem of isolation" (p. 336). Although Whitaker and associates (1965) do not discuss the exact nature of these two areas of difficulty, it can be extrapolated from their writing that overinvolvement occurs when the therapist is too much a part of the family to be objective, and isolation occurs as a result of the therapist trying too hard to maintain distance from the family. The vagaries of balancing intimacy with separation in a therapeutic context have been outlined in the psychoanalytic literature as well, especially with respect to the concept of empathy (Greenson 1960).

Whitaker and his associates hold that the best way to resolve countertransference problems is to prevent them. They suggest that this prevention is related to various strengths and experiences that a therapist should have. Like Freud and many other therapists (Aponte and Winter 1987, Jackson 1956), Whitaker and associates (1965) believe that a therapist must have had an adequate experience of being in therapy to prevent her countertransference reactions from negatively affecting the therapy she provides. They believe this therapy experience is important "so that [one] comes to the treatment process with a maturity and freedom to become involved in the relationship without losing [one's] own integrity or without becoming pathologically transferred to the treatment situation" (p. 336).

Whitaker and associates (1965), like other therapists (e.g., Aponte and Winter 1987), also believe that the family therapist needs an adequate training experience, one in which the therapist has an opportunity to face her own countertransference tendencies as well as work through countertransference affects that help her grow through struggle. They mention the need for a good base of support within one's professional arena and healthy relations within one's own family as well. They suggest that these strengths and experiences prevent countertransference from becoming a problem in that with them the therapist can have the confidence to approach the family honestly with countertransference feelings. Whitaker and associates believe that the honesty the ideal therapist embodies in expressing countertransference feelings works as a model for the family, and thus not only prevents countertransference from becoming a problem but also leads the family members to become more honest with each other.

Although Whitaker and associates (1965) make the point that countertransference feelings should be shared, it is not clear how this helps a family. Paradoxically, they also warn that overt expression of the therapist's "pathology" to the family must be controlled by the therapist's clinical judgment of its danger. "However," they write, "unwillingness to share it is frequently based on the therapist's pride and embarrassment, and in this event only produces a secondary type of confusion in the relating" (p. 325). Thus it appears that the primary purpose of expressing countertransference reactions to a family, according to Whitaker and associates, is to model honesty in relating for the client-family. The expression of countertransference feelings also prevents the therapist from being inauthentic.

Whitaker and associates (1965) do not mention how the therapist might make the clinical judgment mentioned above in deciding whether countertransference feelings, or one's own pathology, pose a danger to the family. However, a contribution for which Whitaker (1958) is well known is his belief that the use of a co-therapist can ensure that the countertransference reactions of one therapist do not get out of control and hurt the treatment. Whitaker and associates (1965) write that "the only effective counter to [strong countertransference reactions] seems to be a co-therapist who can help make the personal needs of the therapist a current problem of the treatment situation" (p. 328). That is, if one therapist believes the other is acting out countertransference feelings, then that issue should be brought up with the family in the therapy. They believe that countertransference acting out is less likely when two therapists are present. When two therapists are present, they believe, one therapist can probably insure that the other therapist is "stable in his own setting and in being himself" (p. 330).

Whitaker and associates (1965) also believe that co-therapy can be helpful in resolving countertransference difficulties because it allows a therapist who finds that he is having a countertransference reaction to retreat into the co-therapy relationship. According to Neill and Kniskern (1982), who chronicled and integrated Whitaker's work, by utilizing co-therapists "the therapists gained power in their ability to reflect and comment on both their own and the family's feelings and activities" (p. 17), which suggests that a form of self-reflection is a part of this approach. Perhaps the stability gained from working with a co-therapist can also help a therapist maintain the level of separateness from a family that Whitaker and associates describe as essential.

One last suggestion given by Whitaker and associates (1965) is that a therapist should maintain an overview of the family as a whole. They believe that the therapist's affective relationship to the family as a whole is one way to keep from having countertransference with individual members or subgroups within the family. They pose this overview as one side of a dilemma, stating that the therapist must also maintain contact with the individuals and subgroups. A resolution of countertransference for the therapist, they write, "necessitates a type of fluidity and strength in his moving in and out of the family situation. To be strong and fluid the therapist must 'be,' and in his 'being' stand and move in his own personal uniqueness and his own spontaneity. Continuity in relating is less valuable than authenticity" (p. 338). Other family therapists also believe that characteristics related to this "fluidity" and "authenticity" are essential in doing family therapy (Ackerman 1966, Keith 1987, Kempler 1965, 1968, Luthman 1974, Skynner 1981). From the perspective of Whitaker and his associates working with such fluidity suggests that there is no problem with countertransference.

This paper by Whitaker and associates (1965) demonstrates that Whitaker had not significantly changed his general therapeutic approach with regard to countertransference since his early work. Yet such an approach would cause many observers to wonder about countertransference difficulties, since so much action is involved in it. It seems Whitaker and his associates do an excellent job in describing how those countertransference difficulties that might be encountered in their approach are prevented or controlled. But more than that, their unintentional use of countertransference is also outlined. Therapeutic cure comes from being "in" the family system but not "of" the family system. Another way of describing their view would be to say that the therapist must be fully a part of the therapist–family system without becoming incorporated into the family system. As part of the therapist–family system, as Whitaker and associates emphasize, and Whitaker has always maintained, the therapist's mental health is of utmost importance. What appears to be lacking in the work of Whitaker and his associates is a comprehensive understanding of how emotions and behavior are passed along and shaped—a theory backing up the therapeutic approach, and one that could lead to a more direct understanding of what kinds of intentional interventions bring salutary change in families. Since their view seems to position the therapist within the therapist–family system, it would seem that a clearer understanding of the therapist's countertransference would provide the type of theory most needed in their approach.

Walter Kempler

Although Kempler (1965, 1968) uses his experience with families broadly, he does not specifically discuss a need to avoid negative feelings with a family. His approach to working with feelings is similar in some ways to that of Luthman (1974) and in other ways to that of Whitaker (Whitaker et al. 1959, 1965). Like Luthman, Kempler looks for ways to bring expression to negative feelings generated in him. Unlike Luthman and much like Whitaker and associates, however, Kempler (1965) is likely to simply mention how he is feeling. His goal, like that of Whitaker and his associates is to remain genuine and to ask that family members be genuine as well. Given the similarities of his approach to those of the other therapists presented in this section, we find that Kempler also shares the same major difficulty in using countertransference. Although the unintentional use of countertransference is clearly an important part of his work, no theoretical understanding is applied in clarifying the interpersonal dynamics involved in such a process. The therapist following his approach would thus lack the awareness of these interpersonal dynamics that is necessary to use them fully for the benefit of the treatment.

Summary and Conclusions

Experiential family therapists have either not discussed countertransference or have used that term only in the classical sense. In general, a comprehensive theory by which therapy can be understood and guided is universally lacking among authors who use the experiential approach. Their work, however, with its emphasis on a "use of self" or authenticity, does seem to indicate a strong unintentional use of countertransference. All of the therapists in this section advocate becoming part of the therapist–family system in which the person of the therapist is essential to the therapeutic action. Although the intentional use of countertransference is de-emphasized by these authors, they differ dramatically in the extent to which they suggest the therapist's self-reflection should be applied. Thus, in the work of Satir and Luthman, the intentional use of countertransference is in evidence even if not emphasized. In the work of Whitaker and associates and Kempler there is very little evidence of an intentional use of countertransference.

The intentional and unintentional uses of countertransference found in the work of Satir and Luthman seem to be directly related to the therapist's desire for empathic responding. The work of Whitaker and associates and Kempler, on the other hand, emphasizes the quality of authentic response much more than empathy. It would appear that the therapist's authenticity, in their view, would often preclude self-reflection since such intentional mental action would interfere with the therapist's authentic personal process. Nevertheless, although Whitaker and associates emphasize unintentional uses of countertransference they also recognize the dangers involved. They discuss becoming too close to the family but feel that, being in the family group, the therapist's natural reactions to the family can be meaningful and must be shared. Their advocacy for a "fluid" use of the therapist's self suggests that the therapist's emotional reactions are used in a totalistic sense. Instead of using self-reflection, which may interfere with authenticity, however, they rely on a co-therapist to reign in the acting out of countertransference reactions, and perhaps to bring some reflective quality to the treatment. Kempler seems to use methods very similar to those of the Whitaker group, but without a co-therapist. Evidence of Kempler intentionally avoiding acting out is not apparent, but it is possible that what he considers an authentic response includes checking his own behavior. Unfortunately, Kempler does not specifically discuss any restraint on his part, and self-reflection cannot be said to be part of his method.

It is possible that the freedom with which experiential therapists work is beneficial to families, even without self-reflection. But it would seem that using self-reflection does give some insurance that countertransference difficulties will be limited and interventions will be more carefully formulated. When applying a totalistic definition of countertransference, it seems clear that all these therapists do advocate a use of countertransference. Such a use of countertransference requires a large amount of faith in the relatively advanced development of the therapist and/or, in Whitaker's case, faith in the co-therapist, since self-reflection is not emphasized. The way these therapists use their personalities is admirable. There is great care evident, and a willingness to truly open the experience of the therapist to even the most difficult aspects of the family's dynamics. But with a guiding theory lacking, it would seem that these authors pass up many opportunities that could only be recognized by directly applying knowledge gained from an explicit description of the way the therapist becomes part of the therapist–family system. Such knowledge would lead to interventions in which the family learns how its members pass on emotions and shape each others' behavior.

THE UNIMPORTANT VIEW

Countertransference, being a psychoanalytic term, has not been much discussed in family therapy. The systems, solution-oriented, and narrative approaches that most family therapists now practice generally do not consider countertransference or similar phenomena important. The fact that most of the adherents of these approaches insist that the therapist's emotions are unimportant, combined with the emphasis they place on action in the therapeutic approach, makes their placement at the action end of the self-reflection versus action continuum obvious. This is true even though systems theory would seemingly necessitate discussion of the therapist–family system, and therefore some use of countertransference, whether the term countertransference is applied or not. That is, an impact of the family on the therapist and vice versa would be predicted by systems theory. Since the systems therapist is trying to have a therapeutic impact, one might guess that systems theory would suggest that the therapist gain an understanding of how she has become part of the therapist–family system and attempt to harness that knowledge to salutary effect. But such thinking, although at times acknowledged (Minuchin and Fishman 1982), has not been well-developed by systems therapists. In fact, the way that systems theory has most often been applied to families excludes the therapist's personality from consideration (Haley 1976, Madanes and Haley 1977). As in systems-focused therapies, solution-oriented and narrative approaches have also not considered the therapist's part in the interpersonal dynamics of the therapist–family system, nor have they used any constructs that might have similar meaning. The powerful impact the family can have on the therapist has occasionally been acknowledged in these approaches, but responses to it have led only to ways of mitigating or nullifying that impact.

Salvador Minuchin

The structural viewpoint, as developed by Minuchin (Minuchin and Fishman 1982) does not have much to say concerning problematic aspects of countertransference. But Minuchin's perspective does not really fit the "unimportant view" position on the self-reflection versus action continuum. It would fit better in a "not very important" category. By extrapolation, Minuchin's approach can be identified as including at least an unintentional use of countertransference. He implies that he operates from within the therapist–family system. From within that system Minuchin's "use of self" (p. 30) is extremely important. He states: "Family therapy requires a use of self. A family therapist cannot observe and probe from without. He must be a part of a system of interdependent people" (p. 2). More specifically, that "use of self" is made up of feeling the family out, knowing when to coach, when to throw oneself into the family fray, or when to be an expert. If the therapist can do that successfully, Minuchin believes the therapist performs her duty well. Given these thoughts, it seems that Minuchin uses countertransference at least unintentionally if not intentionally. It is very unclear, however, why he would not experience any countertransference difficulties, especially when considering the extent to which he operates inside the family.

Don Jackson

Although Jackson's work was discussed earlier, I would like to place it on the self-reflection versus action continuum. It is interesting to observe that although Jackson's (1956) work on countertransference with psychoanalytic patients so clearly indicated how psychoanalytic theory could be modified to fit the family context, he nevertheless was also one of the most fervent advocates of the systems approach and of discarding psychoanalytic theory. What is apparent, however, is that the interpersonal aspects of human communication were very important to him. It is not known why the importance of the therapist as part of a therapeutic system never again became a part of Jackson's work after that time. Taken at surface level, directly from his paper (Jackson and Weakland 1961) that addressed psychoanalytic concepts as they might apply to family therapy, Jackson found no utility in the concept of countertransference when applied to the family therapy paradigm.

It is interesting, however, that his systems view, as propounded in that paper, although aimed at discounting the usefulness of concepts like countertransference, seems to imply that countertransference should be used to bring out communication in family members. That is, the approach to using countertransference that could be found in that paper of 1961 is similar to that which Satir and Luthman advocated. If the therapist feels a strong emotion toward the family, he can find out how others in the family are reacting to the same circumstance that evoked that emotion in him. Such an understanding and interpretation of Jackson's work comes about only with some analysis, however. Jackson's work can be placed at this point on the self-reflection versus action continuum because of his emphasis on action in therapy, as well as his direct statements suggesting that the concept of countertransference is of little utility. Since some evidence of self-reflection in his approach does exist, however, his approach should be placed toward the beginning of the unimportant position.

Paul Watzlawick, Janet Helmick Beavin, and Don Jackson

Therapists working from the strategic position do not discuss countertransference per se. Perhaps this is because they describe themselves as operating on the system of the family from the outside. Operating in such a way allows them to be effective with a family and remain objective. This idea comes originally from the book *Pragmatics of Human Communication* (Watzlawick et al. 1967) in which the authors describe problems in families as "games without end." These authors believe a therapist must be outside the "game" of a family so that they can "change the rules." They write: "In our view [the possibility] of outside intervention is a paradigm of psychotherapeutic intervention. In other words, the therapist as outsider is capable of supplying what the system itself cannot generate: a change of its own rules" (p. 235).

These authors do not discuss the likelihood that this positioning helps them to avoid emotional contact with a family (which leaves room for discussion of whether or not it actually does so), but it would seem to reflect a belief generally held by strategic therapists that operating outside the family system allows them to be invulnerable to the strong emotional pull that families can create.

Considering the therapist to be exclusively outside the family system in this way, however, is not necessarily contradictory to viewing the therapist as part of the therapist–family system. The relational systems perspective would fit with their view in that it recognizes that the therapist is outside the family system, but inside the therapist–family system. These theorists miss the potential for those interventions that can be formulated only if the therapist's emotions are recognized as reflective of the therapist–family system dynamics.

Jay Haley

Although Haley (1976) does not discuss countertransference, his work from outside the system, perhaps partially influenced by the work of Watzlawick and his colleagues (1967), suggests that countertransference would be completely unimportant from his perspective. This is so even though he discusses engagement with a family, a maneuver I believe suggests some emotional connection. Haley's engagement with a family is only at a problem-solving level, however. As with the work of Watzlawick and associates reviewed above, if Haley's work is to be viewed from the relational systems perspective, then the system created between therapist and family in his work constitutes a different sort of system than the one involved in the problem-generating system of the family itself. Haley emphasizes the therapist's ability to engage with the family at an exclusively problem-solving level, and identifies the therapist's inability to disengage from a family that no longer needs help as a typical problem encountered by therapists. In my view such an inability to disengage could be said to be a difficulty with countertransference.

But Haley (1976) does not discuss using countertransference in his work because of his strong belief that introspection is generally useless as a therapeutic tool. If introspection is useless, then, of course, self-reflection is useless as well. Haley does not believe that introspection helps either a therapist or a family (Madanes and Haley 1977). So, in his model, if a therapist is having difficulty in a therapy situation, then that therapist must look for a specific intervention that will remedy that situation. According to Haley, as a therapist becomes more skilled at working with problems, difficulties in working with families become less common. Perhaps the well-trained strategic therapist would not experience such difficulties if training helps her to maintain distance from the family. But such distance would likely interfere with the therapist's engagement of the family. Thus Haley's positioning of the therapist as a skilled expert operating from outside a system could allow for the avoidance of countertransference difficulties. But at the same time, it is clear that, when comparing such a model with practices using therapeutic empathy, or any other emotional attachment of the therapist, this procedure would be likely to preclude many opportunities. In the strategic model, interventions that could only be derived by allowing one's self to experience and notice the emotional push and pull in family therapy have no place.

Mara Selvini Palazzoli, Luigi Boscolo, Gianfranco Cecchin, and Giuliana Prata

The Milan systemic school of Palazzoli, Boscolo, Cecchin, and Prata sets up its therapy very specifically to avoid what appear to be countertransference problems. These authors (1978) postulate that induction always occurs when a therapist interacts closely with a family system. Induction, along with the negative connotation given to it, is a word that suggests becoming too enmeshed in a system to retain effectiveness in changing it. These authors are also very much influenced by the communications theory discussed by Watzlawick (Watzlawick et al. 1967), and "family games" are a big part of their work. In order to prevent the induction they fear, these authors use a co-therapist as well as two observers. They believe that involving themselves with their own group prevents induction into the family. The Milan systemic school seems to believe that the emotional powers of a family are very strong and could pose a large problem for the family therapist. However, the attempt to avoid the emotional power of the family, as opposed to harnessing it, seems to me to be putting the emphasis in the wrong place. By understanding, rather than avoiding the experience of being inducted into the family system, therapists using this model could more directly address systemic difficulties while also using insight to avoid countertransference acting out.

NARRATIVE AND SOLUTION-ORIENTED THERAPISTS

Among the narrative and solution-oriented therapists are Michael White (1991) and David Epston, William H. O'Hanlon, and Steve deShazer. Common among the views of these therapists is the view that the family already holds its solutions within itself. These therapists, sometimes referred to as constructivist (Nichols and Schwartz 1991), attempt to work with families toward co-constructing a different view of the reality that is already in existence but not recognized by their clients. The therapist points out where the family is already succeeding, where it is strong, or perhaps where its weakness has been misinterpreted. Solution-oriented therapies of this kind, like systems models, seem to view the position of the therapist as outside of the family, and consequently terms like countertransference are not discussed. It is hard to imagine, however, that the practitioner of these therapies never had the experience of finding a family hard to work with, or many of the other experiences that could be considered countertransference.

Perhaps part of the reason such experiences are not discussed within these models is that the models position the therapist in opposition to old ways of thinking that oppress the family. In these models, the therapist is on the same side as the family, but does not align with their problem-focused perspective. Discussing a countertransference reaction would be focusing on something the family is doing to maintain a problem (a problem focus) and would make it difficult to demonstrate how the family is handling things well. It is also possible that these narrative and solution-oriented approaches are yet too young to have needed to discuss these aspects of treatment. But as I have stated in referring to systems models, I believe many beneficial opportunities are likely missed due to the denial of emotion as an important factor in treating family problems. That denial probably becomes part of the therapist's experience (or lack of experience) in treating the family, so that the therapist becomes unable to access a part of himself that might be helpful.

Summary and Conclusions

Systems, narrative, and solution-oriented approaches to family therapy have not had much to contribute to the literature on countertransference. With the exception of Minuchin's structural perspective, the therapist in systems therapy is typically thought of as being outside the family system. In fact, positioning the therapist outside the family system has been considered an important way to ensure objectivity in helping families. Perhaps Murray Bowen's influence on systems therapy is important in this regard. His logic for positioning the therapist outside the family system was based on his belief that the therapist's ability to steer clear of the family's emotional system was essential to the work.

In looking at these methods from the relational systems perspective and with reference to the concept of countertransference, several things are apparent. One good way to describe the therapist's approach might be to say that these therapists attempt to close their own intrapsychic system while they attempt to intervene in the open system of the family. Thus the therapist has an effect on the family, but the family does not have an effect on the therapist. Unfortunately, systems therapy has not applied its own theory to itself. The family system is analyzed but not the therapist–family system, which is naturally created by the very fact that the family is seeking therapy. Such an analysis would probably indicate that families do have an effect on therapists and that therapists also have an effect on families. Without the application of any theoretical understanding of these issues, however, systems therapists inevitably miss opportunities to intervene with families in deeply meaningful ways that address interpersonal and intrapsychic experience and are at the same time structural, strategic, solution-oriented, or narrative.

Perhaps with an appropriate application of theory, the therapist's emotional experience when encountering a family could inform her of areas where the structure is collapsing (e.g., if the therapist feels infantilized by a parent), or where intrapsychic phenomena could lead to a strategic intervention (e.g., if the therapist feels controlled by a parent who is complaining that her child is too wild, she might assign "wild" behavior to that parent with the strong feeling that she controls so that she won't feel controlled), and so on. While the intentional use of countertransference is nonexistent in systems, narrative, and solution-oriented therapies, the unintentional use is probably prevalent, as neither the therapist's experience nor the therapist's part in the therapist–family system are often discussed.

CONCLUSION: THE USE OF SELF AS VIEWED IN FAMILY THERAPY

Examining countertransference in family therapy through the lens of the totalistic perspective reveals that its use is ubiquitous, but that countertransference has not been thought of as a tool by many authors in this field. Its intentional use has only been emphasized by a few. Yet the unintentional use of countertransference is important within several schools of family therapy.

In most psychoanalytic family therapy approaches it seems that countertransference is used somewhat indirectly as a consequence of avoiding countertransference problems. Object relations family therapists have attempted a relatively complete integration of the use of countertransference but have failed to examine the impact of the therapist's unique personality within the therapist–family system. Integrationist approaches have shown the greatest potential toward a comprehensive use of countertransference. Among the integrationist approaches, the most promising recognize both the unintentional use and the intentional use of countertransference by emphasizing both an experiential aspect and an application of interpersonal theory to therapeutic process. Experiential therapists, on the other hand, have not applied any theory to therapeutic process and have asserted that the therapist's personality is central to a therapeutic effect; these therapists thus emphasize the unintentional use of countertransference. Systems, narrative, and solution-oriented therapists, comprising the unimportant position, do not describe any use of countertransference. Of course the unintentional use of countertransference cannot be extracted from any kind of therapy, and if systems epistemology is fully applied, the recognition of the therapist's part in a system with the family will also bring recognition of the unintentional use of countertransference. This review clearly demonstrates that the use of countertransference could be enhanced where it already exists and should be introduced where it has not been considered.

Two areas that account for the lack of a thorough integration of the use of countertransference into the family therapy realm need to be addressed. First, therapists have typically not viewed themselves as part of the therapist–family system. Second, no theory of communication that addresses both intrapsychic and interpersonal phenomena has been adequately applied. Many other issues are also related to these two areas, such as the unintentional use of countertransference, the definition of projective identification, and—perhaps the stickiest issue of all—the mental health of the therapist. However, what is essential, and lacking, is a useful integration of theory that takes into account the therapist–family system. That is, an adequate development of theory for the therapist–family system presents a tremendous opportunity for clarifying the therapeutic process in family therapy. The use of countertransference can be a powerful tool. Not yet well-understood or utilized, it has the potential to bridge many approaches to family therapy and to be used in attaining many very different therapeutic goals.

3

Perspectives on the
Therapist's Use of Self

In Chapter 2, several approaches to family therapy were reviewed for the purpose of understanding how each makes use of countertransference. Despite possible weaknesses in each approach, they all share in the following formulation: the family therapist is part of the therapist–family system. In that system, the therapist's experiences are reflective of the interactions among all the personalities involved, her own and those of all the other participants. The use of countertransference occurs unintentionally as the therapist reacts behaviorally, without self-reflection. The intentional use of countertransference occurs when the therapist reflects upon her experience to understand what that experience might mean with respect to the therapist–family and family systems. Because the therapist is involved in the therapist–family system, her personality is of great importance in ensuring mostly salutary effects, intentional or unintentional, within that system. Finally, the therapist's full understanding of her part in the therapist–family system requires application of a comprehensive theory of emotional communication that defines the therapeutic process. Only with such a theory, ingrained in the therapist, is it possible for her to intentionally formulate therapeutic interventions, based on countertransference, that fully address intrapsychic and interpersonal patterns. These core propositions, which represent the essence of the relational systems perspective, are extrapolated from analytic thinking about the concept of countertransference.

This chapter focuses on key notions about countertransference, from its first application by Freud (1910), who used the term to represent problematic emotional reactions in the psychoanalyst, to its modern applications, which unmistakably place the therapist within an emotional system with clients or client-families.

DEFINITION OF TERMS

The concept of *totalistic countertransference*, as discussed in the Introduction, will be utilized throughout the remainder of this book. According to Winnicott (1949):

> One could classify counter-transference phenomena thus:
>
> (1) Abnormality in counter-transference feelings, and set relationships and identification that are under repression in the analyst. The comment on this is that the analyst needs more analysis, and we believe this is less of an issue among psycho-analysts than among psychotherapists.
>
> (2) The identifications and tendencies belonging to an analyst's personal experiences and personal development which provide the positive setting for his analytic work and make his work different in quality from that of any other analyst.
>
> (3) From these two I distinguish the truly objective counter-transference, or if this is difficult, the analyst's love and hate in reaction to the actual personality and behavior of the patient, based on objective observation. [pp. 69–70]

This definition has some great advantages. It makes room for problematic responses as well as the healthy uniqueness of the analyst's personality. At the same time, the personality of the analyst, although unique, does have objective reactions that are informative. These objective reactions, spelled out in the third part of the definition, were considered by Winnicott to be especially important in analytic work. But my own concept, the *unintentional use of countertransference*, primarily involves the first and second parts of Winnicott's definition. It is the first and second parts that allow for discussion of how the therapist has become part of an emotional system with the family. It is the third part that allows for discussion of how the therapist intentionally makes use of the fact that he or she has become part of that system.

ABSTINENCE AND NEUTRALITY

The concepts of *abstinence* and *neutrality* are problematic for the use of countertransference in family therapy for two reasons. First, the use of countertransference, as opposed to only being aware of it, might suggest that the therapist's personality is involved in ways that violate neutrality or abstinence. Defining these concepts in a way that preserves their meaning, and fits with the notion of the therapist as within the therapist–family system, is essential to a discussion of using countertransference. Second, since family therapists are typically more active than individual psychoanalytic psychotherapists, some would argue that the activity level of family therapists makes the use of these psychoanalytic concepts in family therapy impossible. In my view, however, both of these concepts are essential in any kind of therapy.

The discussion of neutrality and abstinence begins with Freud. The following excerpt is the most basic outline of Freud's (1914) thinking on the subject of abstinence:

> The treatment must be carried out in abstinence. By this I do not mean physical abstinence alone, nor yet the deprivation of everything that the patient desires, for perhaps no sick person could tolerate this. Instead, I shall state it as a fundamental principle that the patient's need and longing should be allowed to persist in her, in order that they may serve as forces impelling her to do work and to make changes, and that we must beware of appeasing those forces by means of surrogates. And what we could offer would never be anything else than a surrogate, for the patient's condition is such that, until her repressions are removed, she is incapable of getting real satisfaction. [p. 165]

Freud believed the patient could not work through maladaptive patterns unless the therapist abstained from gratifying the patient too much. Gratification, since it removes the motivation for change, would prevent the development of insight about those patterns of behavior and thinking that cause the patient's difficulty.

The following comment on neutrality further describes Freud's therapeutic stance, in which he advocates that the analyst be like a mirror to the patient (1912).

> The doctor should be opaque to his patients and, like a mirror, should show them nothing but what is shown to him. In practice, it is true, there is nothing to be said against a psychotherapist combining a certain amount of analysis with some suggestive influence in order to achieve a perceptible result in a shorter time—as is necessary, for instance, in institutions. But one has a right to insist that he himself should be in no doubt about what he is doing and should know that his method is not that of true psycho-analysis. [p. 118]

Freud's intention seems clear with respect to the analyst's role. The analyst should be like a mirror in showing the patient only who the patient is, and he should not influence the patient since such influence would get in the way of the patient seeing him- or herself. But as many have pointed out, within Freud's own clinical work the level of abstinence and neutrality he advocated is rarely demonstrated (Giovacchini 1989).

In the larger psychoanalytic literature it is likewise not clear what the concepts abstinence and neutrality mean. Complete abstinence is described, at times, as causing difficulties for an analysis such as premature termination of treatment (Greenson 1967, Schafer 1983) or preventing the formation of the working alliance that is necessary for the patient to gain insight and work through conflicts (Greenson 1967). Many therapists describe their stance of neutrality toward the patient as simply a way to ensure that the patient is at least not gratified too much.

Ralph Greenson's work demonstrated some desire to retreat from the strict definition of abstinence. Greenson (1967) asked the question: "If one shows no sympathy for the patient, how can one expect him to bare the most intimate, most vulnerable aspects of his mental and emotional life?" (p. 280). He then responded: "The answer is complicated. On the one hand, the analyst's therapeutic commitments to the patient should be in the background of all his undertakings. This does not have to be verbalized; it should be felt by the patient's reasonable ego" (p. 280). Having one's "therapeutic commitments" in the background, but available to the patient's "reasonable ego" certainly is not complete abstinence. It seems that the feeling it would engender would probably gratify the patient at least to some extent. The kind of abstinence that Greenson recommended allows this small comfort.

Roy Schafer (1983), in discussing neutrality, also does not advocate absolute abstinence. In an elaboration of this theme Schafer (1983) criticizes Freud's (1912) reference to the analyst being "opaque" and his use of the "mirror" metaphor.

> Freud's recommendation does not legitimize stiff formality, impassivity, and remoteness. The "mirror" refers to the analyst's reflecting back to the analysand, now in neutral analytic form, what the analysand has been showing unconsciously in his or her associations and behavior. It is an active, transformational mirror and so is not a mirror at all. The metaphor is not well chosen. It is better to call this mirroring a psychoanalytic reading of the analysand's text. In the same vein, "opaque" refers to the analyst's not using personal disclosure as a major tool of analysis. "Opaque" would be better called the subordination of the analyst's biography and personality to the task at hand. [p. 24]

While Schafer advocates against the therapist being stiff, impassive, and remote, he does consider neutrality important. His description of neutrality, however, is different than Freud's. Neutrality to Schafer (1983) means that the therapist should not recklessly bring his own personality into the therapeutic situation, nor should he be judgmental. According to Schafer (citing A. Freud [1936]), "in his or her neutrality, the analyst does not crusade for or against the so-called id, superego, or defensive ego. The analyst has no favorites and so is not judgmental" (p. 5).

When therapists discuss psychoanalytic psychotherapy, as opposed to psychoanalysis, there is further room for a different perspective on neutrality. Robert Langs (1973) writes this about neutrality and abstinence in psychoanalytic psychotherapy:

> In all, the therapist operates in a setting of relative abstinence, as Freud . . . termed it. By this, we mean that he offers warmth and neutral,

insight-oriented interventions, but essentially no gratifications beyond those. This is a vital part of his stance; neurotic maladaptations are perpetuated by extratherapeutic gratifications and the patient will not seek nonsymptomatic adaptions if his neurotic needs are satisfied by the therapist. [p. 210]

Langs's viewpoint in this excerpt is essentially like that of Freud, but the addition of words like "*relative* abstinence" (emphasis mine) and "warmth" change Freud's original definition significantly.

For those psychoanalytic psychotherapists who recommend using countertransference within the treatment, the definition of neutrality changes even more. Giovacchini (1989), for example, sets the tone for his point of view by ridiculing the classical analytic pose. He comments on a therapist's ability to integrate the stance Freud proposed, and criticizes Freud's telephone receiver and surgeon metaphors, by stating "I also wonder whether analysts who can act like surgeons and who can, without feeling, electronically decipher messages are able to integrate these capacities within their psyches because they lack other qualities that may be essential to reach the deeper recesses of the patient's inner misery" (p. 13). Giovacchini goes on to compare the classical stance to the development of a "false self" (Winnicott 1965a). "For most analysts, especially because of the types of patients we see, such a neutral stance would be forced. It would be equivalent to constructing a false self, as Winnicott described. Relating at a false-self level would be experienced as oppressive, and the therapist's attitude toward the patient would be strained" (p. 13).

This next excerpt captures the kind of neutrality that Giovacchini recommends:

To be neutral indicates that we are nonjudgmental and that we respect all layers of the mental apparatus. It does not signify noninvolvement or emotional distance . . . At most, as A. Freud (1965) stated, it refers to maintaining equidistance between various parts of the mind; it does not mean, however, that we have to be distant from the patient as a person. On the contrary, to achieve such an equidistance in the realm of psychic structure requires considerable involvement with and feelings for patients.

In general, it is considered desirable that analysts reveal as little as possible about their feelings or personal lives. This helps facilitate the development of the transference . . . [But] it is unwise to generalize when discussing psychoanalytic treatment. In view of the diverse personality types we encounter, it is best to maintain some flexibility. Revealing our personal feelings and attitudes could be helpful in some instances (Boyer 1983, Giovacchini 1979, Searles 1965). [pp. 14–15]

More than anything else, the neutrality Giovacchini advocates is an ever-present attitude toward the patient that fosters insight and growth. The method of the therapist can change but not the attitude.

Among psychoanalysts, countertransference has been most freely used within relational approaches (such as the intersubjective, interpersonal, or two-person psychologies). From this perspective, without a transference–countertransference interchange there is no therapy. Mitchell (1988) puts it this way: "Unless the analyst affectively enters the patient's relational matrix or, rather, discovers himself within it—unless the analyst is in some sense charmed by the patient's entreaties, shaped by the patient's projections, antagonized and frustrated by the patient's defenses—the treatment is never fully engaged, and a certain depth within the analytic experience is lost" (p. 293).

Chused (1992) has emphasized the nonjudgmental attitude, Poland (1981) a respect for the otherness of the patient, Wachtel (1986) the patient's understanding that he or she is valued as a person regardless of behavior, Greenberg (1986) the maintenance of an optimal tension between the perception of the therapist as a new or old object, and Aron (1992) an openness to new and different perspectives. The main point is that, as T. Shapiro (1984) has written, "the analyst is not a non person or a neutral icy being" (p. 281), but rather uses herself in whatever way is necessary for best achieving the "aim of understanding the unconscious" (p. 281). Poland (1981) has distinguished abstinence from neutrality in a way that is suggestive of Greenberg's "tension" as well as Aron's "openness": "Neutrality is global in its statement of the analyst's openness to all experiences and processes in the analysis, in the patient, in himself. Abstinence implies the more narrow limitation, perhaps titration, of transference gratification in order to promote further psychological work, the not giving on one level in order to facilitate regression to a deeper level of hidden meanings" (p. 287).

Some analysts have even suggested that the only kind of neutrality that is worthwhile specifically takes into account the interactional field. Franklin (1990) states:

> From this perspective the analyst tries to maintain an open-minded position, free from stereotyped ideas about the analyst's functioning, about the many possible kinds of analyst–patient interactions that might be beneficial in furthering analytic treatment. A flexible attitude in the analyst toward his selectively bringing into play any aspect of his relatedness to the patient that fosters the patient's self-expression, so that he can better explore and understand himself, constitutes the central aspect of what I term interactional neutrality. [p. 213]

Wachtel (1986) is more specific:

> it is in the very act of participating that the analyst learns what it is most important to know about the patient. And it is in coming to see their joint participation in what is for him a familiar pattern, but a joint participation with the crucial difference of reflectiveness, that the patient too learns what he must in order to begin the process of change . . . If the analyst adopts the pose of neutrality, this crucial aspect of therapeutically useful insight is short-circuited. It is precisely in pointing out how the patient's reactions are not simply a distortion, in examining just how the patient has evoked a familiar reaction (first internal, then overt) from the analyst, that the most therapeutically valuable aspect of the work is achieved. [p. 63]

Clearly, the concept of neutrality has not been abandoned within relational analysis, but it has been modified to accommodate more active therapies.

Neutrality and Abstinence in the Relational Systems Perspective

The functions referred to as neutrality and abstinence have always involved a certain effort of the therapist in being therapeutic. That effort, no matter what name it might be given, is essential in therapy, and the terms neutrality and abstinence have continued in use as an aspect of that effort. In looking at the evolution of these terms, it becomes apparent that psychoanalytic thinking prizes abstinence and neutrality to the extent that they lead to the patient working through his or her maladaptive perception of (and behavior toward) others. Abstinence and neutrality should be upheld to the extent that they maintain enough tension within the therapeutic relationship to foster development. Thus the concepts we are struggling to define here must bridge the tension between being helpful and meddling. With respect to neutrality, the most important component is the nonjudgmental attitude emphasized by Schafer and Giovacchini. The ability to remain nonjudgmental is connected to A. Freud's notion (1936) of maintaining equidistance from id, ego, and superego manifestations. When viewed from a family therapy perspective, perhaps the best way to understand this ability is to say that the therapist must maintain equidistance from the many and various influences within the therapist–family system, while remaining concerned and open to new experience.

In applying the concepts found within this study to family therapy, concern, warmth, and a nonjudgmental attitude reflect the nature of the therapeutic stance I recommend. These characteristics are likely to be independent of the therapist's activity level, but are related to his awareness of pressures within the therapist–family system. I recommend that these characteristics become part of the therapist's ever-present work attitude. As much as possible, they should be integral to the therapist's functioning as an individual. The therapist must maintain neutrality and abstain from gratifying clients too much no matter how active he might be or clients will become dependent upon the therapist's position with them in the therapist–family system, and thus fail to mature and grow without the therapist. Particularly with the high activity level that is necessary in family therapy, the therapist's mental health becomes a primary issue in that neutrality and abstinence must be maintained preconsciously and naturally, without the mask of inactivity behind which to hide bias and gratification.

TRANSFERENCE

Evident in the discussion above is the importance of transference. The reason abstinence and neutrality are so integral within the discourse on psychoanalytic psychotherapy is that they facilitate the development of transference. The working through of transference has become the sine qua non of psychoanalytic psychotherapy. But several questions come up in reference to the working through of transference in family therapy. What is the essential nature of transference? Is it important in family therapy? Does it require the lack of activity advocated by some psychoanalytic therapists, or is the formulation of neutrality described above sufficient to allow its development? Finally, is the only useful definition of transference made in reference to the therapist, or can its occurrence between other people be observed and used in therapies, like family therapy, where more than one person is involved? These are the kinds of questions that must be answered here. The following discussion briefly outlines a view of transference appropriate to the totalistic use of countertransference in family therapy.

Greenson is one of the most well-recognized advocates of the classical position in psychoanalysis. In his book, *The Technique and Practice of Psychoanalysis* (1967), Greenson provides a review of the classical definition of transference, and outlines the continuation of its use in current clinical approaches. According to Greenson, Freud first thought of transference as a resistance to treatment. In the case of Dora, Freud (1905) realized that his failure to recognize and handle the transference led to premature termination. Freud described how Dora experienced feelings toward him that were facsimiles or reprints of feelings she developed toward other significant figures in her early life. Freud declared these "transferences" a necessary part of psychoanalytic treatment. He stated that, although the transference produces the greatest obstacle to treatment, it is also an extremely important ally. The analyst recognizes in the transference what the patient must work through.

Greenson (1967) credited Ferenczi (1909) with being the first to state that transference occurs in other relationships outside the analysis. Ferenczi considered transference to be a special form of displacement. The predisposition toward transference, he believed, existed in the patient. The analyst was only a catalyst for transference, for which the patient hungered. He believed that patients take the analyst into their private worlds, and that the analyst is only a "cover person," or screen for the objects of the patient's infantile past. Although they are not specifically referred to in Greenson's remarks, Ferenczi's views are cited by many authors as constituting the origin of the object relations approach in psychoanalysis (as for example in Slipp [1984]).

Freud (1912a) described the transference as a compromise formation (pp. 102–103). By perceiving the therapist as though he is similar to significant figures of the past, the patient invents a context for his id impulses while defending against the recognition of those impulses. Transference reflects indefensible id manifestations as well as the attempt at defending against them. Freud stated that every conflict of the patient must be fought out in the transference situation of analysis (p. 104). This fight is crucial in an analysis where the patient is allowed to struggle in the present with his important object relations of the past. During this process Freud believed that it was not possible for the patient to overcome these conflicts without reliving them. It was in another paper of the same year that Freud (1912b) used the "mirror" metaphor (cited above) in describing how the analyst could encourage the development of the transference by reflecting only what was presented to him.

Two years later, Freud (1914b) added the concepts of repetition compulsion and transference neurosis. The repetition compulsion simply describes the fact that the patient has little choice but to relive his infantile object relations. The transference neurosis names the process by which the transference is played out with the analyst, and the focus on it makes the working through of transference the paramount treatment objective in psychoanalysis. In 1920 Freud put forth the idea that childhood reactions are repeated in the transference, not because the patient hopes for pleasure through their expression, but because the compulsion to repeat is even more primitive than the pleasure principle and overrides it (pp. 20–23). (This formulation, based on Freud's view of the "death instinct," has drawn considerable debate that extends beyond the scope of this study.) According to Greenson (1967), Freud did not develop the concept of transference beyond this point.

Newer formulations of transference come ever closer to seeing transference as ubiquitous. Here the views of the object relations therapists are crucial. According to Greenson (1967), Kleinians

consider the interpretation of the unconscious meaning of transference phenomena to be the crux of the therapeutic process . . . Transference phenomena are regarded essentially as projections and introjections of the most infantile good and bad objects . . . They do not communicate with a cohesive, integrated ego; they do not attempt to establish a working alliance, but seem instead to establish direct contact with the various introjects. [Heimann 1956, cited by Greenson 1967, p. 169]

Object relations therapists, generally following this pattern, see the relationship as the curative factor. The reliving of childhood experience (transference or transference acting out) is reflected in the patient's personality functioning in the here and now. Remembering is not necessarily as important as insight about how one functions in, and perceives, one's own world. In fact, the differences between classical psychoanalytic and object relations thought can be clarified by distinguishing the emphasis on remembering and transference in classical psychoanalysis from the emphasis on acting out and transference acting out in object relations thinking.

Where traditional Freudian psychoanalysts emphasize remembering the past by understanding the transference the patient develops toward the analyst, object relations therapists emphasize a reworking of the past in the relationship with the analyst, where transference acting out occurs and can be observed and interrupted by the reality of the therapist's personality as well as interpretation. Classical psychoanalysts suggest that acting out is only a part of a therapy when the patient regresses to such an extent that the working alliance is lost. Object relations therapists accept the fact that transference acting out is a part of therapy that must be recognized at all times. Object relations therapists suggest that experience in relationships involves acting out, and that memory comes as a by-product of the patient's recognition that her perceptions and actions do not fit the therapeutic relationship. Similarly, where classical psychoanalysts focus on that part of transference of which the patient must be made aware, object relations therapists focus on transference acting out that can be worked on within the relationship even if the patient never becomes aware of it as transference.

The working alliance, which is essential in classical psychoanalysis, represents work at higher symbolic levels, where thought takes the place of action. Object relations therapists work at presymbolic levels, as well as higher symbolic levels, so that their therapy emphasizes both the cure of the relationship at levels of transference acting out and curing with the working alliance at levels of transference that are easily made conscious and are not acted out. In object relations therapy, the analyst observes and intervenes in the patient's reliving of her past in the present in hope that what is presently automatically transferred to others can be reflected upon. Awareness of and reflection on her perceptions allow the patient to change the nature of her relationships. By perceiving relationships more accurately, the patient significantly alters her own contributions to those relationships.

The first such relationship is with the analyst, whom the patient begins to see as another person with the full potential of many possible feelings and thoughts other than those earlier projected by the patient onto him. Interpretations are aimed at understanding how and why the patient views her world as she does and at allowing the patient to see that her view is not necessarily correct but left over from the past. When a patient recognizes that her perceptions are not correct, remembering may occur (as opposed to false perceptions), as the patient becomes better able to understand why she has come to perceive the world in this false way. Working through involves integrating previously projected and split-off parts of the personality so that they become seen as acceptable aspects of the patient herself as opposed to unacceptable aspects of others.

The work of Hans Loewald is a good demonstration of the mix between object relations and classical psychoanalytic thinking. In a paper titled "On the Therapeutic Action of Psychoanalysis," Loewald (1960) regards the analyst's role with respect to the transference as the most important curative factor in analysis. Neutrality is important in aiding the therapist to accurately interpret transference "roles." Loewald broadens the idea of transference when he refers to the roles assigned to him. The word "role" seems to imply the influence of the patient's expectations, as opposed to merely the perception the patient has of the therapist (which is the classical view of transference). Sandler later (1976) included as part of the transference the pressure from the patient toward behaviorally playing out those roles in therapy.

The goal of treatment, according to Loewald, is for the patient to reorganize his personality in a healthier way. The transference must be both fostered and analyzed for this reorganization to occur. The promotion of the transference can be seen as the utilization of controlled regression. But as a result of this regression the therapist has an opportunity to interpret the infantile aspects of the patient's character, thus bringing on "new discovery of objects" (p. 18) and personality reorganization.

The new discovery of objects to which Loewald refers suggests the growth of the patient's unique potential as a person. The analyst helps in bringing out that potential by reflecting the distortions of the transference back to the patient. Thus there is a new discovery of objects that the patient previously perceived in others via transference and now recognizes as part of himself. The patient can only discover these lost objects by realizing that his view of the new object (the analyst) does not correspond to his view of the old objects about which he had been unaware and had projected on the analyst.

The qualifications for the new object that Loewald considers essential to this process include objectivity and neutrality toward the patient's potential. He states that the analyst must be able to recognize and foster the growth of a core that he recognizes in the patient. He likens this relationship to the parent–child relationship in which the parent is empathic toward the child but also has a vision of the child's future based on prior knowledge of growth and development. The child identifies with this vision of the future, but the empathy the parent has also allows for recognition of the unique core within the child. The child becomes him- or herself but needs the parent's guidance. Referring to the parent–child relationship, Loewald writes, "In analysis, if it is to be a process leading to structural changes, interactions of a comparable nature have to take place" (p. 20).

Loewald's emphasis on the relationship between analyst and patient, and the transference that is part of that relationship, is a good example of the redevelopment of object relations, as opposed to memory of the past, which object relations therapists consider essential. He suggests that the patient is cured, not when "no further transference occurs," but when the patient's transference to the therapist is a close approximation of reality. In concluding his paper he states:

I hope to have made the point in the present discussion that there is neither such a thing as reality nor a real relationship, without transference. Any "real relationship" involves transfer of unconscious imagines [sic] to present-day objects. In fact, present-day objects are objects, and thus "real," in the full sense of the word (which comprises the unity of unconscious memory traces and preconscious idea) only to the extent to which this transference, in the sense of transformational interplay between unconscious and preconscious, is realized. The "resolution of the transference" at the termination of an analysis means resolution of the transference neurosis, and thereby of the transference distortions. [p. 32]

By perceiving others as "objects" Loewald refers to the patient's ability to see others as having both good and bad traits as well as the ability to perceive others as having full potential as persons. Although the patient can become able to have mature object relations, however, that does not mean that the patient has no transference at all. Loewald clearly intends the reader to recognize that transference is a part of every relationship.

A more contemporary author who is well known for his object relations perspective is Otto Kernberg. Kernberg (1989) gives the following view on transference:

The primary vehicle of the treatment is the analysis of the transference in the here-and-now. The patient's internalized object relations are played out vividly in the transference. As these internalized representations gradually become integrated, the transferences shift from primitive to more advanced forms. When more realistic transferences emerge later in the treatment, the therapist begins to interpret genetic antecedents. Thus over time the focus of treatment shifts, as does the mixture of specific techniques. [p. 50]

Kernberg's portrayal of the transference being played out "vividly" is a step closer to the understanding of transference as ever-present in the patient's experience of his relationships.

Transference in the Relational Systems Perspective

It is not a big jump from Freud's repetition compulsion to an understanding of transference as commonplace in the daily functioning of most people. The repetition compulsion is central in understanding how systems models can be integrated with psychodynamic models. Repeated patterns within families and, as I will argue, between the family and therapist, are the glue of systems. Some integrationist authors (Durkin 1972, Slipp 1984) argue that many systems theorists have an erroneous understanding of psycho-analysis as being based on Freud's libido theory from before 1920 when the theory was not yet fully developed. According to these authors, that erroneous understanding has led to the view that psychodynamic thinking is incompatible with systems thinking. But as can be seen, the ever-present nature of transference, as discussed by Loewald and suggested by Kernberg, is a helpful way to view transference in the family therapy situation. The therapist–family system is constructed of multiple transferences, some based in reality and others based in the past experience of the participants. A primary goal of treatment is to foster the development of increasingly accurate perceptions within the family. The use of countertransference, also understood as ever-present, is helpful in distinguishing the nature of mul-tiple transferences. To understand the connection between transference and countertransference it is necessary to discuss another term, projective iden-tification, which can be understood as the behavioral manifestation of repetition compulsion.

PROJECTIVE IDENTIFICATION

The concept of projective identification was first discussed by Melanie Klein (1946). Over time it has become an integral part of understanding psychological processes in the analytic situation. Although it is usually associated with the treatment of character-disordered or psychotic patients, some authors have speculated that it is an important concept in the treat-ment of relatively healthy patients as well (Langs 1978, Malin and Grotstein 1966). Some family therapists also consider it useful (Box et al. 1981, D. Scharff 1991, Scharff and Scharff 1987, J. S. Scharff 1992, Slipp 1984, 1988). For the purposes of this study the work of Thomas Ogden (1979) on projective identification will be outlined. More than any other author, Ogden has clarified the use of this complicated concept. The work of Bion (1959a,b), Malin and Grotstein (1966), Langs (1978), and Bollas (1987) will also be discussed for the purpose of discovering the wide range of transference phenomena that are at times given the name projective iden-tification. This section will focus on the changing definition of projective identification from that of a concept applicable only to relatively severe pathology to one that is applicable to all people regardless of pathology.

Thomas Ogden

Ogden defines projective identification as: "a group of fantasies and accompanying object relations having to do with the ridding of the self of unwanted aspects of the self; the depositing of those unwanted 'parts' into another person; and finally, with the 'recovery' of a modified version of what was extruded" (p. 357). Although Ogden describes these as three separate phases of action (for which he cites Malin and Grotstein 1966), he goes on to explain that considering them as parts of "a single psychological event better conveys the sense of simultaneity and interdependence that befits" (p. 358) the concept projective identification.

Ogden describes projective identification in three phases, which involve projection, pressure on the object to accept the "unwanted 'parts'" that the projector is attempting to deposit into the other person, and reinternalization of the perceived response of the recipient. Ogden states that the difference between projection and projective identification is that "in projection, the projector feels estranged from, threatened by, bewildered by, or out of touch with, the object of the projection" (p. 358). The person involved in projection believes the feelings he has attributed to the other are unrelated to his own feelings. There is a solid boundary perceived between the projector and the recipient. Ogden says "the person involved in projection might ask, 'Why would anyone act in such an angry way when there is nothing to be angry about? There's something the matter with him'" (pp. 358–359). Whereas in projective identification, the person feels at one with the recipient who, he believes, now experiences exactly the same feeling that has been "transplanted" into him via interaction.

Projection and projective identification can be differentiated by the extent to which either intrapsychic or interpersonal phenomena are involved. Projection is purely intrapsychic. The projector feels the need to disavow certain feelings, completely denying them in the self. Projective identification is interpersonal. The projector might disavow certain feelings, but needs the other person to accept them or hold them so that they can be made safe and taken back into the self of the projector. Thus, in accordance with that need, the projector uses interpersonal pressure, albeit unconscious, to bring about the projected feelings in the recipient. The objective of projective identification will be discussed in more detail below. But here it is important to describe how the projector uses pressure to bring about feelings in the recipient.

Ogden (1979) refers to the second part of projective identification as the "induction" phase and is clear about the interactional pressure it involves. He states: "This is not an imaginary pressure. This is real pressure exerted by means of a multitude of interactions between the projector and the recipient. Projective identification does not exist where there is no interaction between projector and object" (p. 359). Ogden gives several examples of this pressure, none of which is subtle. In the first, a young woman incessantly bumps into others with the resultant feeling in the recipients of being constantly intruded upon. In the second, a young man torments his therapist by repeatedly kicking the furniture, ringing the waiting-room buzzer, and ruminating without pause in a high-pitched whine. The resultant feelings in the therapist in this case are extreme tension and helpless rage.

Interestingly, Ogden states that in this second case "the patient was fully conscious of both his attempts to get the therapist to feel angry, as well as the calming and soothing effect that that had on him" (p. 359). Thus, this is an example of the patient's need to feel at one with the therapist into whom he has projected parts of himself. Pressure is exerted because of the projector's desperate need to feel at one with the recipient as well as the extreme need to rid the self of unwanted feelings. Ogden goes on to say that the projected parts are necessary aspects of the patient's personality which, although perceived as noxious agents that must be extruded, must also be preserved in someone else because they are essential for life. For example, the patient needs the emotion, anger, for the self, much as one must have identifications with parental figures, even if those parental figures are tormenting. When these aspects of the self are put into another, they are preserved and possibly perceived as less noxious to the self. These projected aspects of the self are not only gotten rid of. The effect they have on the other is perceived as soothing in that it creates a oneness between the projector and the recipient.

The third phase of projective identification involves the "psychological processing" of the projected parts by the recipient and then the reinternalization of those parts, now modified, back into the projector. "Psychological processing" refers to the reaction of the recipient to having the projected parts put into her. That reaction is not the same as the projector's fantasy since the recipient's personality is her own and has developed differently from that of the projector. As Ogden describes it, "A different set of defences and other psychological processes may be employed by the recipient so that the feelings are 'processed', 'metabolized' (Langs 1976b), 'contained' (Bion 1959b), or managed differently" (p. 360). The reaction of the recipient may exemplify a better or worse handling of the projected emotions. Ogden describes a "successful" processing, however, as a new way of handling the projected feelings that demonstrates that the feelings can be lived with and maybe even enjoyed.

The processed version of the feelings can now be reinternalized through either the more primitive mode of introjection, or the more mature one of identification (Ogden cites Schafer [1968]). In introjection, the projector unconsciously takes on the recipient's reaction as if it were his own way of dealing with the feelings in the moment. With identification, the projector aims to emulate the recipient's effective way of handling the difficult feelings. In the psychoanalytic process the *hope* is that the recipient is more mature than the projector. When this is in fact the case, the processing of projections will be relatively successful and the patient will be able to reinternalize a better way of dealing with the projected affects.

Now that the processes involved in projective identification are clear, Ogden's (1979) views on the objectives of projective identification can be discussed. Projective identification occurs because the projector gets some sort of intrapsychic or interpersonal benefit. Ogden differentiates four purposes of projective identification. The first is defense: the projector rids himself of an unwanted part of the self or keeps it safe in someone else. The second is communication: the projector makes himself understood by pressuring another person to experience feelings like those of the projector. The third is object relatedness: the projector interacts with someone who is separate enough to receive a projection but undifferentiated enough to be misperceived as being in a symbiotic-like relationship with the projector. The fourth is a means of psychological growth: the projector develops psychological structure as a result of recovering a modified version of what was projected after the recipient has processed it. Ogden sees these four aspects of projective identification as a common and essential part of the mother–infant relationship. Likewise, they are considered by some analysts to be central to the therapeutic relationship.

Within a therapeutic context, projective identification can be seen as encompassing all of these purposes at once. For example, a client or client-family might unconsciously use projective identification to avoid certain intolerable affects. Since these affects are intolerable, the person experiencing them cannot possibly understand them at a verbal level. But in the effort to be understood, in the same way that they might have tried to receive understanding in preverbal infancy, clients or client-families try to create in the therapist, through subtle but real pressure, the same feeling state that they fear experiencing. As already stated, Ogden emphasizes that this pressure actually occurs at a behavioral level. Success at creating these intolerable affects in the recipient makes the projector feel at one or in a symbiotic-like relationship with the recipient, who, by taking on the projected experience, has allowed the projector to communicate in a symbiotic-like manner (Winnicott 1960a). With the projector's perception of the recipient's reaction to these seemingly intolerable affects, the cycle of projective identification is completed. The projector either learns a slightly new way of dealing with the affects through identification or introjection, or the recipient confirms for the projector that the feelings are intolerable.

There is one area not covered by Ogden. Ogden's (1979) emphasis on the behavioral aspect of the "induction" phase in projective identification suggests that, in his view, this behavioral aspect is quite pronounced, even if not well understood, in the patient who is using projective identification. But other authors have emphasized the therapist's or recipient's sensitivity or willingness to take on projective identifications in doing the therapeutic work or spending time with the projector. If the recipient's sensitivity is considered, then the severity of pathology in the projector can vary, which suggests that the patient who communicates via projective identification does not necessarily have severe pathology. The next five authors loosen the definition of projective identification, making it possible to cover this area.

Wilfred Bion

Bion is well known for his application of Kleinian theory to group process as well as to individual treatment. Bion used the term *projective identifi-*

cation as it is described by Ogden above. However, he also addressed the issue of how projective identification is related to the extent of the projector's pathology. Bion (1959a) described a normal amount of projective identification in this statement: "I shall suppose that there is a normal degree of projective identification, without defining the limits within which normality lies, and that associated with introjective identification this is the foundation on which normal development rests" (p. 312).

In this excerpt, Bion refers to projective identification as a process similar to the tendency of the child or infant to pass on intolerable feelings to the mother and then introject the ability of the mother to handle those feelings. In fact this paper, entitled "Attacks on Linking," specifically discusses what happens to patients when they have had the experience of being unable, at a very early age, to communicate through projective identification. The result of not being able to use projective identification in infancy is an "*excessive*" [emphasis mine] use of projective identification, as well as "deterioration of . . . developmental processes" (p. 313), leading to pathology in adulthood. In other words, chronic lack of responsiveness to a child's intense crying, for example, can lead that child to efforts at ridding the self of that discomfort through excessive use of projective identification into adult life. Bion's reference to projective identification as "normal" in development may simply suggest that he believed it to be normal in infancy. But his reference to "excessive" projective identification as the result of early deprivation implies that using projective identification is to some extent normal in adulthood. In fact Bion made many references to a normal amount of projective identification throughout his work (1959a,b 1970). Bion did not, however, fully describe what a normal amount of projective identification is. Nevertheless, by referring to "excessive" amounts of projective identification and by mentioning the normality of projective identification, Bion seems to suggest that there is some kind of continuum between its normal and pathological use.

This discussion can be enriched by an addition of one more term given by Bion. Bion (1959b) amplified his description of projective identification by introducing the term "valency" to describe the "unconscious function of the gregarious quality in the personality of man" (p. 170). In other words, valency is the tendency of a person to engage in certain levels of communication, verbal or nonverbal, which have particular kinds of content and emotional qualities. In his view, a person can have "*no* [italics in original] valency only by ceasing to be, as far as mental function is concerned, human" (p. 116).

This term has certain ramifications when applied to the therapist. The therapist's valency is not only a countertransference reaction that must be controlled, but is also a tool. Valency can represent the therapist's sensitivity to the patient. Bion's use of this term suggests more or less valency in people for specific emotions and behaviors being evoked by specific emotions and behaviors of others. According to Bion, the therapist, like any other person, will have more or less valency for specific emotions or behaviors. The patient's transference, from this perspective, would at times include only minor behavioral influence (behavioral influence being a hallmark of projective identification) that, due to the therapist's valency, could successfully induce projective identification. Bollas has discussed a concept called "extractive introjection" that elaborates on the introjective side of "valency," as opposed to the projective side, which has been captured by the concept of projective identification.

Christopher Bollas

Bollas (1987) coined the term "extractive introjection" in describing a phenomenon in which a person not only has valency with respect to projection but actually actively introjects self representations from others.

> I believe there is a process that can be as destructive as projective identification in its violation of the spirit of mutual relating. Indeed, I am thinking of an intersubjective procedure that is almost exactly its reverse, a process that I propose to call **extractive introjection.** Extractive introjection occurs when one person steals for a certain period of time (from a few seconds or minutes, to a lifetime) an element of another individual's psychic life. Such an intersubjective violence takes place when the violator (henceforth A) automatically assumes that the violated (henceforth B) has no internal experience of the psychic element that A represents. At the moment of this assumption, an act of theft takes place, and B may be temporarily anaesthetized and unable to "gain back" the stolen part of the self. [p. 158]

Bollas goes on to give examples of this phenomenon, which include the stealing of mental content, affective process, theft of mental structure, and theft of self. Regarding mental content, Bollas describes a situation in which B has come up with an idea and presented it to A who then takes the idea as his own as though B never had the idea, with the result that A feels he has good ideas and B begins to feel that his ideas have no merit. Regarding affective process, A assumes B does not have normal human feelings at a time when it would be inhuman or insensitive not to have those feelings, with the result being that A feels like a paragon of sensitivity and B develops the inability to have those normal human feelings. Regarding mental structure, Bollas gives an example of A assuming that B does not have some particular human capacity, such as the ability to know right from wrong, with the result being that A becomes the holder of that virtue and B develops less ability to know right from wrong. Finally, regarding theft of the self, Bollas describes a situation in which A deconstructs the history of B such that A feels a stronger identity in relation to B who begins to lose the feeling of having a cohesive identity.

Extractive introjection is a term that denotes an extreme in introjective valency. Rather than having a predisposition toward accepting the projection of others, extractive introjection occurs when one has such strong valency that projection or projective identification need not occur. Elements of another's personality are so badly needed that they are extracted for the purpose of maintaining the personality of the introjector. In cases where extractive introjection occurs it is possible to have no induction aspect of projective identification, and yet parts of one's personality are transferred from oneself to another through the induction of the introjector. If no projective induction is necessary in a phenomenon that involves the transfer of intrapsychic part objects, then obviously, when introjective valency is strong, there is little need for induction in some forms of projective identification. If there is presumed to be a continuum of levels of induction in any communication such that the induction of the communication is either more or less strong and either more related to either the projector or the introjector, then some level of induction is involved in all communications. Even normal interactions involve induction, although sometimes at very low levels, and that induction is a composite of projective and introjective pressures. For further explanation of normal levels of projective identification, I now turn to the work of Malin and Grotstein.

Arthur Malin and James Grotstein

The work of Malin and Grotstein (1966) is interesting because their definition of projective identification clearly places it within the normal interpersonal functioning of the mature adult: "As Freud (1921) has stated, the infant relates by identification prior to making anaclitic object choices. We agree with this and go two steps further; first, we believe that all identification includes projection, as we hope to show; and second, that projective identification is also a normal, as well as abnormal, way of relating which persists into mature adulthood" (pp. 26–27). Malin and Grotstein make this bridge by supposing that identification, a more mature way of learning from others than introjection, is produced by first projecting what one already thinks or feels about the other, and then taking it back through the perception of how well that projection fits with the other's behavior. They assume that the projection itself, after connecting with the reality of the recipient's person, is what is reinternalized, with modifications made by the reality of the recipient's personality. With this viewpoint, the behavioral aspect of projective identification does not need to be so pronounced as is the case with Ogden's (1979) definition. In psychoanalysis, transference changes over time because projections are slowly modified by reality within the relationship to the analyst. This process occurs with all patients, regardless of the degree of pathology.

Malin and Grotstein (1966) believe all transference phenomena are projective identifications to some extent; as they put it, "If we accept a broad view of transference to include all object relations, internal and external, after the primary relationship with the breast-mother which is now internalized, then we are stating that all object relations and all transference phenomena are examples, at least in part, of projective identification. This implies that there must be a projection from within the psychic apparatus into the external object" (p. 28). Although they are not emphasizing the manipulative aspects or induction phase of projective identification, these authors do believe that projective identification is a different process than transference. Transference is the broader term within which projective identification specifies the projection from within the patient *into* the analyst. And they appear to be indicating that transference always has a projective identification aspect, inferring that its existence suggests some influence on its target.

But rather than emphasize the manipulative aspect of the interaction, Malin and Grotstein emphasize the willingness of the recipient to accept the projections. They cite Searles (1963) in stating, with respect to projections, that it is the analyst's receptiveness, without encouragement, that must be emphasized. Through his perception of the analyst's handling of these projections, the patient can find a "new level of integration" (p. 28). By emphasizing the analyst's openness rather than the patient's manipulation, these authors broaden the meaning of projective identification well beyond its usual use. It is clear that this kind of sensitivity to the patient's transference can be helpful where countertransference is employed.

Robert Langs

Langs (1978) also employs a broad definition of projective identification. Within his "adaptational-interactional" framework, Langs considers projective identification a part of many interpersonal interactions between persons at all levels of mental health. This is demonstrated in part by the regularity with which he attributes projective identification to the analyst as well as to the patient.

Like Malin and Grotstein, Langs sees projective identification as a mechanism attributable to relatively healthy persons. He implies, however, that it does involve some unconscious manipulation. Nevertheless, that manipulation is not always considered indicative of pathology. Langs's (1978) definition of projective identification emphasizes its interactional nature and its universality: "Projective identification is specifically interactional, in that it is unconsciously designed to create an intrapsychic effect within the recipient. While its use stems from the earliest mother–child relationship, it is a universal mechanism that may entail fluidity of self-object boundaries or may occur in more sophisticated forms in the presence of intact boundaries" (p. 317). As stated earlier, Langs (1978) often attributes projective identification to the analyst. "Projective identifications are also used at times by the analyst. They are essentially countertransference-based and are conveyed to the patient through his [the therapist's] errors in intervening and mismanagements of the framework.

They are far more common than previously recognized and are the basis for many analyst-evoked disturbances of the [bipersonal] field" (p. 318). Obviously Langs sees the therapist's use of projective identification in terms of the therapist's acting out of a problematic countertransference reaction. Nevertheless, within the interactional framework that he describes, projective identification is a very common means of communication, even if not ideal.

The focus of this study is, of course, on using countertransference to better understand the patient through an understanding of her projective identifications. Langs's work also points in another direction. One reason for making countertransference a priority in any therapy is that the therapist's acting out can often be prevented by awareness of how the patient's behavior influences the therapist's emotions. Another reason is that the therapist's awareness of how he is affecting the patient can prevent the continuation of acting out in which the therapist has already engaged. I pick up these aspects of the discussion in a following section on acting out.

Projective Identification in the Relational Systems Perspective

Projective identification is possibly the most important concept in psychotherapy. It describes the glue of relationships. It connects one individual's intrapsychic dynamics to his interpersonal behaviors and then to the way those interpersonal behaviors influence the intrapsychic dynamics and interpersonal behaviors of others. An understanding of projective identification is integral to an understanding of any human system and will be essential in my own formulation of the workings of the therapist–family system.

The definition of projective identification given by Malin and Grotstein (1966) aids in the discussion of many clinical phenomena. I will use this definition throughout the remainder of the book. But the reader must also assume that where I discuss projective identification as affecting the therapist, I am also suggesting that the therapist, in some way, whether it be through willingness or natural personality style, has some valency toward taking on that projection or projective identification.

Normal transference often involves very minor behavioral inducements that become projective identification as long as there is a willing recipient. Loewald (1960) describes his understanding of the role he plays within the patient's transference as being his clue to what that transference is. Is it not possible that he comes to an understanding of that role partially through projective identification without there being a strong behavioral inducement?

I am not suggesting that projection and projective identification are the same (as might be incorrectly interpreted in reading Malin and Grotstein), but only that where there is projection, there is also projective identification. When we compare projection and projective identification in one situation, their content may be the same or different. For example, if person A projects fear on person B and behaves in a scary way, thus creating fear in person B, then the content, fear, is the same in the projection as in the projective identification. However, if person A projects fear on person B and subsequently avoids person B due to disdain of fear, then perhaps the possibly consequent abandoned feeling engendered in person B when avoided by person A can be seen as the derivative content of the projective identification (as opposed to fear), meaning that person A cannot tolerate the feeling of abandonment that might be experienced if he were to act scared and thus he uses projective identification, with the behavior of avoidance, to rid himself of the abandoned feeling. Nevertheless, it can be seen that projection and projective identification are always related.

Since many therapists use the term projective identification only in referring to character-disordered patients, I would like to clarify that I agree that projective identification is a more forceful part of the regressed patient's interpersonal functioning. Even if projective identification is seen as a mode of communication common to all people that requires the therapist's sensitivity or valency, some people use it more often, and with more force, than others. This view fits descriptively with the work of many authors. As I have already stated, Bion (1959a), in discussing specific patient populations, has mentioned the "excessive" use of projective identification. By using the word "excessive" to describe projective identification, Bion seems to differentiate levels of pathology. Yet the word "excessive" also indicates a view of projective identification consistent with it being a common part of healthy relationships when it is not excessive.

Kernberg (1965, 1989), who emphasizes that projective identification is a regular part of therapy with some populations, describes a continuum of countertransference responses that become less and less determined by the therapist's pathology as projective identification becomes more greatly utilized by patients who are severely regressed (see the Kernberg discussion in the section on countertransference below). Thus, when a client uses projective identification often and with strong behavioral inducement, it can be indicative of severe pathology. (In the example above, where projection and projective identification involved the same content, fear, and the projector used scary behavior to induce that reaction, a more severe level of pathology could be assumed than in the case where the projective identification had a more derivative content than the projection.)

The definition that Malin and Grotstein give, however, allows for the use of countertransference in detecting projective identification with all client populations. And with the addition of the concept of valency it becomes necessary to recognize that when the therapist chooses to use the term projective identification in situations where there is not a strong behavioral inducement, the therapist must take some responsibility for the feelings experienced in the relationship. The term valency, when applied to the therapist, can account for that part of the experienced feeling the therapist has the predisposition toward taking on.

For example, it is even possible that a therapist's choice of profession can be suggestive of particular valencies that are pertinent. In the definition of countertransference used here, Winnicott (1949) has suggested that one level of countertransference involves those aspects of the therapist's personality that aid her in doing analytic work. One personality attribute likely to be common in therapists is the tendency toward taking on the patient's emotions in helping the patient. Thus, the therapist's valency might prime her toward gaining knowledge about the patient's emotional state through countertransference by simply being exposed to the patient.

The phenomenon of extractive introjection, regarded as an extreme of valency, can be applied to the therapist as well. It is important for therapists to understand this process because the extractive tendency can be quite subtle. It could be said, in fact, that one reason therapists become therapists is for the purpose of comparing themselves favorably to their "sick" patients. To the extent that this is true, the therapist is unable to help the patient who, by relational contract, must remain sicker than the therapist in order for the therapist to feel good. The concept of extractive introjection clearly indicates the need for therapists to recognize and encourage the potential for growth within their patients.

Kernberg's (1965, 1989) continuum of countertransference, regarded as being more or less attributable to projective identification depending on the severity of the patient's psychopathology, can be expanded to describe two continua related to projective identification and extractive introjection, both of which fall under the heading of valency. I view projective identification as a continuum with clear communication on one side, projection in the middle, and strong behavioral inducement on the other extreme. I view extractive introjection as a continuum with clear communication on one side, introjection in the middle, and strong behavioral inducement on the other extreme. The closer one's interaction comes to being clear communication, on either continuum, the more indirect, and less immediately effective, the projective identification (as in the example above differentiating projection from projective identification). The combination of tendencies along these two continua, among all members involved within any interaction, determines the extent to which valency, and thus projective identification and extractive introjection, are involved.

For the sake of simplicity, the term *projective identification* as I use it in the remainder of this study will include any unconscious influence of one person or group on any other person or group, including extractive introjection. As part of such an interaction, I will continue to emphasize the recipient person's (or group's) valency toward identifying with or introjecting the particular content of the projective identification, as well as the impact of influence from the projector. The strength of the projective identification concept is in its explanatory power. Projective identification connects intrapsychic dynamics to interpersonal dynamics. As such, awareness of its workings can point to interventions that address intrapsychic and interpersonal aspects of family system and therapist–family system functioning. But if the therapist fails to recognize the extent to which his own valency is involved, that is, the therapist's tendency to use projective or extractive introjection within his own interactions, then the concept of projective identification is nearly useless in explaining the use of countertransference from within the therapeutic system.

CLASSICAL COUNTERTRANSFERENCE

The definition of countertransference has gone through many changes. The topic was written about by Douglas Orr in 1954. The reader is referred to his paper, "Transference and Countertransference: A Historical Survey" for a more detailed discussion. The focal areas of discussion can be listed as: (1) the importance of conscious and unconscious aspects of counter-transference versus unconscious aspects only; (2) the general feelings and attitudes of the therapist versus the therapist's transference to the patient; and (3) the fact that countertransference simply exists and must be analyzed versus the idea that countertransference affects the treatment negatively. What follows is an outline of the major developments in the classical understanding of countertransference up to 1954.

In 1910 Freud first discussed what he called "counter-transference." He described countertransference as arising in the therapist as a result of the patient's influence on the therapist's feelings. He stated that the therapist should be compelled to recognize this countertransference within himself and overcome it: "We have become aware of the 'counter-transference', which arises in [the analyst] as a result of the patient's influence on his unconscious feelings, and we are almost inclined to insist that he shall recognize this counter-transference in himself and overcome it" (pp. 144–145). In reference to this recognition of countertransference feelings, Freud laid out one of his most famous psychoanalytic tenets: "No psycho-analyst goes further than his own complexes and internal resistances permit; and we consequently require that he shall begin his activity with a self-analysis and continually carry it deeper while he is making his observations on his patients. Anyone who fails to produce results in a self-analysis of this kind may at once give up any idea of being able to treat patients by analysis" (p. 145). This view of countertransference gives the impression that it can only cause difficulties for the therapist. Although it might be inevitable, it is an obstruction to the therapist's ability to perform her function in analyzing the patient.

The development of countertransference from Freud's original statements can be followed through the work of many authors. In 1924 Adolph Stern published the first paper dealing specifically with the issue of countertransference. His view was that it was the therapist's transference to the patient. That view is shared by many other analysts (Berman 1949, Ferenczi and Rank 1923, Fliess 1953, Reich 1951). In 1937 English and Pearson published a book that suggested, in contrast to Stern, that everything the analyst feels toward his patient is countertransference. In 1939 Balint and Balint suggested that everything that is related to the therapist (his office, his clothing, and his personality) is included in a transference–countertransference interplay. Balint and Balint believed that countertransference does not necessarily have a negative effect on the patient's ability to develop transference. It seems this viewpoint from Balint and Balint is related to that held by Winnicott (1949), who included within countertransference those aspects of the therapist's personality that aid her in doing therapeutic work. In 1947 Sharpe suggested that there are conscious and unconscious forms of countertransference but that only the unconscious forms are problematic. In 1951 Reich excluded conscious material from her definition and generally saw countertransference as the therapist's transference. She widened the definition, however, in differentiating a more chronic kind of countertransference, associated with acting out, from an acute kind of countertransference that occurred in specific situations. Whereas chronic countertransference was described as occurring owing to some habitual need of the analyst, she characterized acute countertransference as occurring more suddenly, when specific aspects of the analyst's character are evoked. In 1953 Fliess, generally maintaining that countertransference consisted of the analyst's transference to the patient, differentiated the quality of identification necessary for empathy from that of counter-identification, which causes the therapist to act out his countertransference.

Those contributions leading to the totalistic definition will be left for the next section. Here, I would like to present two analysts who represent current thinking with respect to the classical view. For this I turn to the work of Jacob Arlow (1985) and Charles Brenner (1985).

Jacob Arlow

Arlow (1985) does not advocate a totalistic definition of countertransference, but his view is a good representative of the classical perspective. Following from Reich (1951), Arlow discusses three ways in which countertransference is likely to manifest in psychotherapy. First, like Fliess (1953), he describes an identification that is similar to that which is required in empathy, and emphasizes that it can become countertransference if the therapist becomes unable to self-reflect and pull himself out of the identification, in order to give himself the distance to remain objective. Second, he describes a disturbance, like Reich's "acute" countertransference, that arises in response to the patient's material. This disturbance comes from evoked fantasy material in the analyst that is not identical to the unconscious wishes of the patient. Third, he describes something like Reich's "chronic" countertransference, an analytic setting that represents a "theater where the analyst may play out some unconscious role of being the central performer to an admiring audience—an opportunity to display his cleverness or to use the analytic situation as a testing ground for his capacities" (pp. 166–167).

In Arlow's (1985) opinion the most common of these is the first, which interestingly was not directly considered by Reich. Each of these counter-transference manifestations is consistent with the classical view of coun-tertransference within the totalistic view. That is, Arlow considers the re-actions of the therapist that are problematic as constituting the true meaning of the word countertransference. In concluding, Arlow (1985) states that all countertransference reactions "fall under the heading of loss of ana-lytic stance" (p. 173).

It is important to note that Arlow does in part work with countertrans-ference, as is indicated by the totalistic approach discussed in this study. The first type of countertransference he discusses is related to losing ob-jectivity when using countertransference in the totalistic sense. He does not, however, refer to this as using countertransference. Instead he sub-sumes what I call a use of countertransference under the heading of em-pathy. That is, he uses self-reflection to pull himself out of identifications with patients so that he will remain both empathic and objective.

Charles Brenner

Brenner's (1985) views on countertransference include empathy within the definition. Brenner sees countertransference as ubiquitous. He states: "My thesis is this. Countertransference is ubiquitous and inescapable, just as is transference" (p. 156). He goes on to say

> Countertransference is the transference of the analyst in an analytic situation. Becoming an analyst, practicing analysis, necessarily in-volves, for each individual analyst, derivatives of that analyst's child-hood conflicts. There is nothing pathological or neurotic in this. It is,

in fact, as inevitable for the profession of analysis as it is for the choice and practice of any other vocation. The choice of analysis as a vocation is as much a normal compromise formation, a normal outcome of conflict over childhood drive derivatives, as is the choice of any adult occupation. It is when pathological compromise formations appear in an analyst's professional activity that analytic work may be disturbed. Instances of countertransference which interfere with analysis are examples of pathological or neurotic compromise formation. [p. 156]

Despite the fact that Brenner is a drive theorist, he uses a very broad definition of countertransference. However, the viewpoint given here is not very different from Arlow's (1985). Brenner still chooses to discuss countertransference difficulties as those countertransference reactions that are worthy of discussion. His main point is that all reactions, all decisions, all roles, are compromise formations (compromises between drives and their expression, mediated by reality concerns and the defenses that have developed in relation to those concerns). The question is whether or not the compromise formation at work in the here-and-now of a therapy is pathological or relatively benign. When a therapist is reacting to a patient in a way that is relatively healthy there is nothing to worry about from Brenner's point of view.

Brenner does not, however, specifically discuss countertransference as a tool for the analyst. Countertransference is only useful to him to the extent that it is a compromise formation through which the analyst desires to do his work or does his work. Here, again, we see a view of countertransference that corresponds to the second part of Winnicott's (1949) view. That second part represents the therapist's natural tendencies—we might say compromise formations—which help him with the analytic task.

Classical Countertransference in the Relational Systems Perspective

These works from Arlow (1985) and Brenner (1985) represent current classical viewpoints. Although their approaches differ in many respects, neither of them advocates the use of countertransference. Arlow sees empathy as having an important therapeutic function and Brenner, through compromise formations, suggests the same. Thus, it could be said that they do use countertransference. On the other hand, since neither of them discusses the possibility of using it as a bridge to an empathic response or deeper understanding, through an awareness of projective identification, it seems they would not completely agree with the use of countertransference that is advocated here. Nevertheless, their views fit well with the classical part of totalistic countertransference. Especially important from that classical perspective is the question of how the therapist is affected by classical countertransference. That is, as in the descriptions of both Arlow and Brenner, what happens when countertransference is a problem? In reference to the focal areas outlined earlier, the contemporary classical view posits countertransference as a transference to the patient that is unconscious and causes difficulties within the therapy. The method suggested for resolving countertransference difficulties from the classical perspective has not changed since Freud's dictum of 1910. The analyst must either receive more analysis, or self-analyze, to prevent and resolve countertransference difficulties.

One problem with the classical view of countertransference is that there is no room for the concept of projective identification, which adds so much depth to clinical understanding. Perhaps the kind of neutrality used by these analysts obviates sensitivity to projective identification. But sensitivity to the influence of the patient is essential in any work that attempts to intervene in interpersonal dynamics. If the analyst is neutral to the point that she does not feel the influence of the patient but only perceives through empathy how the patient views her, then the self-fulfilling aspect of repetition compulsion is left unanalyzed. (It could be argued that empathy is not even possible in this circumstance, as discussed in a later section.) That is, the patient never influences the analyst in the way he influences others outside of therapy. Sensitivity to that influence, if allowed to occur in therapy, would provide grist for the analytic mill.

The primary concern when considering the classical view is, simply put, that the analyst should not act on his problematic countertransference feelings. And this concern remains when considering the totalistic view. But with the totalistic view, analyzing the self-fulfilling aspect of the repetition compulsion is of primary importance. Since therapists who seek to use their countertransference reactions are concerned about acting on those feelings where they should not, they have had to discuss the difference between acting out with the patient, on one hand, and the useful experience of the pull toward acting out that is brought on by projective identification, on the other.

ACTING OUT

Some analysts have gone so far as to suggest that it is impossible not to be affected by the roles patients attempt to foist on the analyst through projective identification.

León Grinberg

Grinberg (1962, 1979), for example, suggested that the analyst is often unconsciously involved in a projective counter-identification, a role placed on him by the patient through projective identification. According to Grinberg, in projective counter-identification the therapist plays out the role placed on him without even altering the patient's projection with his own personality.

Grinberg (1968), in a paper on the patient's acting-out behavior, makes the following statement, one that indicates that the analyst will at times act out with the patient: "The analyst who succumbs to the effects of the patient's pathological projective identifications, might react to them as if he had actually acquired the aspects which were projected on him (the patient's inner objects or parts of the self). The analyst feels passively 'dragged' into playing the role that the patient in an active, though unconscious, way, literally 'forced' upon him" (p. 172).

Here Grinberg seems to indicate that to "succumb" to this acting out is undesirable but almost unavoidable. In his work, of course, he advocates experiencing the feelings of being pulled in a particular direction but not acting on that feeling. Nevertheless, Grinberg sees acting out as always involving an object relationship. If a person is acting out, there is someone acting out with him. When patients are under the influence of overwhelming intolerable intrapsychic forces, Grinberg says, "patients . . . project the tyrannical relationship into the object, inducing it, in turn, to act out" (p. 177). Although this should not occur in a therapy, the excerpt above clearly demonstrates his view that it sometimes does.

Heinrich Racker

Another helpful viewpoint on the therapist's acting out can be found in the work of Racker. Racker was one of the pioneers of the totalistic approach to using countertransference. One important distinction he described was the difference between countertransference "thoughts" and "positions" (1957). In the case of countertransference thoughts, the therapist does not act out the thoughts that are involved. With countertransference positions, however, the therapist does act out, primarily due to overinvestment of the ego. Racker stated that countertransference thoughts "are characterized by the fact that they threaten no danger to the analyst's objective attitude of observer" (p. 322). Countertransference thoughts "are experienced as thoughts, free associations, or fantasies, with no great emotional intensity and frequently as if they were somewhat foreign to the ego" (p. 322). In contrast, with countertransference positions, "the analyst's ego is involved in the countertransference experience, and the experience is felt by him with greater intensity and as true reality, and there is danger of his 'drowning' in this experience" (pp. 322–323).

Acting Out and the Relational Systems Perspective

Although these distinctions may often seem implicit in discussions involving the use of countertransference, since countertransference is often only associated with the therapist acting on her feelings inappropriately, the distinctions are instrumental in describing how using countertransference is different from having countertransference difficulties. Grinberg's (1968) view, which is at one extreme, points to the power of projective identification to affect the analyst in cases where there is a strong behavioral inducement. One wonders how analysts who deny the importance of projective identification deal with the effects it has under circumstances like those he describes. Racker (1957) offers a view of acting out that is easier to apply to the use of countertransference in less extreme circumstances. Racker's differentiation between countertransference "thoughts" and "positions" is a simple way of distinguishing between the experience of potentially helpful feelings induced by the patient and acting out on those feelings. Racker's contribution in this area will be considered implicit to the remainder of this study. That is, countertransference thoughts will be considered potentially informative, while countertransference positions will remain a concern. But the strong behavioral inducements that Grinberg (1968) discusses will not be considered necessary in causing countertransference positions or acting out. With the focus on the therapist's receptivity to projective identification (Bion 1959a, Malin and Grotstein 1966), taking on countertransference "positions" is of major concern even when clear behavioral influence is not present.

THE ORIGINS OF THE TOTALISTIC PERSPECTIVE

Although Kernberg (1965) coined the term "totalistic countertransference," the concept has its roots in the work of Winnicott (1949), Heimann (1950), Little (1951), and Racker (1953, 1957). This definition is a far cry from the one originally used by Freud (1910). The main impact of using this broader definition is that many countertransference feelings can be recognized as a normal part of treatment (Winnicott 1949) and can provide a fuller understanding of patients as well as an essential tool for formulating interpretations (Bion 1959b, Heimann 1950, Racker 1957, Kernberg 1965). Although in following Freud's definition some therapists aim to avoid countertransference reactions or to analyze them out of their own personalities, in work that utilizes a totalistic definition countertransference is often seen as part of a process in which "holding" (Winnicott 1960a), "containing" (Bion 1959b), "processing" (Bion 1959b), or "metabolizing" (Langs 1976b) projections or projective identifications is paramount, and the therapist is also required to analyze his own reactions. Thus, if therapists use the totalistic definition, then countertransference is implicitly an integral part of their approach to treatment. The following analysts pioneered the use of countertransference.

Donald Winnicott

Winnicott (1949) was the first psychoanalyst to use a broader definition of countertransference. As opposed to limiting countertransference to subjective reactions in the therapist, Winnicott expanded the concept to include "objective" reactions the therapist might have toward the patient. He also included what he termed *subjective countertransference*, which can be viewed as conducive to therapy within his definition (like my view of the unintentional use of countertransference). The "objective" and subjective but beneficial aspects of countertransference, when added to the classical ones, provide the essential framework for the relational systems perspective. Winnicott is one of the primary contributors to the object relations school, which initiated a movement in psychoanalysis toward interpersonal as well as intrapsychic mental health.

Winnicott believed that in analysis with patients who were either psychotic or at least non-neurotic, the patient, by way of projective identification, often unconsciously attempted to recreate a symbiotic relationship with the therapist, patterned after his relationship as an infant with his mother. The reaction of the therapist to these unconscious pulls Winnicott considered "objective." Instead of creating a block in treatment, these reactions could provide information to the therapist. If the therapist could create a "holding environment" (1960a) for the patient who was attempting to recreate this symbiotic relationship, the relationship between the therapist and patient would allow for the reworking of a developmental arrest suffered by the patient. In this way, Winnicott explained how countertransference is a natural part of the therapeutic process that provides understanding of the patient.

Winnicott's ideas correspond to Ogden's (1979) fourth purpose of projective identification as described above. That is, his main emphasis is on the psychological growth that could occur in therapy based on the ability of the therapist to accept the patient's projections and then, by remaining empathic to the patient, to change those projections so that their reinternalization will be healthier for the patient. But he did not yet include the therapist's verbal interpretation of his understanding accomplished through countertransference as part of his therapeutic approach. Rather, Winnicott believed the *end* of a successful analysis was reached when the patient could be told of negative and positive, but objective, feelings the therapist had experienced toward him at an earlier stage of treatment.

Paula Heimann

Heimann (1950) described a more elaborate way to use countertransference. Kernberg later used her words in coining the "totalistic" definition of countertransference. In a paper, "On Countertransference," she wrote: "For the purpose of this paper I am using the term 'countertransference' to cover all the feelings which the analyst experiences towards his patient" (p. 81). She was also the first to advocate that therapists become aware of their countertransference reactions so that such reactions could be used as a therapeutic tool. She believed that "the analyst's countertransference is an instrument of research into the patient's unconscious" (p. 81). Whereas Winnicott (1949) described feelings that he could not help but experience when with a patient, Heimann recommended that the therapist analyze her own inner state, thus consciously uncovering feelings toward the patient as a way of understanding the patient. Her view constitutes a more intentional use of countertransference feelings than had been advocated by Winnicott.

Margaret Little

Little (1951) had the iconoclastic idea, originally advocated in certain situations by Ferenczi (Heimann 1950), that countertransference feelings should be discussed with the patient. She was not willing to limit her discussion of the awareness of countertransference to those aspects considered to be objective reactions to the reality of the patient, as Heimann had before her. Rather, Little described the origin of countertransference as reactions to a patient's particular way of being as well as the analyst's subjective way of perceiving the patient.

Another difference between Little and Heimann is that Little concerned herself only with countertransference that interfered with treatment. But because Little felt that countertransference was widespread and often normal, she also felt that these interfering reactions must become a constant consideration in analytic treatment. She suggested that transference and countertransference are so inextricably interwoven as to make their disentanglement extremely difficult. In describing her approach, Little (1951) wrote:

> The whole patient–analyst relationship includes both 'normal' and pathological, conscious and unconscious, transference and counter-transference, in varying proportions; it will always include something which is specific to both the individual patient and the individual analyst. That is, every counter-transference is different from every other, as every transference is different, and it varies within itself from day to day, according to variations in both patient and analyst and the outside world. [p. 33]

Countertransference is thus part of a dynamic between therapist and patient. According to Little, the therapist's countertransference can be the product of a behavioral interaction that is designed to evoke responses similar to those of the patient's parents.

The therapist's countertransference is even more likely, however, to be her unconscious reaction, based on her own unresolved and repressed conflicts. To the extent that the therapist acts out these feelings, as the parents of the patient did, the patient's projection onto the therapist becomes a reality in the therapeutic relationship, rather than transference. Thus the therapist is left unable to interpret the patient's transference because, rather than appearing as transference, the patient's perception has actually become manifest in the relationship between analyst and patient.

For this reason, Little believed the therapist must self-analyze before acting out countertransference feelings, and then, when the time was right, reveal openly to the patient the feeling that would have made her act like a parent. Likewise, when the patient is able to correctly perceive an action or feeling in the analyst, Little advocated admitting openly the feeling or action and taking responsibility for it. Only with this kind of straightforward honesty, she believed, would the patient's sense of reality be bolstered enough so that actual transference distortions could be explored and worked through.

Heinrich Racker

Racker (1953, 1957) described processes similar to those discussed by Little (1951). Racker believed that transference and countertransference acted upon each other reciprocally. Where a transference neurosis develops, so does a countertransference neurosis. In this way the therapist's perception of the patient could become as distorted as the patient's perception of the therapist. Furthermore, the therapist's responses under the influence of this distortion lead to increased distortion of the patient's perception. He believed that a therapist must closely analyze and accept his own countertransference reactions to ensure minimal interference with the patient's progress. He also believed, like Heimann, that the analyst's analysis of his or her own countertransference would lead to insights about the patient.

Racker (1957) differentiated between countertransference that can be helpful to the patient and countertransference that is the responsibility of the analyst alone. As discussed earlier, he distinguished between countertransference "positions" and countertransference "thoughts." Of course, countertransference thoughts, too, can originate in the analyst's unresolved conflicts. And so all countertransference reactions must be analyzed to assess their usefulness. In the following paragraph on the "ideal of the analyst's objectivity," Racker describes the complication inherent in differentiating the origin of countertransference and also elucidates his own impression of how this should be handled by the analyst. He begins by stating that it is a distortion to think that analysis is an interaction between a "sick person and a healthy one."

The truth is that it is an interaction between two personalities, in both of which the ego is under pressure from the id, the superego, and the external world; each personality has its internal and external dependencies, anxieties, and pathological defenses; each is also a child with its internal parents; and each of these whole personalities—that of the analysand and that of the analyst—responds to every event of the analytic situation. Besides these similarities between the personalities of analyst and analysand, there also exist differences, and one of these is in "objectivity." The analyst's objectivity consists mainly in a certain attitude toward his own subjectivity and countertransference

. . . True objectivity is based upon a form of internal division that enables the analyst to make himself (his own countertransference and subjectivity) the object of his continuous observation and analysis. [pp. 308–309]

Thus, according to Racker, the therapist and patient interaction combines two personalities. But the therapist's ability to subordinate his own countertransference and subjectivity to the analytic task makes his understanding of those reactions available to the treatment in a salutary way. As will be seen, this viewpoint bears remarkable similarities to the relational understanding of the transference–countertransference system (Aron 1992, Atwood and Stolorow 1984, Greenberg 1986, Mitchell 1988, Ogden 1994a,b, Stolorow et al. 1994, Wachtel 1986).

Perhaps Racker's most distinctive contribution to the discussion of countertransference was his differentiation of two kinds of countertransference, concordant and complementary identification. Concordant identification is the empathic response of the therapist to an aspect of the patient's self-representation. In complementary identification, the therapist identifies with a part of the patient's object representation. Thus if a patient is feeling like a victim, the therapist in a concordant identification will empathize with that feeling. The complementary identification in that same situation would consist of the therapist feeling like a victimizer.

According to Racker, in cases where the therapist might reject the concordant identification, complementary identifications are likely to become intensified. Thus, following Racker, if a therapist refuses to accept and empathize with a patient's perversity, for example, he is likely to identify with a complementary, punitive stance toward the patient, often characteristic of the patient's object representation. The patient will perceive this reaction in the therapist and it will confirm the patient's transference (in this case, a view that others condemn her).

Racker distinguished self and object projections of patients based on which feelings he became emotionally identified with under the influence of projective identification. He believed that patients worked through their traumas by recreating both the self (victim, for example) and object (aggressor, for example) roles in themselves and the therapist. Racker elaborately described processes much like those Little had discussed; however, he was hesitant to recommend revealing countertransference feelings to the patient. He also viewed countertransference as informative about the patient's conflicts, whereas Little limited her view of countertransference to its creation of problems in the analysis. I will return to Racker's work as it pertains to empathy in a later section.

Harold Searles

Searles is well known for the complete integration of the use of counter-transference. His early work with schizophrenics best demonstrates the many viewpoints on the use of countertransference that he continues to advocate in his recent writing. I will base this brief review on four papers he published between 1958 and 1963, all of which can be found in his book *Collected Papers on Schizophrenia and Related Subjects* (1963).

Searles considers more fully than any analyst before him the full extent of the impact made by the therapist's thought and behavior. He (1958) views the schizophrenic as especially vulnerable to perceiving the unconscious thoughts of the analyst. According to Searles, the patient sometimes perceives the analyst's unconscious processes as part of the patient's own personality, and sometimes experiences those unconscious processes in the form of hallucinations. Searles also sometimes considers the patient's acting out to be a manifestation of the therapist's unconscious processes. He commonly sounds the theme that these processes can only be dealt with if the therapist makes himself aware of the fact that the conflicts or attitudes demonstrated by the patient actually originated in the therapist. Only by becoming more comfortable with his own unconscious tendencies, even though they may be somewhat disturbing at times, can the therapist help the patient.

One good example of this necessity for the therapist to be aware of his tendencies occurs in what Searles (1959a) calls the "effort to drive the other person crazy." According to Searles, the schizophrenic patient is especially prone to enter into relationships where he and the other person are attempting to drive each other crazy. This process originates in the patient. But Searles explains that it is so common, and so compelling, that the therapist must become part of it. That is, the therapist must at least recognize the pull toward acting this way, and recognize that the tendency also exists in him, although it is perhaps not as pronounced as it is in the patient.

Searles (1959a) believes that this process is a necessary part of treating the schizophrenic and that the therapist does often, in attempting to drive or keep the patient crazy, "utilize (largely unconsciously . . .), just as do patients, the whole gamut of modes or techniques" (p. 277) that are utilized by the patient in attempting to drive the therapist crazy. Searles considers the therapist's acceptance of his dependent relationship (that part of him that wants the patient to remain ill so that the relationship will continue) especially important to the treatment. The avoidance of this relationship, and its symbiotic nature, is viewed by Searles to be part of what caused the difficulty for the patient in his original parental relationship.

Searles is even quite verbal with his patients about his countertransference feelings. Especially with schizophrenic patients, Searles (1959b) believes it is necessary to be open about his thoughts and attitudes because they are so perceptive and vulnerable. In other words, if the schizophrenic patient is perceiving something in the analyst, her vulnerability makes it necessary to validate the veracity of that perception. Since schizophrenic patients struggle with reality testing, letting them know when they have correctly perceived something bolsters their understanding of what is real. Searles is not as likely to be so open with the neurotic patient. With the neurotic patient it is more important for the therapist to simply be comfortable with his feelings. Neurotic patients, as they increasingly become able to see the therapist as a real person, will know that the therapist had certain feelings toward them but was able to cope with those feelings safely.

Searles (1963) brings many of these ideas together in his paper "Transference Psychosis in the Psychotherapy of Chronic Schizophrenia." In this paper, he emphasizes the symbiotic nature of the transference. Most important, perhaps, Searles suggests that the therapist's acceptance of the patient's projections is absolutely essential to treatment. Using the mother–infant pair as his example, he suggests that the therapist, like the mother, must be able to handle the patient's intolerable affects. He states that the therapist's task with the schizophrenic is constructed of three major elements:

First, the therapist must become able to function as *part* [italics in original] of the patient and to permit the patient to be genuinely, at a deep level of psychological functioning, a part of himself. Secondly, he must be able to foster the patient's individuation (and, to a not insignificant degree, his own re-individuation) out of this level of relatedness, a level which is conceptualized variously by several workers in this field . . . and by most writers, including myself, as being a phase of symbiotic relatedness between patient and doctor. The therapist's third task is to discern, and make interpretations concerning, the patient's now differentiated and now integrated whole object, that is to say neurotic, kind of transference manifestations. [p. 661]

Searles (1963) most emphasized in this process the ability of the therapist to "endure the explicit emergence of [the delusional, symbiotic] transference on the part of the patient towards him" (p. 674). He goes on to say that the experience of this transference is difficult to describe:

The extent to which the therapist feels a genuine sense of deep participation in the patient's 'delusional transference' relatedness to him during the phase of therapeutic symbiosis . . . is difficult to convey in words; it is essential that the therapist come to know that such a degree of feeling-participation is not evidence of 'countertransference psychosis', but rather is the essence of what the patient needs from him at this crucial phase of the treatment. [p. 705]

Thus Searles clearly emphasizes the ability of the therapist to handle strong countertransference feelings as part of what is crucial to the patient's treatment. But beyond this ability to handle the patient's projections, it is also clear that Searles views the acceptance, and almost a welcoming, of these affects, along with the symbiotic relatedness with the patient, as essential in the treatment of schizophrenics.

Summary: The Origins of Totalistic Countertransference

Searles's work has some similarities to the work of the analysts before him. He advances the idea that the therapist must be somewhat like the mother to the patient, as did Winnicott. Like Heimann, Searles learns about the patient's psychodynamics by recognizing a pull on him to behave in certain ways. Like Little, he views the verbalization of countertransference feelings as sometimes necessary. Like both Little and Racker, he sees the processes between therapist and patient as being in need, at times, of an arduous self-analytical process aimed toward differentiating whose conflicts are whose. But in several ways Searles also adds to the work of these other authors. He readily admits to the influence the patient has on him and is concerned with the influence he has on the patient. Although these other analysts express similar concerns, Searles is far more open to suggesting that his own pathology (which he regards as similar to the underlying pathology in all neurotic personalities) is part of the treatment. In this way, Searles's work is a move toward viewing the patient–analyst relationship as involving a whole that is greater than the sum of its parts. I will refer to this whole as the transference–countertransference system in reviewing more current additions to the literature on countertransference.

TOWARD A TRANSFERENCE–
COUNTERTRANSFERENCE SYSTEM

Since the time of Winnicott's 1949 paper, "Hate in the Countertransference," which marked a transition within psychoanalytic thinking to a view of countertransference as useful data, there have been many contributions to the literature that indicate wide acceptance of such thought. Of special interest to this study is the work of several authors who have taken the use of countertransference to new levels. The work of these authors expands on the contribution of Racker (1953, 1957), who wrote that for every transference there is a related countertransference. The most important factor connecting these works is the presentation of the psychoanalytic situation in a new light, one in which the nature of the therapist's unique personality is integral to the patient's treatment. Building upon the ideas advanced by psychoanalytic thought, the dyad formed by the patient and therapist can be construed as forming a transference–countertransference system. In this study, which focuses on the therapist's part in family therapy, these ideas about countertransference are especially enlightening. Several of these ideas will be discussed here in the order of their development within psychoanalytic theory.

Otto Kernberg

Kernberg has been highlighted in this study as the analyst who named "totalistic" countertransference (1965). Within that same paper, however, he goes beyond simply summarizing the work of analysts before him. I cited Kernberg earlier as an author who differentiates the extent of pathology in the patient based on the storminess of the patient's transference. That is, the severely character-disordered patient utilizes projective identification in a rapidly fluctuating and somewhat forceful way that manifests in the therapist's countertransference. This idea is important here because I view projective identification as an interpersonal phenomenon that is common at all levels of pathology. But, nevertheless, it is obvious that, with more severely disturbed patients, projective identification takes on a powerful flavor that is much more difficult for the therapist to handle. Kernberg (1965) describes a continuum:

> As we proceed from the "neurotic pole" of the continuum toward the "psychotic pole," transference manifestations become increasingly predominant in the patient's contribution to the countertransference reaction of the therapist, displacing the importance of those countertransference aspects which arise from the therapist's past. When dealing with borderline or severely regressed patients, as contrasted to those presenting symptomatic neuroses and many character disorders, the therapist tends to experience reactions having more to do with the patient's premature, intense and chaotic transference, and with the therapist's capacity to withstand psychological stress and anxiety, than with any particular, specific problem of the therapist's past. In other words, given reasonably well-adjusted therapists, all hypothetically dealing with the same severely regressed and disorganized patient, their countertransference reactions will be somewhat similar, reflecting the patient's problems much more than any specific problem of the analyst's past. [pp. 42–43]

According to Kernberg, then, with more severe pathologies, countertransference is more likely to be the manifestation of the patient's projections. In fact, Kernberg is well known for discussing the particular manifestations of countertransference with particular patient populations.

Joseph Sandler and Colleagues

In their 1973 book, *The Patient and the Analyst: The Basis of the Psycho-analytic Process*, Sandler and his colleagues Dare and Holder extended the concept of transference from the projection of aspects of the past or figures of the past onto the analyst, to all the patient's attempts to manipulate or provoke situations with the analyst. In his 1976 paper, "Counter-transference and Role-Responsiveness," Sandler discusses the importance of the analyst's response to those transferences that include the patient's "attempts to manipulate or to provoke." He considers these responses as part of a relationship, or interaction, that develops between the two parties in the analytic situation. Referring to the way the roles of patient and analyst combine in the analytic situation, Sandler clarifies the way in which his behavioral responses can be construed as transference manifestations. "What I want to emphasize is that the role-relationship of the patient in analysis at any particular time consists of a role in which he casts himself, and a *complementary* [italics in original] role in which he casts the analyst at that particular time. The patient's transference would thus represent an attempt by him to impose an interaction, an interrelationship (in the broadest sense of the word) between himself and the analyst" (p. 44). Since this manifestation of transference so strongly represents the past relationships of the patient, Sandler does not believe that the opportunity to use his own response to that transference can be left out of an analysis.

As an indicator of the patient's transference that has not yet become conscious for the therapist, the behavioral response of the analyst becomes important in Sandler's work. He suggests that the therapist should maintain a "free-floating role-responsiveness" just as he should maintain free-floating attention. Sandler (1976) says this about free-floating role-responsiveness: "My contention is that in the analyst's overt reactions to the patient as well as in his thoughts and feelings what can be called his 'role-responsiveness' shows itself, not only in his feelings but also in his attitudes and behaviour, as a crucial element in his 'useful' countertransference" (p. 45).

This view of countertransference makes the therapist very much a part of an analytic dyad. Perhaps with free-floating role-responsiveness Sandler is less neutral than other therapists would suggest being. But his use of this concept is essential to his perspective on working with transference. And the term "free-floating" seems to denote exactly the kind of neutrality that is essential within the relational systems perspective.

Perhaps a primary reason for Sandler's emphasis on this point is that many analysts do continue to see countertransference reactions in more of a classical sense. Sandler (1976) believes analysts need to be aware of the countertransference reactions that truly are the result of their own unresolved conflicts or defenses. Yet Sandler also cautions against maintaining a narrow view of countertransference reactions. He clearly views his countertransference reactions as a product of the interaction between patient and analyst. He refers to these reactions as a "compromise formation" between the analyst's tendencies and "his reflexive acceptance" of the role projected upon him. This view could be a very useful way for family therapists to understand their countertransference reactions with families.

Robert Langs

Langs (1976a) suggests that the analyst and patient together create a "bipersonal field," a concept that is almost identical to the transference–countertransference system. Within the bipersonal field, Langs brings the personality of the therapist into the analytic picture more clearly than any analyst before him. In Langs's paper specifically addressing countertransference (1983) he describes the "bipersonal field" as

> the temporal-physical space within which the analytic interaction takes place. The patient is one term of the polarity; the analyst is the other. The field embodies both interactional and intrapsychic mechanisms, and every event within the field receives vectors from both participants. The field itself is defined by a framework—the ground rules of psychoanalysis—which not only delimits the field, but also, in a major way, contributes to the communicative properties of the field and to the analyst's hold of the patient and containment of his projective identification. [p. 72]

Although this field involves two contributing personalities, it is clear in this excerpt that Langs advocates the classical posture of the analyst in maintaining the ground rules of psychoanalysis. In doing so, Langs indicates, as Racker (1953, 1957) had before him, that it is the analyst's attempt at objectivity that differentiates his input from that of the patient. Nevertheless, it is also clear in his further descriptions of this field that he does not discount the influence of the analyst on the therapeutic dyad.

Within the interactional field, Langs considers the major communicative mechanisms to be projective and introjective identification. He attributes these mechanisms to both the analyst and the patient within the typical analysis. It could be said, in fact, that Langs's most remarkable addition to the understanding of countertransference is on the therapist's side of the bipersonal field. That is, he writes about the value of understanding the therapist's momentary inability to handle certain actions of the analysand. The value of the countertransference is in discovering the potentially adaptive context of one's defenses and then understanding how that adaptation came about in the interaction with the patient. Ideas similar to those of Searles can be seen in this next excerpt, in which Langs (1983) focuses on the patient's introjection of the analyst's countertransference in an interactional context.

> The interactional approach proves to be of special value in these pursuits in three important ways: (1) by establishing the finding that the patient's communications and symptoms may be significantly derived from the countertransferences of the analyst; (2) by indicating that through the process of introjective identification the patient becomes a mirror and container for the analyst, in the sense that the patient's communication will play back to the analyst the metabolized introjects derived from his countertransference-based interventions (and his valid, noncountertransference-based interventions as well); and (3) by directing the search for the form and meaning of countertransferences to the sequential interactions of each session. [pp. 75–76]

That Langs feels strongly about the analyst paying attention to his influence on the patient is clear in this excerpt. Unlike other analytic writers who suggest that their own strong emotions are more largely attributable to the patient than to themselves, Langs's approach seems to put responsibility back on the therapist. Yet the emphasis is still on using those emotions to better understand the patient.

The concept of the bipersonal field, more than any other ideas put forth before it, describes the psychoanalytic dyad as a system. The connecting factors in that system are transference and countertransference. Langs (1983) goes on to indicate just how important countertransference is within the bipersonal field: "The bipersonal field concept directs the analyst to the investigation of his countertransferences when any resistance, defense, symptom, or regression occurs within the patient or himself. Since the adaptational-interactional view considers all such occurrences as interactional products, it generates as a technical requisite the investigation of unconscious factors in both participants at such moments in therapy" (p. 77). The reference here to "any resistance, defense, symptom, or regression" is so inclusive that Langs's use of countertransference seems universal. The analyst must reflect upon countertransference manifestations continually throughout an analysis.

George Atwood and Robert Stolorow

Stolorow and Atwood (1979) picture psychoanalysis

as a science of the *intersubjective* [italics in original], focused on the interplay between the differently organized subjective worlds of the observer and the observed. The observational stance is always one within, rather than outside, the intersubjective field or "contextual unit" (Schwaber 1979) being observed, a fact that guarantees the centrality of introspection and empathy as the methods of observation (Kohut 1959). Psychoanalysis is unique among the sciences in that the observer is also the observed. [pp. 41–42]

Even though they refer to the analyst as the observer, and in fact recommend, in general, a stance of neutrality for the purpose of fostering the patient's transference, they maintain that the analyst's personality is important to the dynamic between analyst and patient. In the intersubjective relationship, Atwood and Stolorow see the uniqueness of two individually formed personalities together contributing to the analytic situation.

They describe the intersubjective approach as a "direct outgrowth" of the interplay between transference and countertransference. The transference is seen as a microcosm of the patient's psychological life. Its analysis allows for the clarification of the patient's patterns. Countertransference, on the other hand, is viewed as being related to the way in which the analyst's subjectivity shapes his experience of the analytic relationship and the patient's transference.

Two primary types of countertransference are specifically discussed by Atwood and Stolorow (1984). Intersubjective conjunction and intersubjective disjunction arise from the interplay of transference and countertransference. Intersubjective conjunctions represent instances in which the therapist either maintains identification with the patient (empathy) or fits into the patient's view of others. Disjunction occurs when the therapist assimilates the presentation of the patient into patterns from his own personality which significantly alters the subjective meaning of the material for the patient. Both of these types of countertransference occur inevitably as a reflection of differently organized subjective worlds.

Intersubjective conjunctions, much like Racker's (1953, 1957) concordant identifications, are often associated with empathic responding, but are not always beneficial. Intersubjective disjunctions include Racker's complementary identifications, and can be associated with problematic countertransference reactions, but can also lead to beneficial changes in the patient's perceptions, or the empathic use of countertransference.

Atwood and Stolorow (1984) explain that with a conjunction the therapist may reflect on similar experiences of his own that allow him to understand the patient. However, if those experiences are, as is the case with the patient, still unconscious, unresolved, and unintegrated, the analyst is unable to see the conjunction as part of the transference. In this case the analyst and the patient may simply not examine an important aspect of the patient's experience. It is also possible that the conjunction that is unconscious for both the analyst and the patient can lead to both of them unconsciously acting out together or to the therapist encouraging the patient in defensive ways of viewing the world that are similar to her own.

Atwood and Stolorow state that it is the continual and unresolved intersubjective disjunction that is more likely to cause countertransference difficulties or even "negative therapeutic reactions." With an intersubjective disjunction, by incorrectly assimilating the patient's experience into her already existing structural configurations, the therapist misunderstands the patient. Atwood and Stolorow (1984) are particularly interested in the results that occur when a therapist mistakenly views as resistance the patient's true archaic transference needs. They state that "the patient will experience such misinterpretations as gross failures of empathy" (p. 53).

Atwood and Stolorow offer an example of a happening of this kind in which a patient's childhood experience consisted of almost complete unresponsiveness from her parents with the exception of her father's sexual interest. She had developed a coquettish style that her analyst mistook as resistance. Atwood and Stolorow (1984) explain that the analyst used an overly literal interpretation of the rule of abstinence because of his own need to maintain control lest he feel as though he were a slave to the oppressive will of others. The analyst had, in fact, experienced his mother as tyrannical. Here, "The patient's desperate demands for mirroring responsiveness were unconsciously assimilated into his emotionally charged themes of power and control, evoking a reaction of stubborn resistance and entrenching his already withholding and unresponsive style" (p. 54). The result of the analyst's inability to recognize the patient's selfobject need in her coquettishness was a vicious spiral in which the analyst believed her demands to be a need for dominance. Thus, her needs continued to be invalidated. The analysis ended after eighteen months when the patient attempted suicide.

So it becomes clear that both intersubjective conjunction and disjunction require self-reflection of the analyst to be used effectively as therapeutic tools. As the authors (1984) comment, "Whether or not these intersubjective situations facilitate or obstruct the progress of analysis depends in large part on the extent of the analyst's reflective self-awareness and capacity to decenter (Piaget 1974) from the organizing principles of his own subjective world and thereby to grasp empathically the actual meaning of the patient's experiences" (p. 47). The process of decentering, or self-reflecting, is required when the analyst has already gotten involved in the intersubjective conjunction or disjunction. Since Atwood and Stolorow see these phenomena as constantly occurring within the transference–countertransference intersubjectivity, it becomes clear that continuous self-reflection is necessary in their approach.

Atwood and Stolorow's (1984) contribution to the psychoanalytic understanding of transference and countertransference is most distinctive in its emphasis on the responsibility of the analyst for what occurs in the treatment. They believe that the analyst must always be aware of her own process as inputs into the analytic whole. This belief is similar to Langs's view as described above. But even more than Langs, Atwood and Stolorow maintain that the psychopathology of the analyst leads to problems within treatment. Where Langs seeks to be aware, Atwood and Stolorow believe the therapist must take responsibility for her part in the process. Their emphasis on the analyst's psychopathology will become clearer in a later section of this study devoted to the therapist's character. I now turn to another analyst who views the analyst's personality as integral to transference and countertransference.

Peter Giovacchini

Giovacchini (1989) refers to what he calls the transference–countertransference interaction or the transference–countertransference axis. His work differs somewhat from that of other analysts in that he presents this transference–countertransference interaction outright as the essence of psychoanalytic psychotherapy. He explains this as a "re-creation of the infantile environment, a process that is inextricably bound to and revolves around the transference–countertransference axis" (p. viii). He believes, therefore, that the connection between transference and countertransference is primary in any discussion of psychoanalytic treatment.

Perhaps at the time that this particular book was written Giovacchini was able to address these issues as integral to the psychoanalytic process without fearing criticism from classical analysts, as had not been the case with the other analysts thus far presented. The integration of a use of countertransference, at this point in time, had become quite acceptable to many analysts. In a way similar to the other analysts I have presented, Giovacchini (1989) sees the analyst's personality as central in the psychoanalytic interaction. He stresses that treatment success or failure often hinges upon the "irrational parts of both the therapist's and the patient's personalities" (p. 1).

Unlike the other analysts whose views were presented earlier, however, Giovacchini presents his ideas to a wide audience (as can be shown by his inclusion of psychoanalytically oriented psychotherapy in the excerpt above) in a clear and concise language not obfuscated by the need to defend his views. According to Giovacchini, clinicians no longer believe that countertransference reactions necessarily constitute the therapist's mishandling of the treatment. He stresses that treatment is not a unilateral process and that all therapy should involve the analysis of countertransference.

Just as he believes the consulting room must become a re-creation of the infantile environment, and that it is the infantile in the patient that will be analyzed, Giovacchini also believes "clinicians must consider the countertransference as a counterpart of infantile factors in the therapist with which the patient is getting in touch" (pp. viii–ix). He stresses the infantile part of the therapist's personality more than any other analyst since Searles. Searles (1975) believes that the analyst is best off recognizing that what is touched on in her is truly her own conflict that, although worked through better than the patient's, remains incompletely worked through.

Although Giovacchini (1989) recognizes the impact on therapy of the therapist's unresolved past, he emphasizes the fact that countertransference represents some way in which the patient has stimulated the infantile past of the therapist. It is the fact that the stimuli may not be entirely determined by elements in the analyst's infantile past that makes them potentially useful. Giovacchini feels that the analyst must take responsibility for his emotions. But he sees the countertransference feelings that the analyst does experience as a balance between what the patient stimulates and what emerges spontaneously from the analyst. Because of that balance he divides countertransference reactions into two broad categories, homogeneous and idiosyncratic countertransference reactions.

Giovacchini describes homogeneous countertransference reactions as those that would be stimulated by the patient in any mentally healthy person who experienced the patient's behavior of that particular moment. Idiosyncratic countertransference reactions are those that involve the unique reaction of the analyst to the particularities of the patient. "Homogeneous reactions, as is true of all responses, have infantile elements, but they are minimal. They are average expectable reactions that will cause most of us to react in a similar fashion . . . In other instances, the analyst may react in an exaggerated or unique fashion to a situation that most therapists would consider innocuous. I call this type of transference idiosyncratic because the therapist's reactions are idiosyncratic" (pp. 21–22).

Giovacchini states that the distinction between homogeneous and idiosyncratic countertransference stresses the extent to which infantile elements are involved. Infantile elements are involved more when trauma and conflict are involved. He presents parallels in transference, stating that perhaps the main purpose of an analysis is to have the patient's idiosyncratic transference become homogeneous transference. By this he means, as some other analysts have suggested (Loewald 1960), that there is a certain amount of transference that is healthy and necessary in human attachment, but that the patient's transference should move ever closer to a true perception of reality.

How much disruption of the treatment a countertransference reaction may cause is another important distinction Giovacchini makes. He explains that both homogeneous and idiosyncratic countertransference reactions can be disruptive or valuable: "The homogeneous variety can also be nondisruptive, and idiosyncratic countertransference can, in some instances, become a valuable asset to the therapeutic process" (p. 25). The important factor with all countertransference reactions is whether or not the therapist is able to make use of them.

The emphasis in Giovacchini's work is on how countertransference is useful in treatment. In fact, in much of his work he demonstrates how he uses countertransference with specific populations (1975a, 1979). That view of countertransference has become a regular part of the psychodynamic epistemology. Authors like Masterson (1983) and Kernberg (1965, 1975, 1976, 1989), for example, have specified the kinds of countertransference that can be expected with borderline and narcissistic patients (as well as others). This way of using countertransference is currently the mainstream among psychodynamic therapists who work with character-disordered patients.

But Giovacchini's work is more distinctive than these other authors in terms of the therapist's part in the process. The work of Kernberg and Masterson does not focus as much on the therapist's own personality, instead concentrating in great detail on what feelings can be expected with specific patient populations.

Theodore Jacobs

Jacobs's work (1991) is often referred to by modern relational analysts even though he does not encourage the relatively free activity found in some of their work. Like Sandler (1973, 1976), Jacobs focuses on the role played by the therapist's role-responsiveness. With that focus, he emphasizes the therapist's ability to grasp how countertransference has affected his behavior. He calls such behaviors "countertransference enactments" and suggests that, if attended to, they can be especially useful. Without a constant effort on the therapist's part toward understanding why he is acting as he is, he runs the risk of becoming involved in a mutual acting out with the patient. By understanding how such entanglement has occurred, and what part was played by the therapist, the process of a therapy can be more fully comprehended.

One particularly important aspect of the therapist's role-responsiveness discussed by Jacobs concerns the therapist's bodily movements. He notes that "While it seems self-evident that an analyst, while listening, utilizes his entire self in the process and that bodily movements are an integral and essential part of the 'analyzing instrument,' the degree to which bodily reactions are both available and useful to the analyst unquestionably differs from individual to individual" (p. 116). He points out that acting out can be silence and stillness as well as gregariousness and movement, and he analyzes such behavior in both the therapist and the patient. Such a viewpoint can be seen as a transition to the relational approaches now becoming popular.

Darlene Bregman Ehrenberg

Ehrenberg (1992) has contributed to relational analysis in her description of work that seems especially humanistic, authentic, and cognizant of the therapist's addition to the analytic whole. Her work is especially useful here in demonstrating the extent to which the use of countertransference has become integral in understanding relational systems within an analysis. She describes the "intimate edge" in analysis, the intersection where patient and therapist boundaries meet, clash, or cross. Ehrenberg describes the place of countertransference in a way that fully depicts the relational approach:

> There is no way to avoid countertransference, and attempting to deny its power can be dangerous. The question at this point is not whether to use countertransference but *how* [italics in original] . . . In considering how best to use countertransference I believe it is useful to distinguish between the *reactive* [italics in original] dimension of

countertransference, which has to do with what we find ourselves feeling in response to the patient that is often a surprise rather than a choice, and the kind of *active* [italics in original] response that takes into account this reactive response as data to be used towards informing a considered and deliberate clinical intervention. Silence, or any other reaction, can fall into either category . . . The point is that active use of countertransference requires a thoughtful decision process with regard to how to use awareness of one's "reactive" countertransference responses to inform what will then become a considered response . . . In some instances the analyst might actively decide to express the countertransference impulse in some direct way. In other instances an active decision may be made to remain silent . . . I do not mean to imply that every response must be a considered one. There are times when our inability to stay on top of our reactions—even our losing it with a patient—may be useful. As Winnicott (1949, 1969) notes, the unflappable analyst may be useless when it is essential for the patient to know that he or she can make an impact . . . Nor do I mean to imply that the analyst must "understand" his or her countertransference reactions to use them constructively. In some instances willingness to let the patient know what the analyst is experiencing, even if the analyst may not at the time understand his or her own reaction, can facilitate the analytic work, simply because of the kind of collaborative possibility it structures. [pp. 95–97]

Thus the effort at some objectivity in self-reflection is maintained in Ehrenberg's work, but the idea that objectivity is always possible is dispelled, along with the view that lack of objectivity in one's response necessarily creates a negative outcome. Ehrenberg seems to suggest that the analyst's job is to become part of the system with the patient and try to be aware of the system as much as possible. There is room for subjectivity and mistakes, but they are then grist for the therapeutic mill.

Thomas Ogden

Ogden recently published a paper entitled "The Analytic Third: Working with Intersubjective Clinical Facts" (1994a). In it he expands on the intersubjective view of psychoanalysis. Ogden emphasizes the importance of all the analyst's thoughts as having value in an analysis, not only those emotions felt strongly when with the patient. He includes even the mundane reveries concerning everyday details of the analyst's own life.

In discussing the fleeting thoughts that enter his mind during an analysis, Ogden indicates how, within what he terms the "analytic third," he is able to find clues to his own unconscious, which he is then able to use in better understanding the patient. He describes the particular thoughts or experiences that become conscious for him during the analytic hour as a function of the combined experience of himself and the patient.

One important message that can be extrapolated from this paper is a further refinement of the meaning of neutrality. Ogden (1994a) states that these inner thoughts are typically thought of as something that the analyst must get through or put aside in the effort to be emotionally present and attentive. Seen as obstacles, these thoughts threaten the neutrality of the therapist. But, Ogden argues, these thoughts are viable clinical facts that should not be ignored. Although he thinks his views will be resisted, Ogden insists that ignoring these fine details will result in an incomplete analysis.

> This realm of transference–countertransference experience is so personal, so ingrained in the character structure of the analyst, that it requires great psychological effort to enter into a discourse with ourselves in a way that is required to recognize that even this aspect of the personal has been altered by our experience in and of the analytic third. If we are to be analysts in a full sense, we must self-consciously attempt to bring even this aspect of ourselves to bear on the analytic process. [pp. 12–13]

Thus, with the threat of the disturbing effect that paying attention to one's innermost thoughts might have, many analysts would certainly worry about their ability to focus on the patient. But these inner thoughts are, according to Ogden, often related to what has developed between the analyst and patient. To ignore these inner thoughts is to ignore a significant part of the analysis. It is not a long jump from Ogden's theme to say that it is essential that the analyst find a way to be neutral in analyzing even this material. But neutrality would have to mean, in this context, a particular attitude that is integrated within the analyst's personality.

Ogden's theme leaves no room for a belief that the analyst is not affected by the patient.

Ogden's viewpoint as discussed here demonstrates not only the importance of the transference–countertransference system but also its expansion in current psychoanalytic thinking. Perhaps a simple way of expressing Ogden's theme would be to say that when two people meet, they affect each other down to the deepest psychic levels, even if only unconsciously. One's own thoughts are always connected to the other, even if the connection is unknown. For Ogden, our unconscious experience becomes conscious in very subtly connected thoughts that, if attended to, signify particulars of our own and the patient's experience while together. If we ignore these thoughts, we lose an important aspect of the treatment. But being self-conscious of these thoughts, which indicate the influence of others on what we believe to be our core selves, challenges our very sanity.

It is also interesting to understand what the patient's experience of the "analytic third" might be. Ogden explains that the experience of the analytic third is different for the patient than it is for the analyst. Ogden's own keen sensitivity allows him to recognize an experience that, although shared by the patient, is not as available to the consciousness of the patient. The patient's role does not permit her to become aware of the analytic third to the same extent as does the analyst.

> As a result, the unconscious experience of the analysand is privileged in a specific way, i.e. it is the past and present experience of the analysand that is taken by the analytic pair as the principal (although not exclusive) subject of the analytic discourse. The analyst's experience in and of the analytic third is, primarily, utilized as a vehicle for the understanding of the conscious and unconscious experience of the analysand (the analyst and analysand are not engaged in a democratic process of mutual analysis). [p. 17]

The idea that the analysand, as the focus of the analysis, contributes in a different way to what occurs between analyst and patient is a common theme among authors who use countertransference. Similar statements have already been mentioned in the work of Racker (1957) and Langs (1976a,b). The difference between analyst and analysand in this input, it seems, will always be a concern where human systems are observed. For example, systems therapists often use the term "hierarchy" to describe the obvious difference in roles and functions of father and son within a family. The therapist also has very different roles and functions than does the patient. But one major difference between other approaches and the intersubjective approach is that the analyst is able to view aspects of his own, and the patient's, contributions to the analytic third, without necessarily attributing those contributions to pathology. This difference is most evident in Ogden's use of the term projective identification.

Describing intersubjectivity, Ogden (1994b) writes about projective identification in a different way than he has in the past. He puts less emphasis on its behavioral inducement aspect and considers projective identification to be a part of all communication and a process in which two participants are mutually involved. He states: "I view projective identification as a dimension of all intersubjectivity, at times the predominant quality of the experience, at other times only a subtle background" (p. 99). He goes on to say:

> The vitalization or expansion of the individual subject is not exclusively an aspect of the experience of the projector; the "recipient" of a projective identification does not simply experience the event as a form of psychological burden in which he is limited and deadened. In part, this is due to the fact that there is never a recipient who is not simultaneously a projector in a projective identificatory experience. The interplay of subjectivities is never entirely one sided; each person is being negated by the other while being newly created in the unique dialectical tension generated by the two. [p. 102]

Further, he states that when one is involved in this kind of communication "one finds oneself unconsciously both playing a role in and serving as author of someone else's unconscious fantasy" (p. 103). Projective identification in the intersubjective mode is occurring at all times, but to varying extents. Thus, the intersubjective approach as described by Ogden (1994b) does not require pathology in either participant for countertransference to be used. Yet the use of countertransference does depend on the analyst's greater attention to such experience and also is affected by the role the analyst has in this particular dyad.

Summary: The Transference–Countertransference, Therapist–Family System

Up until relational approaches were considered, other approaches were limited with respect to how they might be applied to systems thinking. The work of each of the authors in this chapter can be thought of as contributing to a systems view in psychoanalysis, but only the relational therapists truly recognize the full impact of both the analyst and patient. Nevertheless, each of the analysts presented in this chapter contributes an essential element to the full understanding of the transference–countertransference system. When combined, these contributions create a perspective that is essential for using countertransference in family therapy. The following review outlines the importance of each contribution.

Kernberg (1965) has discussed countertransference in depth and coined the term "totalistic" to define the kind of countertransference earlier described by Heimann (1950) as including all the emotions of the therapist. The continuum of countertransference reactions posited by Kernberg is especially useful in demonstrating that although the system of a therapist and a severely regressed patient will be dominated by the patient's pathology, the perception of projective identification at healthier levels would require an acknowledgment of the therapist's part in the process of emotional exchange. The therapist's sensitivity in that emotional exchange can result from something as simple as the therapist's desire to become part of a system with the patient, but it can also involve the therapist's psychopathology.

Sandler's work is helpful in demonstrating that the analyst's *behavior* can be, in a meaningful way, a reaction to the patient and that what some would call acting out can be used to enrich and deepen a treatment. Sandler's (1976) concept of the use of "free-floating role-responsiveness" is an essential one in working with transference if one is to acknowledge that transference has an effect on the therapist. The term "free-floating" denotes exactly the kind of neutrality necessary in the relational systems model. Sandler's idea that the therapist's thoughts and behavior reflect a compromise-formation between the analyst's tendencies and "his reflexive acceptance of the role which the patient is forcing on him" (p. 46) is a very useful way for family therapists to understand their countertransference reactions with families. Such a viewpoint makes possible a description of the transference–countertransference system within an active therapy where role-responsiveness is likely to be common and the therapist's true personality would be difficult to hide. Furthermore, Sandler's work is interesting in that he is the first author who seems to suggest that the therapist's *behavioral* countertransference reaction, as opposed to mere thought, can be used productively *after* it occurs.

Langs's work demonstrates the necessity for examination of the reverberating projections and introjection that move both ways between analyst and patient. And it fully reflects an acknowledgment of the therapist's responsibility in creating the system that is formed between patient and analyst. But in limiting his understanding strictly to pathological aspects in both participants, however benign, Langs fails to include healthy, but deep, communication within his descriptions of the bipersonal field.

Atwood and Stolorow are the first authors who I consider part of the relational school, in which there is full recognition of the therapist's influence. The relational approaches posit that what occurs between people is the result of the combined effect of both parties' ongoing structuralization of events. In other words, there is an impact from both (two or more) personalities, constructed from the tendencies in each to perceive, interpret, and interact with the world in particular ways. The impact from each personality is determined by how the accumulated experience, including unique aspects and present role of each person, affects and is affected by the other. This perspective is far different from those before it because, while it views pathology as playing a part, it regards all personalities, regardless of pathological level, as impacting each other differently. The work of Atwood and Stolorow has been instrumental in defining the relational perspective. Their most distinctive contribution to the use of countertransference has been their view that the patient's behavior and thoughts in therapy cannot be analyzed without considering the effect of the therapist's personality.

Giovacchini's work has been presented primarily because it shows how integral the use of countertransference has become to psychoanalysis and psychoanalytic psychotherapy. He sounds many of the themes already presented. The analyst's contribution to an analysis cannot be denied. There are some countertransference reactions that mostly originate with the analyst and some that mostly originate with the patient. Giovacchini's approach is reflective of a particular mainstream of psychoanalytic psychotherapists that is also represented by authors like Kernberg and Masterson.

Jacobs's work, which is often cited in the work of relational analysts, is perhaps the earliest that fully integrates the effect of the therapist and the patient within a transference–countertransference system. His use of the phrase "countertransference enactment" is similar to the use of the word "enactment" in the work of Minuchin (Minuchin and Fishman 1982): it describes sequences of behavior in family therapy that represent patterns of behavior in a family's daily life. The countertransference enactment he describes involves the whole sequence of activity that occurs between analyst and patient. Jacobs's viewpoint is distinctive in emphasizing the behavior of the analyst, to the extent that even slight bodily movements are considered part of countertransference.

Jacobs's work represents one of several relational approaches that are so interactive that they seem to beg the question of authenticity: What can be gained by acting in any way that does not come naturally? If one is to comprehend one's part in the therapeutic relationship, one can only complicate matters by adding unfamiliar actions to the relationship, for example by intentionally remaining silent. In order to interact with the patient in a way that fully demonstrates responsibility for his actions and their effects, it would seem the therapist would need to consider authenticity essential.

Ehrenberg's work demonstrates the extent to which authenticity is essential to the use of countertransference in relational approaches. Her approach clearly makes authenticity central. She describes the "intimate edge" in analysis, the intersection where patient and therapist boundaries meet, clash, or cross. The "intimate edge" is one way of describing activity that occurs where countertransference can be used to detect projective and introjective identification. In Ehrenberg's view it is impossible to determine when boundaries have been impinged without authenticity in the therapist.

Ogden's work emphasizes just how subtle some countertransference reactions can be. He has modified his original description of projective identification so that it now accommodates very mild behavioral influences and takes into account the therapist's own psychological tendencies. Ogden fully appreciates interpersonal influence, bringing our understanding to a point where we can say that every interaction affects us, even if only in minor ways, to the very core of our being. In fact, he modifies the definition of neutrality to include the seemingly random thoughts of the analyst as long as those thoughts are considered as occurring for a reason related to the therapy. Such a perspective leaves nothing out of the transference–countertransference system.

From a view that considers the therapist–family system to be a kind of transference–countertransference system, family therapy can be viewed as the totality of all personalities involved. This chapter has dealt intensively with the therapeutic dyad, but the concepts developed can be equally applied in the family therapy context. The transference–countertransference system can be viewed as the result of the psychological need to project and introject within each individual of the group as group members interact with various levels of pathology and different levels of intimacy. This understanding of the transference–countertransference, or therapist–family system, will be developed throughout the remainder of this study.

4

The Clinical Intersection of Intrapsychic and Dyadic Systems Functioning

The major topics of this chapter, activity versus insight, self-disclosure, the therapist's personality functioning, and the therapeutic functions of the therapist, are essential elements in an understanding of how countertransference can best be used in the therapist–family system. They represent the clinical manifestations of the intersection between intrapsychic systems and systems that consist of at least two persons.

The activity-versus-insight debate has been an area of contention between systems and analytic models since systems therapies first began to evolve. Despite its controversial nature, this debate brings with it a unique opportunity for integration. That is, combining the argument that the therapist plays an important interpersonal role in the therapy system, regardless of activity level, with the argument that his role is governed by intrapsychic and interpersonal phenomena all of which have been well elaborated in the psychoanalytic literature, naturally leads to a psychoanalytic systems approach to psychotherapy.

An assessment of the therapist's activity level naturally leads to a discussion of self-disclosure. The therapist's part in the therapist–family system includes the extent to which he is revealed to the client or client-family, either verbally or non-verbally. Relational approaches have argued that the therapist's perceptions and beliefs should be used to full potential with explicit disclosure included.

A full understanding of the therapist's part in the therapist–family system, especially within a system that encourages the therapist's activity and openness, requires that the therapist's mental health also be discussed. Functioning therapeutically in such an open and potentially stressful interpersonal environment might be very difficult even for the healthiest of therapists. What is meant by "mental health," however, is typically not made clear. In this section I will elaborate on the therapist's mental health, and its centrality for the therapist, especially with regard to the concept of boundaries.

The therapist's ability to function therapeutically involves many facets of his personality. Analysts have long considered the importance of these functions, specifically with respect to the use of countertransference. The use of empathy is quintessential in therapeutic functioning. How countertransference is related to empathy will be discussed in detail.

INSIGHT VERSUS ACTION

Although insight and action are both important, insight has largely been ignored in family therapy, while in analytic therapies action has been practically forbidden. The insight-versus-action debate requires review here because the likelihood of family therapy models recognizing the intentional use of countertransference seems so connected to the argument that the therapist's insight and self-reflection are important even when the therapist is active. The major arguments contributing to this debate from family therapy and psychoanalytic therapy, with a particularly useful integration of analytic and behavioral therapy, will be introduced and examined.

In this study of countertransference, where attention is focused on the therapist, these differences in emphasis lead one to ask: What is the mental process used by the therapist in formulating interventions that promote insight or action? Are the mental processes involved in formulating interventions similar in psychoanalytic and systems models, or completely different due to the differential emphasis on action and insight in the two?

It is clear that some psychoanalytic therapists emphasize self-reflection, and interpretation that is arrived at partially through self-reflection, as the therapist's analog to the client's insight. From the psychoanalytic perspective, with insight being associated with cure, therapist self-reflection is typically given high regard. Although the caricatured classical psychoanalyst might be expected to derive interventions from an intellectual understanding of psychoanalytic theory, any analyst who prizes empathy is sure to be an advocate of self-reflection. This emphasis can be seen in articles already cited pertaining to countertransference phenomena in which self-reflection is always considered an important part of the therapist's role (Atwood and Stolorow 1984, Bion 1959a, Heimann 1950, Kernberg 1965, Langs 1976a,b, 1978, Little 1951, Ogden 1979,1994a,b, Racker 1957, Winnicott 1949).

Systems therapists, on the other hand, seem to emphasize the action and directiveness of the therapist as analogs of the action of the family. Yet it is unclear how the systems therapist formulates directives. In systems therapy, it often appears that the lack of regard for insight makes the process involved in formulating interventions a nonissue. However, an understanding of the process involved in formulating interventions is an essential part of the attempt to integrate systems theory with an intentional use of countertransference that relies on the therapist's awareness of such processes.

Criticism of Insight from Active Therapists

Cloe Madanes and Jay Haley

"Dimensions of Family Therapy," a paper by Madanes and Haley (1977), specifically outlines areas of controversy between different schools of therapy from a systems perspective. They title one area of controversy "interpretation vs. action." According to their view, psychodynamic therapies emphasize the use of interpretation to effect insight in the client or client-family. However, they do not discuss how the psychodynamic therapist arrives at that interpretation. In their own approach Madanes and Haley emphasize action and directives. It is interesting that, just as they do not discuss the process by which psychodynamic therapists arrive at interpretations, they also do not discuss how therapists using the strategic method arrive at directives. Perhaps it makes sense that the de-emphasis on insight in general would lead to a lack of interest in insight with respect to the way interventions are formulated. But because these authors do not discuss formulation, speculation about their process is necessary.

Perhaps strategic therapists refer to their intellectual knowledge of systems in place of the self-reflection that is involved in some psychoanalytic methods. From much of the strategic literature, analysis of systems appears to be primarily an intellectual pursuit that leads the therapist to an understanding of how to *act upon* the family system. For example, in their paper, Madanes and Haley (1977) describe their approach as "digital" in being problem focused and "analogical" in its view of symptoms as communication. When they have comprehended what communication is occurring as a result of a symptom, they use a directive with the intention of making the symptom impossible. This process of referring to one's intellectual knowledge seems quite different from the self-reflection used by psychoanalytic therapists.

As will be demonstrated later in a review of the work of Tansey and Burke (1985), in psychoanalytic therapy, although the therapist's intellect is important in understanding emotion, it is the emotion, both of the client and the therapist, that is important to the working through that comes with insight. In other words, the therapist uses emotional self-reflection in helping the client achieve emotional self-understanding. In fact, it is clear that no matter what systems therapists say they do, formulation of interventions from within a human system will always involve emotions. Nevertheless, it seems that systems therapists prefer not to discuss the emotional component of formulating interventions.

Don Jackson and Jay Haley

In their 1963 paper, "Transference Revisited," Jackson and Haley comment on transference as well as countertransference in discussing the therapeutic factors of insight and action in therapy from a systems perspective. These authors argue that although working through transference distortions, with self-understanding as the curative factor, is the stated goal of psychoanalytic psychotherapy, the actual curative factor is the change in action of the client within the "strangeness" of the psychoanalytic situation.

First, using the classical definition of countertransference, these authors argue for a change in the understanding of both transference and counter-transference.

[I]n recent years the focus on countertransference has indicated that the personality of the psychoanalyst can be a distorter of "pure" transference and the patient may react to these new elements. With the inclusion of the analyst in the description, the point of view about transference must inevitably change. As Ackerman has pointed out, when countertransference was introduced as a concept, the psychoanalytic situation became a dyadic one even though the terminology remained monadic. [p. 117]

It would seem, given the interactional viewpoint forwarded within this excerpt, that these authors might arrive at a totalistic view of transference and countertransference from their discussion. However, their argument is that transference is not important in therapy, because therapy should be viewed interactionally. Since transference does not represent the client's "pure" misperception of the therapist (meaning that the actual therapist is involved in the client's perceptions), the understanding through insight that it offers is seen as less worthwhile. In psychoanalytic therapies, however, even though many authors believe that a client's transference is partially influenced by the therapist's personality or countertransference (Atwood and Stolorow 1984, Little 1951, Ogden 1994a,b, Racker 1957), they do not reach the conclusion that these concepts are unimportant. Psychoanalytic authors often discuss the interactional effects of transference and countertransference and, using a totalistic definition of countertransference, find that concept especially useful given the interactive nature of the therapist–client relationship.

Jackson and Haley (1963) appear either to ignore or to be unaware of this emphasis in the countertransference literature to which they refer in the above excerpt. As stated above, the argument made by these authors is that the primary therapeutic factor in psychoanalysis is the change in behavior brought on by the "strangeness" of the analytic situation, and not by the insight generated by working through the transference.

Instead of emphasizing the interpretation of the transference with consequent insight to the patient, it is possible to regard the analytic situation itself as largely responsible for a change in the patient, with self-understanding an accompanying but not necessarily crucial factor. This notion arises because when both analyst and patient are included in the description of the analytic situation, one discovers that they have a very unusual communication context. [p. 120]

Perhaps these authors are simply reframing the curative factors of therapy in their work. But in their failure to address the therapist's self-understanding in this interactional context, they miss a primary aspect of psychoanalytic therapy. In fact, with reference to transference and countertransference, some psychoanalytic therapists might agree that the primary therapeutic factor in psychoanalytic therapy is the "strangeness" of the therapeutic situation. What the therapist does with both transference and the countertransference feelings associated with transference, however, is integral to that psychoanalytic situation. Countertransference, when understood, becomes a clue to understanding the emotional process between therapist and client. Its use by the therapist is one of the things that *is strange* about the therapeutic relationship, and that also makes it curative.

An Integrative Model

Paul and Ellen Wachtel

Two authors who advocate an integrative approach are Paul and Ellen Wachtel. In his book, *Action and Insight* (1987), Paul Wachtel discusses the integration of active behavior therapy and psychoanalysis. In their book together, *Family Dynamics in Individual Psychotherapy* (1986), the Wachtels discuss the potentially valuable contributions of family theory in the work of individual therapists. They also discuss their own view of working with transference.

In *Action and Insight* (1987) Paul Wachtel discusses what he believes to be a very useful way of understanding transference. This understanding of transference, although behavioral, does not necessitate the deprecation of insight as is found in the Jackson and Haley (1963) paper described above. Using Piaget's (1954) concepts of "schema," "assimilation," and "accommodation," Wachtel fits transference into an interactional view of therapy. According to Wachtel, with transference the client assimilates who the therapist is into already existing schemata that she has developed in her personality. When the therapist does not fit the already existing schemata, the client may continue to view the therapist as though he fits those schemata (assimilation). Wachtel explains that people often create a self-fulfilling prophecy by believing others to be a certain way. He explains that the reactivity of other people to our perceptions of them maintains assimilation and accounts for the difficulty in accommodating to people being different than we expect them to be. He writes, "even if we are 'wrong' [in what we think about others], the cumulative effect of our acting over and over in a trusting, or a suspicious, or a sexy, or whatever kind of way tends eventually to lead other people to act in ways that prove we were 'right'" (p. 50).

When it is impossible to fit the therapist into already existing schemata, however, accommodation must take place. Schemata already existing are either modified or new schemata are developed. Wachtel associates the change in or new development of schemata with the development of personality structure. With this view he is able to argue that the action of therapy is important without dismissing the importance of insight. His view is that developing insight is one way to change behavior. Where the transference is challenged, accommodation, and therefore behavior change, must occur. This view does not seem very different from that of Jackson and Haley (1963), who argue that the strangeness of the situation in psychoanalysis is what brings about change. As stated above, however, and unlike Jackson and Haley, Wachtel is not willing to throw out the value of transference or insight.

Also important to note is that Wachtel believes that the therapeutic relationship need not be so "strange" as might be inferred from psychoanalytic writing that emphasizes passive neutrality. Neutrality, of course, is often associated with complete abstinence. But even "relative neutrality," which is sometimes suggested in psychoanalytic writing, is considered impossible by Wachtel. At one point in his book he even mentions how "family therapists are fond of saying, one can never 'not communicate'" (p. 177). His general argument is that a therapist cannot be neutral and that being "neutral" is actually a particular way of being active. "Indeed, to call 'neutral' someone who offers himself as a source of help to distressed souls, who frequently as well requests a substantial portion of the person's income, and who then avoids giving a direct answer to questions, refuses to give any sort of advice or reveal anything of his own life or his own opinions, and otherwise vetoes the everyday rules of social exchange is to stretch the word 'neutral' beyond recognition" (p. 49).

However, he also does not suggest that the therapist should be as active as the client. Wachtel emphasizes the asymmetry of the relationship, that the patient is there for therapy and the therapist's role is to help. So, even though both participants are equal in standing, that is "equally deserving of respect and human dignity" (p. 182), their roles and responsibilities differ and the therapist cannot simply "let it all hang out" (p. 182). "Consequently, where one of the two people (the patient) is free to say and reveal whatever he wants, the other (the therapist or analyst) does so only judiciously, when he thinks it will be helpful" (p. 183). But consistent with his views on schemata, Wachtel argues that the client will assimilate, or view within his already existing schemata, most of the therapist's behavior no matter how the therapist acts. It is up to the therapist to be appropriately empathic, interpretive, confrontive, and directive so that the client will accommodate to both a truer understanding of the therapist and the other people in his life.

For Wachtel, then, action and insight stand in a kind of balance different from the one typical of either psychoanalytic therapists or behavior and family therapists. The balance that he advocates he terms "noncontingent responding." Wachtel holds this view in spite of his belief that it is almost impossible, and not even advisable in some situations, to respond completely noncontingently, "despite the wide range of ways in which the therapist can be found inadvertently to contingently reinforce his patient's behavior, and the not infrequent occasions when it is important that he take responsibility for guiding the patient in directions more likely to get him what he wants, there remains a substantial range of therapeutic interactions where a noncontingent, accepting attitude seems desirable and is likely to be feasible" (p. 172). Noncontingent responding seems roughly similar to the position that sees the therapist's neutrality as balanced between remaining nonjudgmental with respect to the client's actions and thoughts, and at the same time not acting out in response to the patient, which would inadvertently encourage assimilation.

Wachtel advocates activity reined in by noncontingent responding. With respect to transference, his emphasis is on demonstrating to the client how the client has replicated his experiences by thinking of his relationships in a particular way. Thus, the client's insight is considered helpful. Insight is fostered with noncontingent responding because a situation is created in which accommodation must occur as a result of the realization (insight) that what was expected was attributable to one's own perspective and not entirely to the reality of the situation. However, Wachtel wants the patient to go beyond mere recognition that he has transferred something old onto the therapist. He wants the patient to realize by the example of the therapeutic situation that he sets up relationships in such a fashion that old patterns are repeated. Noncontingent responding is desirable when the therapist wants to point out the assimilation involved in the transference that has developed. It is inevitable, however, that some of the therapist's responding will be contingent, and will be a part of how the patient replicates his view of others through the subtle (or not so subtle) behavioral pressure he enacts within the therapy. To Wachtel this is not as unfortunate as it may at first seem. "For it is in the very act of participating that the analyst learns what it is most important to know about the patient. And it is in coming to see their joint participation in what is for him a familiar pattern—but a joint participation, with the crucial difference of reflectiveness—that the patient too learns what he must in order to begin the process of change" (pp. 178–179). The process described here sounds much like the workings of projective identification and countertransference as well as transference. It also sounds very much like the views of Sandler, Atwood and Stolorow, and Ogden discussed earlier, except that Wachtel advocates a much more active stance.

It appears that Wachtel (1987) is advocating an active therapy in which self-reflection is key. The therapist must self-reflect before making an interpretation so that the role she is enacting can become part of the intervention. Transference and insight are essential concepts in understanding such a therapy, despite the directiveness Wachtel also advocates.

In their book on family dynamics in individual psychotherapy (1986) the Wachtels use a very similar viewpoint. With respect to insight, they state that it is overemphasized in some therapies. However, they also state " . . . we do believe that insight plays a significant role in therapeutic change. In our view, however, it is but one of a number of aspects of the change process, rather than its heart and soul" (p. 28).

Their view of transference, again, is very interactional. The Wachtels (1986) state: "we regard transference manifestations as always best understood in relation to some action or quality of the therapist" (p. 40). Thus transference and countertransference are intertwined. In the next excerpt they (Wachtel and Wachtel 1986) describe the salutary effects of responding more fully to clients than "neutrality" implies. They believe that a therapist cannot consider her natural impact as exclusively negative. In discussing neutrality they state:

> We do not believe that the therapist can ever avoid influencing the patient (certainly not if he is an *effective* [italics in original] therapist!); nor do we believe that avoidance of influence is to be desired. There is appropriate influence and inappropriate influence, to be sure; some matters are more the therapist's business than others, and some methods are more coercive. But to confuse the effort to sort out salutary and baneful influences (even if such an effort is always only partially successful) with the possibility of ruling out influence altogether is a pursuit of folly. [pp. 39–40]

The Wachtels recognize the interactional aspects of the therapeutic situation as an assumed aspect of the interpretations that would address transference phenomena.

> Within our framework, transference interpretations remain an important part of the therapeutic process. But they are interpretations that recognize the therapist's actions as a crucial element. They are thus contextually oriented interpretations, which are fully consistent with a general emphasis on understanding people in relation to others. As should be clear, they are also interpretations for which the illusion of neutrality is not necessary, and hence the therapist is permitted to entertain a wider range of therapeutic efforts without having to give up the special advantages of focusing on the transference. [pp. 41–42]

Thus, the Wachtels recognize aspects of the therapist's contribution of which she is unaware, as well as a self-reflective component.

The use of transference interpretations within a relational context as described by the Wachtels requires self-reflection. The therapist must be conscious of her part in the transference manifestations of the client. Whether or not this is referred to as projective identification, clearly the Wachtels are advocating a use of countertransference. The discussion of a use of countertransference is limited to one short statement in Paul Wachtel's (1987) book. This statement criticizes even what is considered a relatively broad view of countertransference because it does not go far enough.

> It is certainly useful and important, but it is not enough. Usually it accompanies, in a classical approach, a concerted focus on the patient alone. There is rarely if ever a confirmation of the patient's experience, even where it is correctly apprehended. So long as the analyst hides behind a "neutral" self-presentation, so long as his own participation in the session's events does not become part of the focus of what he discusses with the patient, it is difficult for the patient to understand not just his own experience but how he goes about creating and recreating it in his daily life. [pp. 179–180]

Nevertheless, Wachtel seems to be advocating exactly the view of countertransference that is advocated within this book. This view, it seems, would be the view most useful to family therapists. Although not explicitly stated, it is clear that the therapist must be aware of her countertransference to follow the Wachtels' approach. At the same time the therapist does not eschew the possibility that she influences the client.

Activity and Insight in the Relational Systems Perspective

Countertransference, as described in the work of authors like the Wachtels, would seemingly add much to family therapy and it is clear, in their view, that insight or therapist self-reflection are not impossible even when activity is seen as an important curative factor. In fact, the Wachtels would seem to consider activity essential before self-reflection in the therapist will have meaning. Activity helps in bringing about a therapeutic situation that reflects how the patient naturally interacts in relationships, and that, when reflected upon via the therapist's countertransference, can be very helpful to the patient. The patient, with the guidance of the therapist's observations, can observe and gain insight about her behaviors, which then leads to behavioral change within the relationship to the therapist.

Although systems therapists do not discuss the process involved in formulating interventions, perhaps an analysis of their work would reveal that they not only reflect on a knowledge of systems but also process emotions in a way that is salutary to the treatment situation. Such processing, which is not likely conscious, is emotional to the extent that it involves the personality structure of the therapist. This processing may harness the emotional strength of the therapist, and put that emotion to use in finding appropriate interventions. That is to say, countertransference is used to some extent by therapists of all kinds, so it is clear that making that countertransference conscious through self-reflection would be valuable to family therapists in strengthening interventions and avoiding countertransference difficulties.

Whereas self-reflection and action appear to have at times been viewed as antithetical, it seems likely that it is precisely in the case of high-activity family therapy that self-reflection is crucial for avoiding the damage of countertransference acting out. It also seems that the intense emotions associated with family therapy are likely to bring about projective identification, and thus an intentional use of countertransference could be invaluable. Certainly the family therapist would benefit from reflecting on what purpose she might be serving within the projections of the therapist–family system.

SELF-DISCLOSURE

Wachtel and Wachtel (1986) advocate interacting relatively freely with the client so that enactments, to use the term proposed by Jacobs (1991), can be used as examples of how the client re-creates her perspective of the world in present relationships. Such a viewpoint is quite different from that advocated by classical analysts and thus leads to questions about self-disclosure, as the therapist is revealed much more than has previously been considered acceptable. What is self-disclosure? To what extent does a therapist self-disclose by being with the client, by talking to the client, by crossing his legs, by using his experience of the patient to formulate interventions, by reporting his experience of the patient, by talking about his own experiences outside the therapist–family relationship? To what extent does the therapist maintain focus on the client or client-family if he is attempting to allow enactments to develop? To what extent does the therapist aim to be spontaneous and authentic? What does it mean to be spontaneous and authentic? These questions have recently been discussed in the psychoanalytic literature, where increasing numbers of analysts are advocating relational therapies. Three concerns have become central in the discussion: (1) the therapist described as a "participant-observer" (Sullivan 1954); (2) the relative asymmetry inherent in the therapeutic relationship as well as the aim for a certain level of symmetry and mutuality; and (3) the level of spontaneity or authenticity advocated.

Participant Observation

The therapist was first referred to as a "participant observer" by Harry Stack Sullivan (1954) who emphasized that the analyst both participates in and observes the therapeutic process. If one accepts that view, then neutrality, as I have been suggesting, cannot ensure an absence of influence on the client or client-family. Interpretations of transference cannot be made as though it develops within a vacuum. Rather, everything about the therapist affects the client and the therapeutic relationship. Jay Greenberg (1995) attributes the earliest thinking in this vein to Ferenczi:

> Ferenczi (1988) argued his position on pragmatic and empirical grounds. Analytic anonymity is a myth, he believed, or perhaps a conceit of those who prefer to stay aloof from their patients. Patients, especially those who are the most disturbed, know their analysts very well; we reveal ourselves in everything that we say and do. Self-disclosure is inevitable; our only choice is how we accommodate to this fact of our professional lives. [p. 194]

Greenberg, in agreement with this thinking, concludes, "The decision, then, is not whether to reveal something or not; rather it is whether I choose to reveal something deliberately" (p. 201). When such a stance is considered, one must rethink the value of maintaining silence or anonymity.

One might even consider the possibility that intentional silence or the conscious decision to remain anonymous might add more to the therapeutic situation than it manages to leave out. Owen Renik (1995) puts it this way: "Far from diminishing the analyst's presence, a stance of non-self-disclosure tends to place the analyst center stage. It makes the analyst into a mystery, and paves the way for regarding the analyst as an omniscient sphinx whose ways cannot be known and whose authority, therefore, cannot be questioned" (p. 482).

We are left with the idea that the therapist cannot consider himself a "blank screen." The therapist is in the thick of things, and if transference is to be used, perhaps the therapist makes the most of the client or client-family's transference by not adding more to the situation in attempting to be other than genuine.

Ehrenberg (1992) has even said that the outcome of a therapy cannot be attributed to the therapist's skilled interventions because the interpersonal influence between therapist and patient is so potent. Some aspects of the interaction will always elude the analyst. But these views are in almost complete opposition to standard clinical practice. Thus discussion has been generated about the difference in roles played by therapists and clients.

Asymmetry, Symmetry, and Mutuality

The fact that the client or client-family comes to the therapist for help is, of course, a consideration. Analysts have attempted to reach a balance in activity level with the knowledge that there must be some crucial difference between the professional therapist and the clients he serves. Some degree of asymmetry has been accepted but discussion about the degree to which an analyst should attempt to engender a symmetrical relationship with the patient has been central. Aron (1992) has suggested that a balance can be attempted but that it cannot be governed by any particular rules.

Some degree of asymmetry is a necessary, although certainly insufficient, condition for analysis. The optimal balance or tension between participation and nonintrusiveness, between symmetry and asymmetry, cannot be established in advance by a standard set of rules or by a "model technique," but rather must emerge from the analytic work between a particular patient and a particular analyst and will likely change even from moment to moment within a given analysis. [p. 491]

Although perhaps no standard rules can guide the extent to which asymmetry or symmetry is prominent within a relational therapy, most analysts maintain many aspects of the classical structure.

Even the most radical of relational analysts have maintained the idea that the analyst's position is much different than that of the patient. Irvin Hoffman (1992b) emphasizes the fundamental features of the analyst's position even in his relatively radical social constructivist view. "Whether the analyst is reacting emotionally, talking about the weather, or talking about the patient's childhood, the stamp of the analytic situation should never be lost on the participants" (p. 302). The focus, nevertheless, is different than in the classical stance (as can be noted in Hoffman's reference to the analyst, not the patient, talking about the weather), and relational analysts have struggled to find a way to express that difference.

One word that has been used to describe that different focus has been "mutuality," which refers to the idea that the analyst and patient are two emotional beings in a room together, even if their roles within that room might differ. Burke (1992) has described the tension between asymmetry and mutuality this way:

If the primary focus is on understanding the patient's perceptions, then an emphasis on asymmetry keeps the therapist's influence in check and assures patients the latitude they need to create a picture of themselves through their influence on the relationship. When, however, the relationship between participants is given priority as the unit of analysis, the principle of mutuality is ascendant and emotional information from the therapist's side of the equation becomes not simply an option but rather a technical necessity. [p. 246]

Thus the asymmetry between patient and analyst is recognized, but since the unit of analysis is the mutual influence of one upon the other, mutuality makes self-disclosure necessary.

Bollas (1983) does not use the word "mutuality," but he does assert the mutuality of patient and analyst. According to Bollas, it is our current understanding of transference that another source of the patient's material is the therapist's countertransference. He believes this is true to the extent that the therapist cannot fully understand the patient without looking within himself. He writes, "This process inevitably points to the fact that there are two 'patients' within the session and therefore two complementary sources of free association" (p. 3).

The crucial difference between analyst and patient, however, has something to do with asymmetry which is best summed up in what Wachtel (1986) called the "crucial difference of reflectiveness" (p. 63). Although he believes "it is in the very act of participating that the analyst learns what is most important to know about the patient" (p. 63), "reflectiveness" of the therapist adds understanding to the natural process of involvement with the patient. Burke and Tansey (1991) discuss this crucial difference within the context of the ultimate importance of mutual participation. "The therapeutic action emanates from a cycle of becoming caught up in the old forms of relating with the patient followed by understanding and working through these moments" (p. 375). Burke and Tansey go on to emphasize the therapeutic leverage that develops when mutuality and reflectiveness are combined. "The very fact that the therapist has been caught up in the patient's relational matrix contributes to his therapeutic leverage. The experience of being within the role-relationship allows him the possibility of understanding the patient in a very powerful way and of 'finding a voice' (Mitchell, 1988, p. 295) with which to engage the patient in useful collaboration" (p. 375). Interventions from within the role-relationship might be very powerful, but such a perspective requires a certain understanding of one's subjectivity.

Several analysts have discussed, recognized, and even embraced their subjectivity as part of the analytic process. Bollas (1983) recognizes that his emotional states are subjective, but related to the patient's presentation, and thus must be brought forth within an analysis. Because his subjective state is at least partially determined by the influence of the patient, Bollas believes it is possible to disclose selected subjective states for observation within an analysis. Even if the clinician may not understand the complete meaning of his experience, Bollas argues that the therapist can give expression to his subjective countertransference states as long as the patient knows that such disclosures are reports from within the therapist, expressed for the purpose of benefiting the treatment. It should be noted that Bollas appears to carefully select the subjective states he chooses to discuss with the patient, even though he suggests that he is not always aware of the unconscious meanings they might represent, which indicates that he emphasizes asymmetry within the relationship.

Irvin Hoffman (1992b) has emphasized the importance of the sort of uncertainty mentioned by Bollas above, in fully accepting the extent of subjectivity he brings to analysis. He asserts that it is not possible for therapists to transcend their subjectivity and that recognition of this fact leads to a kind of "uncertainty" that frees analysts to "be themselves," at least as far as is permitted by their analytic role. Hoffman sees the analytic role as constraining the therapist to critical reflection upon the nature of the interaction. He does not, however, see his natural responsiveness as precluding the analysis of the interaction that is allowed by that critical reflection.

Ehrenberg (1992) also embraces subjectivity. She feels there is simply no other way to work except from within subjectivity. Acceptance of this fact, she says, frees the therapist from illusions he may have about being objective and enables him to "appreciate both the interdependence of patient and analyst and the necessity for collaboration: (p. 65). According to Ehrenberg, the analytic field is vastly expanded through such acceptance because it brings with it recognition of the importance of attending to the subtlest emotional nuances.

With the acceptance of the analyst's subjectivity, mutuality is fully recognized. Analysts are coming ever closer to using the relationship between patient and professional to its greatest potential. Asymmetry must always be recognized. The patient comes to the analyst, after all, for help, and with certain expectations about the analyst's expertise. Efforts toward helping the patient make the relationship asymmetrical as the analyst utilizes her expertise and reflects upon the emotional effect of being in a relationship with the patient. However, it is in the analyst's effort toward viewing the relationship as symmetrical where mutuality is found, and an acceptance of the analyst's subjectivity must take place so that the power of mutual influence may be fully harnessed through the understanding of how such influence works. In an attempt to better understand mutual influence, many analysts are now discussing the importance of spontaneity and authenticity.

Authenticity and Spontaneity

Questions concerning the therapist's authenticity and spontaneity are naturally evoked by the idea that mutuality between therapist and patient is desirable. Although these concepts are discussed in the analytic literature, some reticence is always detectable, probably due to the great likelihood that acting out on countertransference will occur, without the necessary ingredient of reflectiveness. Nevertheless, to varying extents, analysts have advocated an authentic and spontaneous stance.

A good example of the caution with which authenticity and spontaneity have been discussed is offered by Bollas (1983), who has differentiated two types of countertransference use: direct (a statement of feeling that has been engendered within the relationship) and indirect (a use of the feeling engendered within the relationship as information in the formulation of an intervention other than a direct use of countertransference). Bollas states, "I must stress that I am not referring at any point, with either an indirect or direct use of the countertransference, to the clinician's thoughtless discharge of affect . . . Any disclosure on the analyst's part of how he feels must be experienced by the patient as a legitimate and natural part of the analytic process" (p. 12). Harmful acting out thus remains a concern when an active use of countertransference is encouraged. Although such concern is common among analysts, several have nevertheless been forthcoming in advocating a spontaneous approach.

But being thoughtful, as is suggested by Bollas' (1983) comment above, is not synonymous with omniscient knowledge of all the reasons for one's actions. Ehrenberg (1992) has been clear in stating that the therapist need not be aware of the reason for her feelings when making use of them in a valuable way. Like Hoffman, she believes that the spontaneity afforded by relatively open expression can facilitate a collaborative effort between patient and analyst. She has also suggested that being spontaneous is of vital importance to being playful in a therapeutic way. She reports that working playfully requires spontaneity, which in turn requires a trust in one's intuitive clinical sensibility. She believes there is a decision to be playful, but that such a decision often precedes more conscious clinical consideration. Ehrenberg points out that such decisions involve complex clinical judgment that is related to the question: "Do we think a particular response will be technically facilitating? rather than: Do we understand exactly what is going on with the patient, the treatment or ourselves, at any given moment?" (p. 120).

Again, the importance of restraint and asymmetry, here referred to as intuitive clinical sensibility, are important. However, Ehrenberg's emphasis is on spontaneity and trusting oneself rather than on such restraint and asymmetry.

Perhaps the most lucid proponent of a spontaneous and authentic approach is Hoffman. He describes the analytic attitude necessary to his "social-constructivist view of the psychoanalytic situation" (1991) as a "combination of personal openness and a particular perspective on the process" (1992a). He states (1992b): "With the elimination of the standard of doing just the 'right' thing according to some external criterion, there is more leeway for a spontaneous kind of expressiveness than there was before . . . " (p. 292). The essential point Hoffman makes with regard to spontaneity incorporates open expression with a sense of transference and countertransference interplay and a form of neutrality he calls "disciplined interest in the patient's experience" (1992a). "Short of the extremes, the analyst's openly expressive participation, integrated with a sense of the continuous interplay of transference and countertransference, and ultimately subordinated to a disciplined interest in the patient's experience, can be a great boon to the analytic work" (p. 14). Hoffman indicates, however, that openly expressive participation requires authenticity. He (1992b) dismisses the objectivity of classical analysis, replacing it with authenticity, but also differentiates his view of authenticity from that advocated by humanistic-existential therapists. "Displacing objectivity as the ideal to which the analyst aspires is a special kind of authenticity. Unlike the authenticity that is encouraged in a humanist-existentialist orientation, however, authenticity in the social-constructivist model is continuously the object of psychoanalytic skepticism and critical reflection" (Sass 1988, pp. 295–296). His view is that all occurrences within therapy are subject to reflection and analysis even if such reflection and analysis are not present at every moment.

Hoffman (1992b) describes his perspective on spontaneity and authenticity as "naturalness" (p. 298), and admits that giving examples of behaving naturally is awkward and cannot possibly reflect the spontaneous quality he is trying to describe. Although it might be awkward to discuss behaving naturally, Hoffman sees this orientation as essential in ensuring that the therapist does not add or subtract from the process in a way that complicates a therapy beyond comprehension.

Hoffman goes on to suggest that behaving in any way other than authentically, especially when aiming for a certain kind of mutuality, can be damaging. While maintaining that asymmetry is always present and necessary, and that certain actions might well be damaging to such asymmetry, Hoffman is respectful of the incredible complexities of the therapeutic process, and argues that authentic activity can incorporate the discipline necessary for preserving asymmetry. The analytic function of the therapist is then, according to Hoffman, best accomplished with authenticity and spontaneity.

Self-Disclosure and the Relational Systems Perspective

From the relational perspective, self-disclosure is inevitable because the therapist is in a participant-observer role. Although asymmetry between therapist and patient must be present due to the therapeutic role of the therapist, mutuality is aimed for, and the crucial difference between therapist and patient with respect to asymmetry is the therapist's reflectiveness. Thus many analysts now suggest that a certain kind of freedom of activity on the therapist's part is necessary. The therapist must be authentic and spontaneous, trusting his own clinical judgment, but not forgetting the asymmetrical nature of the role relationship. Unlike the authenticity encouraged by humanistic-experiential therapists, analytic therapists maintain a reflectiveness that integrates the intrapsychic and the theoretical with the interpersonal and observable process, as part of the authenticity they advocate. This authenticity is essential in making it possible for the therapist to differentiate what he has added to the therapeutic process, as inauthentic action could only increase complexity by adding behavior from the therapist's side that is not integrated into his personality and therefore cannot be fully understood. This relational orientation on self-disclosure is essential to the relational systems perspective where the therapist must be authentically active in the transference–countertransference system, yet reflective as well. The demands such an orientation puts on the therapist, however, would seem to require a certain degree of mental health in the therapist.

THE THERAPIST'S CHARACTER
AND ITS FUNCTIONING

As suggested above, a therapist might have a natural tendency to react to clients or client–families in salutary ways. Of course the therapist might also have a natural tendency to react to clients or client–families in deleterious ways. The therapist's natural tendencies in reacting to others can be described as being the result of his or her character structure. To the extent that it is beneficial to the therapeutic effort, I consider these natural tendencies to be roughly equivalent to the second part of Winnicott's (1949) definition of countertransference.

I would like, however, to expand on this issue in several ways. First, I will discuss the definition of character structure as given by Schafer (1983) and use Atwood and Stolorow's (1984) concept of "prereflectively unconscious functioning" to explain how character functions in relationships. Another concept that has significant implications for any systems view is that of "boundaries," and I will discuss the psychoanalytic concept of "ego boundaries" (Landis 1970) as an aspect of character that functions prereflectively, in focusing on the therapist as an individual who is herself a system. Several specific process concepts will then be discussed, including "holding" (Winnicott 1960a), "containment" and "processing" (Bion 1959a), and "metabolization" (Langs 1976b, 1978), which have evolved in the literature to describe what occurs between therapist and client, and can be understood as the manifestation of various levels of mental health and prereflectively unconscious functioning. This discussion will lead to an acknowledgment of the need for mental health among psychotherapists in general.

Character Structure and the Prereflective Unconscious

Character structure has been defined by Schafer (1983): "It is the name given to the particular way in which a person may be said to organize and stabilize his or her actions. Consequently, character *development* [italics in original] is not the development of an entity, but a progressive change in the way someone both defines and acts in his or her problematic situations" (p. 141). Schafer's definitions of character structure and character development are useful for understanding personality in an interpersonal context.

Atwood and Stolorow (1984) directly discuss the ongoing interpersonal aspects of character structure or "structuralization of experience." In keeping with the developmental nature of character structure, the usual psychoanalytic constructs for development, including self and object differentiation (Jacobson 1964), the rudimentary establishment of self-object boundaries (Mahler et al. 1975), and experience of others as whole objects and the self as a whole self (Kernberg 1976), are used in their descriptions. They also emphasize that the Piagetian (1954) terms "assimilation" and "accommodation" are helpful in deriving a psychoanalytic theory of personality development. These Piagetian terms are emphasized by Atwood and Stolorow, especially with reference to the ongoing structuralization of the environment, in a way that shares similarities with Wachtel's (1987) approach. In describing "optimal structuralization" or psychological health, Atwood and Stolorow state that the ideal can be thought of as the maintenance of an ultimate balance between self-organization and openness to new experience. With such health a person can assimilate many different kinds of relationship experiences and retain stability. At the same time, such health would allow the person to accommodate to new experiences, thus allowing for ever-greater psychological growth. Structuralization is roughly equivalent to transference. But Atwood and Stolorow make a point of stating that the process involved in this structuralization is unconscious even though transference often includes conscious perceptions of others.

Atwood and Stolorow (1984) use the term "prereflective unconscious" to describe how a person structuralizes experience, or responds to the world, in an ongoing way. They suggest that character analysis, which they advocate, involves making what is currently prereflectively unconscious conscious. "Now we add that as psychoanalytic treatment has evolved from symptom analysis to character analysis, the time-honored aim of making the unconscious conscious has increasingly come to apply to the organizing principles and dominant leitmotivs that prereflectively shape a patient's experiences and conduct" (p. 42). Thus, in any way that the patient's perception of the environment or action within that environment is unconscious, that perception or action can be considered prereflectively unconscious. Atwood and Stolorow specify that this form of unconsciousness is not necessarily defensive since it applies to all perceptions of the environment. Its attribution to even nondefensive ways of being means it is applicable even to healthy aspects of a person's personality. The only thoughts or actions that are not prereflectively unconscious are those that are being reflected upon.

The goal of therapy, according to Atwood and Stolorow, is to make the structuralization of the environment available to consciousness for the client. Similarly, as the therapist's own structuralization of the environment becomes clear to him, it is available to consciousness, is no longer necessarily prereflectively unconscious, and can be utilized within the therapy. Atwood and Stolorow suggest that great effort is required to overcome preflective unconsciousness. With respect to therapy, the great effort required to overcome defenses applies to the client in gaining insight and the therapist in self-reflecting on his experience within his role.

This concept applies equally to analyst and patient. In Atwood and Stolorow's (1984) view of transference and countertransference, for example, the prereflective aspects of the analyst's personality are always in action. Atwood and Stolorow do not necessarily attribute complete psychological health to the analyst. And even the relatively healthy analyst is not always aware of all that he is experiencing. Those aspects of a therapist that are functioning in a prereflectively unconscious way are, in part, a reaction to the patient. At the same time, the analyst's work is prereflectively affected by his own level of character development. The analyst's current ability to structuralize his environment in a healthy way is prereflectively determined and thus the therapist's mental health is essential to a positive therapeutic effect.

Atwood and Stolorow include the analyst's character as an important factor in his accurate experience and perception of the patient's psychopathology. They go so far as to suggest that "psychological disturbances can no longer be viewed as resulting solely from pathological mechanisms located within the patient. Like 'negative therapeutic reactions,' psychopathology in general cannot be considered apart from the intersubjective context in which it arises" (p. 55). This logic leads Atwood and Stolorow to take responsibility for their part in working with patients. For example, in working with borderline patients they believe that if the analyst is able to maintain an empathic relationship to the patient, then the typical disintegration and splitting that such a patient may often experience subsides. The patient has already experienced so much empathic failure that a particular kind of relatedness is necessary within the treatment.

It becomes clear when looking at the views of Atwood and Stolorow that the analyst must have a well-developed character structure and prereflectively structuralize perceptions and experience in a healthy way if the patient is to be helped. The analyst's personality must be able to assimilate aspects of the therapeutic situation, like empathizing when the patient's experience seems similar to his own. Yet the analyst's personality must also accommodate to those aspects of the patient's experience that at first may seem alien. The healthy analyst will prereflectively mediate much of this process.

Prereflective Character Structure and the Relational Systems Perspective

Self-reflection, which makes conscious otherwise prereflectively unconscious aspects of the therapist's functioning, can serve to monitor part of the prereflective process so that the analyst does not act out. But the therapist's character and her prereflective responses cannot be erased by self-reflection, nor should anyone want them to be. Self-reflection can bring many aspects of the therapist's character and its functioning to consciousness but, I would argue, never all aspects. And it is in the therapist's humanity, in her ability to react as another person, that she can be of use as a therapist. The concept of prereflectively unconscious functioning allows for a distinction between intentional and unintentional uses of countertransference. Intentional uses of countertransference can result in empathic responding in situations where the therapist initially does not feel empathic. Such a use of countertransference will be discussed below in the section on empathy. The unintentional use of countertransference can be said to be prereflective. It is no less important—and may be more important—than the intentional use of countertransference. For the remainder of this study, I will use the concept of *prereflectively unconscious functioning* to represent the unintentional aspects of the therapist's processing of therapeutic inputs. An especially crucial part of prereflectively unconscious functioning is known as the maintenance of ego boundaries.

Ego Boundaries

For a definition of the term "ego boundaries," I refer to the work of Bernard Landis (1970), who provided a thorough literature review on the topic. He writes: "The term *ego boundaries* [italics in original] is a structural conception that refers to the boundaries that differentiate the phenomenal self in varying degrees (1) from those aspects of the personality not represented in consciousness, and (2) from the world of reality external to the person, as psychologically experienced" (p. 1). I apply this concept to the therapist in her ongoing interaction with the client or client-family. A discussion of human systems requires the concept of ego boundaries in describing how emotions are passed from within one person into another.

Landis (1970) begins his discussion by focusing on the "openness" versus the "closedness" of the ego–non-ego demarcation. He states that this dimension can be "expressed as the 'permeability' or 'impermeability' of the boundaries between the ego and the inner and outer worlds" (p. 1). The "ego" he says, "refers to the total awareness a person has of the subjective contents of his own existence. But this awareness excludes consciousness of his ego boundaries per se; a person is not ordinarily aware of this demarcation" (p. 2).

"Ego boundaries," then, function prereflectively. That is, a person is not generally aware of them. Ego boundaries negotiate the flow of emotionally valued aspects of the unconscious or the external world into or out of consciousness. Prereflectively unconscious functioning, being much more inclusive, however, represents all unconscious processing based on the person's internalized structures, and includes the ego boundaries. The ego, held in by variously permeable and impermeable boundaries, is variously affected by internal unconscious material and external reality.

Landis sites Federn (1952) in stating that two ego boundaries exist. One of these boundaries separates the ego from the non-ego within the personality. The other boundary separates the ego from the non-ego external to the personality. It is this latter boundary that is most important in describing how a person's boundaries affect his interactions with others. But to the extent that the boundary between unconscious and conscious impinges on the ego, thus affecting how it will mediate perception of, and activity in, reality, it too is essential to the understanding of a person's ongoing interpersonal functioning. I will refer from now on to the *inner boundary* when discussing the boundary between ego and non-ego within the personality, and the *outer boundary* when discussing the boundary between ego and non-ego external to the personality.

The balance that must be maintained in the ego by the ego boundaries is discussed by Landis, who states that one must attempt to balance relatedness and separation or belonging and individuation. "In boundary terms this means, optimally, that the demarcation of ego from nonego should be neither too permeable nor too impermeable. The former state leads to fragmentation or to symbiosis, and the latter to isolation; both involve a loss of selfhood" (p. 3). Both boundaries are involved in the balance. According to Federn's (1952) writing, when the inner boundary is too permeable, the person will not be able to differentiate between his inner fantasies and reality, as in psychotic disorders. The outer boundary would thus also be permeable as the person's interactions in the environment would reflect this lack of differentiation. Federn believed that if the inner boundary was impermeable, the person would be walled off from his emotions and would no longer sense his affects as part of the ego. The outer boundary, according to Federn, refers to the "point beyond which the ego does not extend" (1952, p. 331). The person invests narcissistic value in things and people outside the ego. Those things and people with narcissistic value are within the outer ego boundary and everything and everybody else is outside the outer ego boundary. The more permeable the outer ego boundary, the more the narcissistic investment in the outside world. If the outer boundary is impermeable, the person is isolated from others.

Following Federn's views, a few working examples could be useful here. It is possible for a person with an excessively permeable inner boundary (but not completely permeable as in Federn's example above) to also have an excessively permeable outer boundary, as in the inadequate personality. It is also possible that a person with an excessively impermeable inner boundary (again, not completely impermeable as in Federn's example above) also has an excessively impermeable outer boundary, as in schizoid disorders. The outer boundary can, however, have a different level of permeability than the inner boundary, and in many cases it is regulated in such a way as to compensate for the level of permeability of the inner boundary. For example, some narcissistic disorders could be said to be marked by a relatively permeable inner boundary that requires a relatively impermeable outer boundary to defend against psychic damage. Anger, typically invoked by the narcissistic part of an individual but not exclusively associated with narcissistic disorders, is an example of defensive shifting regulated by the outer boundary, which protects the inner self when narcissistic value has already been assigned to aspects of the environment that the inner boundary perceives as potentially harmful. As will be seen in Chapter 6, where I develop the concept of boundaries more fully, I am not in complete agreement with Federn's views on what constitute levels of permeability in the inner and outer boundaries. However, his descriptions are the first developed in attempting to clarify this difficult but common and necessary concept. Throughout the remainder of this chapter, boundaries will be discussed within the general guidelines of Federn's views. Although further development of the ego boundary concept is necessary in specifically describing the systemic influence of particular disorders, the functioning of ego boundaries within the therapeutic system does not necessitate description beyond that given by Federn.

Ego Boundaries and the Relational Systems Perspective

Landis does not discuss how the healthy ego functions. It seems, however, that the healthy ego would have much in common with the description of "optimal structuralization" given by Atwood and Stolorow (1984) above. That is, the healthy ego would maintain a "balance between the maintenance of . . . psychological organization on the one hand and . . . openness to new experience on the other" (Atwood and Stolorow 1984, p. 39). In describing optimal structuralization, Atwood and Stolorow emphasize the sufficiently consolidated psychological structure that can assimilate a wide range of experience while maintaining integrity. They also emphasize that psychological structure should be flexible enough to accommodate new experiences. The concept of ego boundaries is specifically descriptive of the manner in which the personality maintains that balance. In other words, ego boundaries determine how much new experience, either from currently unconscious material or from external reality, the ego or the character structure of the person will attempt to assimilate or accommodate. The healthier the person's ego, the better developed is the person's ability to maintain a balance. Thus, when the personality is healthy, the ego boundaries are functioning well. But how does a person develop a healthy personality?

The Therapist's Mental Health

With the addition of ego boundaries that function prereflectively, yet another aspect of this discussion becomes central. If the therapist's prereflectively unconscious structuralization of the therapeutic process partly defines his or her use of countertransference, then it is imperative that the therapist be mentally healthy. "Mental health" requires some definition if it is to be useful. I propose that the best way to view mental health is in terms of what Kernberg (1976, 1984) calls identity integration. According to Kernberg, in an ideal environment, identifications and introjections (in other words, the generalized perception of others and how one makes those perceptions part of one's self) become increasingly functional over time, eventually resulting in identity integration. A person with relatively complete identity integration has succeeded in integrating self and object representations into a coherent identity. That identity, embedded confidently within the person, allows him to react fluidly to the environment without self-reflection and also allows him to self-reflect when necessary.

More phenomenologically speaking, it might be the tendency of such a therapist to recognize when a client is impinging on his boundaries and to defend those boundaries accordingly. Defense of those boundaries may lead to a confrontation, which allows the patient to recognize boundaries more clearly and internalize an aspect of the therapist that is able to recognize boundaries. It might also be the tendency of such a therapist to empathize with the client without encouraging the client to continue in a self-destructive pattern. The important question about the way that countertransference affects treatment is: Do the therapist's emotional reactions enhance the therapy or interfere with it? The prereflective, unintentional use of countertransference must add more health than pathology to the system. Even the self-reflective, intentional use of countertransference relies on a lack of pathology in perceiving the process of therapy relatively accurately.

Depending on the therapist's level of identity integration, the prereflective reaction that takes place in him, first internally and then behaviorally, could be either traumatic or therapeutic for the family. When the therapist reacts to the family's behavior and attitudes in a way that is defensive and/or a repetition of the family's previous traumatic experiences, the family's perception of their effect on the therapist is not therapeutic but instead a perpetuation of traumatic experience. To the extent that a client or family experiences a therapist as being able to tolerate and/or understand their intolerable feelings, however, his reactions will be perceived by the family in a way that is therapeutic. It is therapeutic because the family is then able to take up part of the therapist's ability to handle their actions (his confidence, understanding, and so on) as their own, thus partially changing within themselves what they project on (or into) others. So, the prereflective use of countertransference can be credited for a therapeutic response.

An intentional, self-reflective use of countertransference can have a negative effect to the extent that the therapist's self-reflection has been influenced by prereflective, pathological elements of the therapist's personality. Even when the therapist attempts to be aware of his emotional reaction, his prereflective reaction to the client-family's perceptions allows for feedback to the family of which he is unaware. If the therapist's pathology does influence his self-reflection, then even the feedback provided by such self-reflection could add pathology to the therapist–family system. If the therapist's pathology does influence his reaction, his feedback is not necessarily very different from that which was originally perceived by the family, since the therapist may have prereflectively reacted to the perception in a way that was consistent with what was perceived (i.e., in a way that confirmed the idea and emotion behind the family's perception).

Going even one step further, this feedback could also be the result of a pathological reaction by the therapist such that the therapist's own faulty perception is then internalized by the family and added to their other faulty perceptions. The main point is, however, that no therapist is able to prevent him or herself from prereflectively reacting. With a high degree of identity integration, however, the therapist's prereflective reaction is more likely to be beneficial to the family.

The Therapist's Mental Health and the Relational Systems Perspective

If the therapist does not use self-reflection as part of her work, then it is especially important that her prereflective functioning be consistent with a high degree of identity integration. This prereflective processing (processing is a term often used in psychoanalytic literature, originating in the work of Bion [1959a], to be discussed in Chapter 5), must be relatively nondefensive, in part involving containment (another Bion term), meaning that the therapist is able to manage the experience of strong emotions evoked in her, and projected by the family, without undue reaction. That is, the therapist does not assign undue value to external phenomena, and is able to tolerate experience to the extent that it is valued. The outer and inner boundaries are maintained at levels of permeability appropriate to the situation. These aspects of therapeutic functioning, especially when they occur prereflectively, require relatively advanced identity integration in the therapist. Integrated identifications and representations give the therapist the necessary strength to maintain her knowledge of self while not rejecting those parts of herself that, although painful, might be similar to the patient's self. The therapist can have a healthful effect on families when affected by their projections, even without self-reflection, if her identity integration allows her to naturally function in such a way as to contain and respond to those projections without the defensiveness that they typically evoke.

From Holding to Metabolization

Healthy therapeutic functioning with respect to projective and introjective identification is described by a group of processes, including what Winnicott (1960a) called "holding," Bion (1959a) called "containing" and "processing," and Langs (1976b, 1978) called "metabolization." Winnicott (1960a) suggested that the therapist must be able to create an atmosphere, in his office and in his relationship with the client, which recreates a holding environment similar to the wished for relationship with a good enough mother. When a client uses projective identification that would lead to the therapist having, for example, hateful or persecutory feelings toward the client, the therapist's ability to respond to those feelings while remaining empathic is very important. If the patient is allowed to relive, now with the analyst, the symbiotic-like situation in which her original traumas with a poor maternal figure occurred, then the "good enough" therapist's "holding" will work to make the client feel adequately cared for. Also, through the therapist's unavoidable mistakes in perfect mothering, the client differentiates the analyst from the fantasy of the perfect mother, and thus individuates. (If the therapist fails to be "good enough," meaning that his capacity for holding is not sufficient, then instead of individuating, the patient's progress will stagnate or regress.) Most important with respect to holding, however, is that nontherapeutic situations, in which the client has become accustomed to receiving reactions to her behavior that might re-create trauma or perpetuate lack of understanding, are not repeated if the therapist is able to adequately "hold" the client. Within the therapeutic relationship the therapist must be able to let the client continue feeling safe and understood. The other processes discussed in this section must all occur in a context of holding to be effective.

With Bion's "containment" and "processing," and Langs's "metaboliz-ing," the therapist's ability to maintain an empathic attitude toward the client, while experiencing the client's intolerable affects via projective identification, allows the client to have a therapeutic experience in which she has not evoked the lack of understanding or abandonment that would usually occur in a similar situation outside of a therapeutic relationship. Important differences between holding, containment, processing, and metabolizing must be understood, however.

Langs (1978) describes metabolization as

a term first used by R. Fliess (1942) to describe the processing by the analyst of temporary trial identifications with the patient. The concept is used more broadly to refer to all efforts to work over sen-sory and nonsensory inputs from the patient, ultimately processed toward cognitive understanding and insight. This last sense of the term may also be applied to the patient's efforts to introjectively identify and contain projective identifications from the therapist, so long as efforts are made toward understanding. [p. 699]

Although attributed to the patient in this excerpt, the term "containment" is, of course, typically linked with the ability of the therapist to handle having the feelings associated with a projective identification (Bion 1959a,b). (In Langs's work, as was discussed earlier, projective identifica-tion is often also attributed to the therapist.) As can be seen in this excerpt, with containment it appears that the ability of the therapist to maintain empathy or neutrality is emphasized. With processing and metabolizing, emphasis is on the change in form of the projection that is brought about after it has had its impact on the therapist. Metabolizing, but not necessarily processing, is associated with the development of understanding. Processing, although it emphasizes an alteration of the projection, refers to everything that happens to the projection, including containment and eventually metabolization, but also the reflexive reaction caused by the projection in the recipient.

Holding and containing refer to the therapist's ability to handle affects that are intolerable to the client. The therapist's ability to handle those affects is first and foremost dependent on his personality. The therapist's holding capacity, similar to that of the "good enough mother" (Winnicott 1960a), is related to the therapist's ability to be soothing and understanding toward the client. That is, the therapist's holding capacity depends specifically on his ability as a person to make others feel safe and secure. Activity level is important only to the extent that it interferes with self-reflection, because self-reflection is so central to the therapist's ability to observe his own feelings and behavior. It is even conceivable that a therapist's inactivity, to the extent that it represents withdrawal from the client, demonstrates a lack of holding or containment. If the therapist is able to address a situation in which the client is using projective identification by accepting the projection and allowing the issue it involves to become part of the active therapy in a safe way, it can be said that the projection has been effectively contained and that the therapist has done an adequate job of holding the client. It seems clear, then, that equanimity of character is a part of the holding and containment functions.

A therapist cannot help but process and sometimes metabolize whatever occurs between him and the client. For example, Langs (1976a) describes the situation between therapist and client as one in which projective identification can fail, but nevertheless the projection is processed. Langs says that "the object has a full opportunity to accept or reject what is being placed into him, and to process these contents according to his own needs" (p. 26). Thus, according to Langs, containment, and therefore holding, does not necessarily occur. When the therapist does respond to his own needs without fully accepting the contents of a projection, he still processes the inputs of the encounter, but metabolization does not occur. Later in the same book, Langs makes a statement about the adequacy of a therapist's containing and metabolizing functions in which it is clear that metabolizing is associated with generating understanding but that more pathological types of processing also occur.

> I had said something earlier about the therapist who, based on coun-
> tertransference needs, offers himself as a nontherapeutic or patho-
> logical container for the patient's disturbed inner contents. I want to
> counterbalance this by noting that the therapist also has an appropri-
> ate function to contain the patient's pathological contents in order to
> introject these contents and metabolize them in a manner that gener-
> ates understanding and interpretations. [Langs 1976a, p. 153]

Thus, according to Langs, the therapist can process projections from a client in a way that involves containment, with metabolization being the ultimate goal. But also, the therapist might process projections in a way that meets his own pathological needs.

Ogden (1979), who discusses these constructs in explaining projective identification, emphasizes the difference in ways of handling strong affects between the projector and the recipient. If the recipient handles the feeling differently than is possible by the projector, then different feelings are generated within the relationship. The recipient may handle the feelings in such a way that communicates to the projector that such feelings can be "lived with, without damaging other aspects of the self or of one's valued external or internal objects" (p. 361). Ogden includes the possibility that these feelings might even be shown to be valuable or enjoyable. If handled well, the process can be extremely beneficial. Ogden states, "to the extent that the projection is successfully processed and re-internalized, genuine psychological growth has occurred" (p. 361).

This statement reflects what ideally happens when a client uses projective identification. It is important to notice that whatever reaction occurs in the recipient of the projective identification, it is available to the projector for reinternalization. Ogden emphasizes the successful processing that will lead to psychological growth, because the reinternalization of what has been successfully processed has a salutary effect. The important ingredient in successful processing, however, is not self-reflection or lack of activity by the therapist. What is important to successful processing is whether or not the object is able to deal with what has been projected into him or her.

Of course, being behaviorally active is also not always the appropriate response. The so-called "silent interpretation" (Ogden 1979, Spotnitz 1969), in which the therapist formulates but does not verbalize an interpretation, may also lead to understanding and thus metabolization. By the ability to "deal with the feelings projected 'into' him in a way that differs from the projector's method" (p. 361) it appears that Ogden is referring to the therapist's lack of defensiveness or relatively healthy character structure. The contained and then metabolized version of the client's projections is the ideal of processing. But processing is inevitable, and containment can occur without full metabolization.

Therapeutic Functions and the Relational Systems Perspective

It is the therapist's ability to "hold" the client and "contain," "process," or "metabolize" the client's projected affects that can lead to a reinternalization by the client of modified versions of those affects. These concepts are especially important to this study because they help differentiate the ways a therapist can use countertransference with families. These concepts all represent, to varying extents, the ability of a therapist to make therapeutic use of a client's difficult affects and projective identifications. Each concept infers a different amount of self-control and a different degree of self-reflection on the part of the therapist. How effective they are depends on the therapist's mental health.

The Therapist's Character and Its Functioning in the Relational Systems Perspective

In this section I have discussed the functioning of the therapist's character in some depth. The concepts and processes discussed demonstrate various ways that the therapist becomes involved interpersonally at an emotional level within the therapeutic system, and it is this emotional involvement that I call use of the self, or using countertransference. Character structure was defined as the way in which a person functions in her environment, based on developmental level. Aspects of a person's character structure were said to function in a prereflectively unconscious way, meaning that a process of accommodation and assimilation structuralizes perceptions of the environment in an ongoing way without awareness. Although self-reflection can be used to become aware of this process, a person cannot become completely aware of all her prereflectively unconscious functioning. The concept of boundaries, which function prereflectively, was discussed as an essential element in human systems. The individual person is a system with emotional boundaries that can be thought of as the inner boundary and the outer boundary. The inner boundary that separates extremely threatening affects from consciousness can be understood as having a direct effect upon the outer boundary that decides what in the environment should have narcissistic value. Thus, how the therapist reacts to her environment is determined by whether or not the environment has managed to impinge on extreme inner affects, and then on how the therapist's personality as a system reacts to that experience. I discussed the concept of identity integration as well, in explaining how a person could be envisioned as developing greater and greater ability to modulate responses to the environment. As a person's experiences increasingly represent an infinite number of interpersonal possibilities, with past experience leading to ever greater ability to perceive reality as it is rather than limiting views, and as a person's confidence that his needs will be met without undue hardship grows, so does identity integration. All of these concepts were discussed as integral to understanding how the therapist processes the emotional influence of clients, as represented by the terms "holding," "containment," "processing," and "metabolization." Perhaps the best way to understand how these concepts differ is to present them together in relation to each other. Simply put, processing ideally occurs in a context of holding and progresses in degree of benefit from containment to metabolization.

Throughout the discussion in this section I have consistently juxtaposed the false idea that therapist activity necessarily leads to harmful acting out with the idea that the therapist's mental health benefits treatment no matter how much activity occurs. Consideration of all the concepts discussed in this section brings us to two essential facts. One of these facts is that it is not activity, but defensiveness, that threatens the therapist's ability to be therapeutic. Nevertheless, activity does diminish the therapist's ability to self-reflect and so it becomes necessary to be aware that where the therapist's identity is not well-integrated, and the therapist is active without being self-reflective, prereflectively unconscious action can be damaging. The necessity for the active therapist's identity to be well-integrated, therefore, is especially pronounced in that she must respond prereflectively in a healthy manner.

The second fact brought forth here is that the therapist functions as a system both when alone and as part of a larger system with clients. A therapist's character structure and development are at issue here because his actions and reactions within the therapist–client (or therapist–family) system are inextricably connected to the effect the client or clients have on him. That effect involves the therapist's intrapsychic system and how it responds to various external pressures, given its boundary definitions and flexibility. Similarly, clients too are systems and function in relation to other systems accordingly. Thus the therapist's defensiveness or lack thereof defines the kind of effectiveness he will have within the therapeutic system. To the extent that the therapist functions prereflectively or self-reflectively in a healthy way, his use of countertransference will be beneficial to therapeutic goals, whether it is intentional and reflective or unintentional and prereflective.

EMPATHY AND COUNTERTRANSFERENCE

The potential strength harnessed in countertransference is best demonstrated in the empathic response. By using countertransference with self-reflection the intuitive kind of empathy, associated with what Racker (1957) called concordant identifications, is controlled so that the therapist does not "lose control of empathy" (Greenson 1960). Empathic responses are also formulated from what Racker called complementary identifications, despite the initiation of such empathic responses in emotions dissimilar from those of the client that at first evoke the opposite of an empathic response.

Many authors have written on the importance of empathy in psychoanalytic psychotherapy. The discourse on empathy has largely focused on what I will, following Racker (1957), refer to as concordant identification. Empathy has been defined by Schafer (1959) as "the inner experience of sharing in and comprehending the momentary psychological state of another person" (p. 345). Schafer also states that empathy "is a sublimated creative act in personal relationships which combines the gratifications of intimate union with the recognition and enhancement of separateness and personal development of both persons involved" (p. 370). Kohut (1959) called empathy "vicarious introspection." Greenson (1960) called it "emotional knowing." Fliess (1942) referred to empathy as the therapist's "trial identification" with a patient. And, of course, Racker has considered empathic reactions in the therapist as derived from "concordant identification." The kind of empathy discussed by these authors does not, at first, appear to be of primary importance to this study. As will be seen, however, the mechanisms involved in using this kind of empathy are closely related to the use of countertransference.

In the psychoanalytic view of empathy a distinction is consistently made between two parts of the therapist that must be active for empathy to be of value. Those two parts are the ability to identify with the client, and the ability to pull away from that identification enough to self-reflect. All of the authors listed above recognize the necessity of separateness in empathizing. In Schafer's statements, the use of the words "momentary" and "separateness" seem to indicate some danger in sharing the feelings of the patient too closely. Kohut's idea that "vicarious introspection" is the primary tool used in psychoanalysis implies the ability to observe its functioning in a relatively objective way. Fliess, in referring to this phenomenon as "trial identification," suggests the need to understand the patient's position but also the need to step away from that position in order to objectively analyze it. Fliess has emphasized that failure to pull out of that identification will lead to a "counter-identification," and thus possibly to countertransference acting out. And Racker has emphasized the difference between countertransference "thoughts" and countertransference "positions," the latter of which are avoided by consistent self or countertransference analysis. In psychoanalytic theory it appears that such separateness is important because it allows for therapist self-reflection in the therapeutic process.

Greenson (1960), in talking about the use of empathy, states:

Since to empathize means to share, to participate partially and temporarily, it means that the therapist must become involved in the emotional experiences of the patient. This implies a split and a shift in the ego functioning of the analyst. In this process, it is necessary for the analyst to oscillate from observer to participant and back to observer (Sterba 1960). Actually, the role of observer is shorthand for designating the different functions of analyzing, i.e. observing, remembering, judging, thinking, etc. [p. 420]

The attributes at the end of this excerpt are included within self-reflection, a quality that is, to some, implicit within the role of the psychoanalyst. As with empathy, self-reflection is particularly important in the use of countertransference. Self-reflection helps avoid the acting out that is of major concern in discussions of countertransference but that is, evidently, necessary even in the most common uses of empathy. It also helps transform complementary identifications (feelings experienced in the therapist that are projected by the client but are not parallel to the client's feeling state) into empathic interventions.

In the sections that follow, I will refer briefly to the work of Heinz Kohut (1971, 1977), whose self psychology made empathy central to the therapeutic role. Greenson's (1960) views will be used in elaborating on the idea that countertransference acting out is more likely if a person does not self-reflect on empathic countertransference feelings. I will refer to the work of Tansey and Burke (1985) to demonstrate that the use of self-reflection, which is required for any effective use of empathy, also makes possible the transformation of otherwise negative countertransference feelings into empathic responses.

Heinz Kohut

Empathy's importance can be connected to the working through of transference. As has been discussed, through a metamorphosis in the client's transference toward increasingly realistic perceptions of the therapist (and others in the client's life), the client functions better (Loewald 1960). The empathic intervention plays an important role in this process. By understanding how the client is feeling, toward the therapist and in general, the therapist helps to change the client's perceptions. The patient sees that the therapist understands her views (and associated feelings), and the very fact that the therapist understands indicates that the client is not isolated in those views, and that where no understanding was expected, understanding does exist. Therefore, the view that one is isolated and that others cannot understand must change. A common thread among fears of sharing one's perceptions boils down to exactly that—a fear that the other will not accept, or will reject, our core self when it is revealed.

Such a view is most specifically discussed by Kohut (1959), who has posited that the therapist, rather than being a screen for projection of the patient's transference, is a substitute for the patient's psychological structure. Considering the therapist to be a substitute for the patient's psychological structure makes empathy central to Kohut's view because the therapist must understand the patient even when the patient is unable to understand herself. Since the etiology of missing psychological structure is found in the context of early care-taking, when the patient was not adequately understood, the therapist's empathy, in Kohut's (1971) view, helps the patient to slowly replace missing psychological structure. In other words, a patient develops an unrealistic transference in therapy based on her incomplete past experience. One way that the therapist helps the patient work through that transference is to be empathic, which will not fit with the patient's transference because the transference includes the idea that others are not empathic. The patient internalizes the understanding reality of the therapist (along with other attributes) as different from her prior experience and is changed by the therapeutic relationship as she slowly begins to understand herself and others more readily. Thus empathy is central to change in psychotherapy. Kohut also viewed the therapist's *failures* in empathy as essential in that they afforded an opportunity for the patient to see the therapist as a real person, as opposed to the wished-for, perfectly understanding and appreciative parent of whom the patient was deprived as a child.

Ralph Greenson

Greenson's paper "Empathy and its Vicissitudes" (1960), outlines the importance of empathy as well as the problems associated with it. Before describing the problematic aspects Greenson discusses, it is essential to review his formulation of the strength involved in the ability to empathize. Greenson believed that the therapist who is able to be empathic also has, in general, a certain amount of self-restraint in reacting to countertransference. In this paper, he posited that there is reason to expect that therapists who are highly empathic are also very sensitive to the nuances of their own emotional life. That is, the wish to make contact with and partake of other people's feelings, learned very early, is closely aligned in the psyche with the need to be sensitive to one's own feelings. According to Greenson, such sensitivity allows the therapist to deal effectively with conflictual or irrational internal reactions to clients without acting on them.

Conversely, unempathic therapists are less likely to be open to their own experiencing and, therefore, might be expected to act out these internal reactions irrationally. The central assumption here is that empathic therapists, as part and parcel of their empathic ability, are more receptive to their own internal processes. Therefore, when confronted by conflictual or irrational reactions triggered by material from the client, the empathic therapist is better able to understand and modulate these internal responses. Accordingly, he is less likely to exhibit them in manifest behavior. The unempathic therapist is more likely to do so. Greenson also made the point, however, that the proper use of empathy is not necessarily practiced by empathic therapists, who might need training in that use.

Greenson (1960) discusses two ways that empathy can become problematic. The therapist might experience "inhibition of empathy" or "loss of control of empathy." Although Greenson attributed the inhibition of empathy to the student therapist who is passive due to fear of making an incorrect intervention, he also stated that chronic inhibition of empathy "is frequently found in those who have a chronically precarious mental equilibrium, or [who have] a deep mistrust of their feelings, impulses, and their unconscious" (p. 419). Inhibition of empathy would seem to limit the therapist's ability to help the patient. That is, if empathy is viewed as instrumental in the working through of transference, and the therapist's work is marked by inhibition of empathy, then the evolution of the transference that relies on empathy will not occur.

Self-reflection is necessary for preventing the "loss of control of empathy." In reference to the loss of control of empathy, Greenson (1960) wrote: "in such situations the therapist begins by being able to empathize with his patient, but this empathy does *not* [italics in original] lead to understanding and then to the proper confrontation of the patient" (p. 419). As suggested above, Greenson believed that the ability to become both involved and detached when with the client is essential for the development of empathy. With the lack of control of empathy, Greenson stated, the therapist becomes "too intensely involved and therefore cannot readily become uninvolved" (p. 420). The therapist becomes "uninvolved" via self-reflection. The work of Tansey and Burke further elaborates on the use of empathy and clearly connects it to countertransference.

Tansey and Burke

Tansey and Burke have written several papers on the relationship between countertransference, empathy, and projective identification. Their work describes the intricacies involved in using countertransference and empathy. I will summarize their view as it is presented in their 1985 paper "Projective Identification and the Empathic Process," and in their 1989 book, *Understanding Countertransference: From Projective Identification to Empathy*. With their elaboration on the work of Racker, they discuss how projective identification can lead to empathic response in the therapist. They also demonstrate, step-by-step, how the complementary identifications typically associated with problems in countertransference can also be used to formulate empathic responses. The work of Tansey and Burke makes clear how projective identification is involved in empathy, the loss of control of empathy, and moving back from complementary identification to empathy.

Tansey and Burke (1985) see both the concordant identification and the complementary identification as constituting the "trial identification." They emphasize that the concordant identification is within the traditional view of the trial identification but that the complementary identification can be viewed similarly. Because the therapist is able to transform the complementary identification into an empathic intervention through self-reflection, Tansey and Burke reason that even though the therapist's initial feeling state will not be similar to the patient's, it can be viewed as a trial identification. When the goal is the empathic response, the initial feeling available for transformation in the therapist can be viewed as trial identification, whether it constitutes feelings similar to those in the client or their complement.

Projective identification is central to Tansey and Burke's (1985) views on empathy. They emphasize its interactional, communicative aspect.

Projective identification, although having intrapsychic characteristics, represents an interactional phenomenon in which the projector unconsciously attempts to elicit thoughts, feelings, and experiences within another individual which in some way resemble his own. As such, there can be no "successful" projective identification without a corresponding introjective identification on the part of the recipient of the projective identification. [p. 46]

Their view of projective identification comes very close to the definition given by Malin and Grotstein (1966) in that they emphasize the receptivity of the therapist.

The centrality of receptivity in their view of projective identification is clear. Tansey and Burke see all empathy as involving projective identification. That is, projective identification is involved in empathy in the concordant identification as well as the complementary identification, both of which, as stated above, are seen as potential paths to empathy. According to Tansey and Burke (1989), in fact, all empathic responding is the result of projective identification.

The experience of empathy on the therapist's part always involves the reception and processing of a projective identification transmitted by the patient. Previous examinations of empathy have not sufficiently recognized that the empathic trial identification, whether concordant or complementary, that takes place within the therapist during the empathic process is an experiential state induced through the interaction with the patient. Empathy in the therapist does not take place in isolation, nor is it primarily an intrapsychic phenomenon. Empathy is the outcome of a radically mutual interactive process between patient and therapist in which the therapist receives and processes projective identifications from the patient. This formulation is applicable to projective identifications from the patient that are difficult to contain and that involve considerable introspective work on the therapist's part as well as substantial pressure from the patient . . . This formulation also applies to easily and smoothly processed projective identifications involving minimal work by the therapist and little or no pressure from the patient. [pp. 195–196]

Because concordant identification is not typically as problematic for the therapist, and because this kind of identification is part and parcel to the therapist's feeling that he is doing a good job, it is not often thought of as being related to projective identification and the problems involved in countertransference.

Tansey and Burke (1989) do not explain in detail what they mean by the concordant identification being the result of projective identification. But with the definition of projective identification given by Malin and Grotstein (1966), it is possible to see what they might mean. Perhaps the patient induces the concordant identification in the therapist through a process of (1) identifying with the therapist, (2) presenting material in a way that is consistent with making such a person understand, and (3) the therapist making himself available to receive the identification by desiring to understand the patient. I use the Malin and Grotstein definition of projective identification in explaining this process because the behavioral aspect of the inducement is not very strong, and because the therapist's availability for introjection is so necessary in allowing the empathy to occur. Such a definition of projective identification is implied in Tansey and Burke's work.

Tansey and Burke (1985) describe three phases that bring the therapist from initial trial identification to an empathic intervention: "reception," "internal processing," and "communication." Each of the three phases has three subphases. At any one time the preponderance of the therapist's efforts will be in one of the three phases but, Tansey and Burke explain, "it is virtually always the case that some work is being done in all three phases simultaneously" (p. 51). Likewise, the subphases are subject to much overlap. Nevertheless, for the sake of simplicity, Tansey and Burke outline the sequence from the beginning of the projective identification through to the formulated intervention.

In phase I, the "reception" phase, there is an arousal within the therapist of certain self-representations and their associated affective states. In the first subphase, the therapist's mental set is most important. To what extent do matters outside the therapy preoccupy the therapist? Or conversely, to what extent is the therapist able to approach what Bion (1967) termed "freedom from memory and desire"? The second subphase is marked by pressure in the interaction. Tansey and Burke emphasize the therapist's ability to tolerate the pressure of this interaction. They explain that therapists might attempt to reduce the pressure by changing topics or addressing non-transference-related issues. The patient is thus denied the opportunity to communicate through projective identification. But if the therapist is able to tolerate, and accept within himself the incipient feelings that are being evoked, the communicative process continues. The third subphase is called "identification-signal affect," which indicates that the therapist has now experienced a full identification with the projection of the patient. Whereas in the second subphase, the therapist may attempt to block the communication, in the third subphase the therapist may attempt to block awareness of the experience. But an increase in awareness may also occur, alerting the therapist to the possibility that an identification has been made. The therapist's awareness of the possible identification demonstrates his capacity to tolerate these "trial identifications" and not feel them to be overwhelming threats to his own ego.

Phase II, the "internal processing phase," is concerned with the step-by-step handling of the communication once it has been received. In the first subphase, the therapist must both contain the identification and recognize his separateness from the identification. Tansey and Burke (1985) cite Bion's (1959b) use of the word "containment" as describing the therapist's continuing efforts to tolerate thoughts and feelings without needing to deny or reject them. Important in this subphase is the therapist's ability to suspend potential superego criticism (Fliess 1942), realize that the current experience does not constitute an unmanageable threat to self-esteem, and understand that the experience is a trial identification and not an enduring representation of self. Tansey and Burke go on to explain that the regaining of separateness greatly reduces the behaviorally induced pressure, both intrapsychic and interpersonal. It also helps the therapist feel that he is in control of his own emotions. In the second subphase the therapist refers to a "working model" (Greenson 1960) of the patient and a "working model" of himself in interaction with the patient. By doing so the therapist attempts to make sense out of his emotional experience. In the third subphase empathic connection is accomplished. That is, the therapist is now able to grasp how his unique feelings fit this unique situation with this particular patient. The hypothesis at which the therapist arrives is based on "three primary considerations: the nature of the immediate interaction, the history of the interaction, and the degree of 'compromise' (Sandler 1976) between the therapist's own 'propensities' and the extent to which his self experience has been projectively 'determined' " (p. 59). When the therapist has reached a complete empathic hypothesis he is ready for the third phase.

Phase III, the "communication phase," is described as beginning the moment the therapist experiences the identification with the patient (which is in phase I, subphase 3, called "identification-signal affect"). It concerns "verbal and nonverbal communications on the therapist's part that convey in either an explicit or implicit manner the extent to which the projective identification from the patient has been processed through the Reception and Internal Processing phases" (p.59). Thus the communication phase should be thought of as the perceptible effect of the patient's projections on the therapist, beginning with the therapist's reception of the projection. Tansey and Burke (1985) choose to focus primarily on "explicit" communications. But all three subphases of the communication phase can also be viewed as different degrees of processing in the therapist rather than sequentially ordered stages. In the first subphase, "silent communication," the therapist conveys that he can tolerate the patient's projections through facial expression, tone of voice, consistency, and the like. This communication begins before the therapist has a full understanding of the patient's communication. Tansey and Burke caution that in less-than-ideal circumstances the therapist can also silently communicate feelings like withdrawal or anger, which reflects a disturbance in the overall processing of the communication. In the second subphase, Tansey and Burke describe a "single participant communication." The therapist verbally recognizes either his understanding of what has occurred from the patient's point of view, or what has happened from his own point of view. Often when this intervention is used the therapist has not yet come to an understanding of the full interactional nature of the situation. Tansey and Burke give an example of a "therapist-interaction communication" and a "patient-interaction communication." A therapist-interaction communication might be, "I feel as though you might be trying to put me on the spot and I think it would be important for us to understand what would motivate you to do this" (p. 62). A patient-interaction communication might be, "It's as though you feel I am attacking you by looking at you" (p. 62). The third subphase is considered a relatively complete intervention. Tansey and Burke call this the "therapist-interaction-patient communication." These interventions range from observing how both participants are feeling in a way that clearly communicates the connection between the two, to those that specifically state how the therapist's understanding has been deepened by the communication. Interpretations at this level always comment on either the similarity or the complementarity of feelings between therapist and patient.

Three other issues that are implied in their material but not directly discussed by Tansey and Burke (1985, 1989) are pertinent to this discussion. First, the trial identification, if it does not become conscious in the therapist, can lead to acting out in the form of either what Fliess (1953) calls "counter-identification" or in acting on complementary feelings. Second, the therapist's ability to self-reflect is a strength that is necessary in any kind of effective use of empathy. Third, the behavioral responsiveness of the therapist while he is processing must communicate to the patient that the therapist is able to handle the patient's projections. Each of these issues is integral to the use of countertransference in any kind of therapy. These issues require discussion in bridging the gap between the views of these authors and those of Greenson.

The problems that could occur if the therapist does not become consciously aware of the concordant or complementary identifications are most clearly indicated by Tansey and Burke (1985) in the first phase of their sequence. The therapist can respond to the "pressure from the interaction" by trying to block communication. The therapist can respond to the "identification-signal affect" by blocking awareness. Thus, allowing communication from the "pressure from the interaction" phase requires openness or "freedom from memory and desire" (Bion 1967). Becoming aware of the "identification-signal affect" requires self-reflection. What occurs when the therapist is not "open" is akin to what Greenson (1960) called an "inhibition of empathy." What occurs when the therapist does not self-reflect is more complicated. With the concordant identification the therapist is likely to either lose control over empathy (Greenson 1960) and become "counter-identified" (Fliess 1953) or become vulnerable to a complementary identification in taking care of the patient (Racker 1957). Not self-reflecting on the complementary identification might lead the therapist to acting out complementary feelings of an even more severe nature, such as victim or victimizer.

One of the issues discussed by Racker (1957) but not by Tansey and Burke (1985, 1989) is that a complementary identification is likely to become intensified when a therapist blocks awareness of a concordant identification. Since some concordant identifications can be quite painful, it is likely that a therapist might take on the complementary identification as a result of being unable to tolerate the concordant identification. If the concordant identification that could be received by the therapist is "victim," for example, and the therapist is unable to contain that projection, the client will then project the "victimizer." The sequence might be explained in this way. In the concordant identification situation the client may have looked for empathy in the therapist for his victimized feelings by inducing the therapist to feel like a victim. If the therapist is unable to contain the victim projection and act empathically to allow the client's reinternalization of the projection, then the client might project an object-representation of victimizer by acting like a victim in some subtle way (e.g., by perceiving the therapist's lack of response as aggressive or disdainful and blaming the therapist for hating him or her, thus evoking in some therapists aggressive or disdainful feelings).

Without self-reflection empathy loses its value, since in its absence the therapist is so likely to take on a countertransference position. Because they do use self-reflection, Tansey and Burke (1985) prevent themselves from taking on countertransference positions. The "internal processing" they use ideally results both in prevention of acting out and in the maintenance of empathy with the client. This processing also includes the therapist's ability to "contain" strong affects and communicate to the patient, either verbally or nonverbally, that these strong affects are contained and understood. Most importantly, however, self-reflection makes it possible to turn complementary identifications, which would otherwise result in countertransference difficulties, into deeply empathic interventions. The process involved includes openness to experiencing the patient's projections (which includes valency within the therapist), the ability to become aware of the experienced feeling without defensiveness, and the ability to process the experience in such a way that empathy (either verbally communicated or not) is reached. I will return now to the previous discussion on "loss of control of empathy" where I will apply Tansey and Burke's (1985) model.

Another Look at "Loss of Control of Empathy"

With the work of Tansey and Burke (1985), the process involved in Greenson's (1960) "loss of control of empathy" becomes clear. Racker's

(1957) view that the therapist's inability to identify with certain self-representations can intensify the therapist's identification with object-representations has some similarities to Greenson's view on the loss of control of empathy. In Greenson's article, it is clear that he was referring to what would be considered, by Racker, a countertransference "position." The comparison I would like to highlight here is that the complementary "position," known as the loss of control of empathy, can be understood as the result of a lack of self-reflection, at first, on concordant identification "thoughts," and second, on complementary identification "thoughts" that occur owing to the therapist's vulnerable state, or valency, when the concordant identification is firmly established.

Greenson (1960) gives an example of a therapist's loss of control of empathy in which the switch from concordant to complementary identification is clear even though Greenson himself did not make this point. The example begins with the therapist having a good empathic response to a patient who had been hinting about some sexually provocative behavior she had engaged in with her child. The client suddenly asked the therapist whether or not sexual contact with a child is harmful. The therapist responded to the patient by impulsively reassuring her that "a parent's sexual feelings towards a child [are] natural and even good for a child" (p. 419). The therapist later stated that he had acted out with his patient the role he would have liked his therapist to play with him—that is, to absolve him of his guilt for sexual impulses and feelings he had toward his own child. With the application of Tansey and Burke's model, Greenson's "loss of control of empathy" becomes the inability to identify with the concordant identification and an acting out of the complementary position.

To look at this process step by step, it could be surmised that the therapist was able to identify with the anxiety of having sexual impulses toward a child. But this identification might have made him vulnerable to the patient and to his own conflicts. When the patient asked a question about the ramifications of having sexual feelings toward one's child, the therapist, already identified with the anxiety of having sexual feelings for a child, could not tolerate identifying with the fear of being unable to manage his sexuality. He had opened his inner boundary to the idea of having sexual feelings toward a child and his outer boundary was open to caring about his patient. He did not, however, expect to find his patient discussing the possibility of harm that could come to a child if such feelings were acted upon. This possibility led to a sudden constriction of his inner boundary in the form of the need to jump to conclusions about the appropriateness of sexual feelings toward children. His vulnerability caused him to momentarily lose the capacity for self-reflection. The patient's fear was suggestive of her inability to handle her own sexuality, which as a projective identification with valency in the therapist as a necessary component, made the therapist, in complementary fashion, reassure her. He soothed the fear for her because he needed the fear soothed for himself, a concordant identification. But he also soothed this fear because the patient had communicated her need for help, a complementary identification. His lack of self-reflection during an empathic response led to a valency for a projective identification, with mild induction, of soothing the patient's fear. Thus in this example empathy might actually predispose a therapist to projective identifications that lead to complementary identifications. As a possible precursor for acting out countertransference feelings, empathy without self-reflection can at times be counterproductive if not harmful for the patient.

Even if the therapist in this situation had already become counter-identified and vulnerable, self-reflection on his ensuing complementary thoughts could have led to the ability to hold the patient's fear and the formulation of an empathic response. Considering the high activity level in the therapist–family system, the therapist is likely to find himself in a complementary *position* that developed interactionally. There are situations where this would happen not because the therapist had been unable to empathize initially, but because he became overly identified at first, leading to a valency to complementary identification. But the therapist, no matter how active, should be able to recognize his complementary position, and formulate an empathic intervention. The therapist must be able to observe his own part in creating the interactional sequence that led to his complementary position and use it within the intervention so that authenticity is maintained and blaming is avoided.

SUMMARY: THE CLINICAL INTERSECTION OF INTRAPSYCHIC AND DYADIC SYSTEMS AND THE RELATIONAL SYSTEMS PERSPECTIVE

The topics of this chapter—activity versus insight, self-disclosure, the therapist's identity integration, therapeutic functions of the therapist, and empathy—are essential adjuncts to an understanding of how countertransference can best be used in the therapist–family system. A discussion of how these processes are related is necessary. Difficulties involving these areas of functioning are more likely to occur in family therapy, where activity and self-disclosure are inevitable. Counteridentifications, concordant identifications, and complementary identifications, all of which play a part in empathy or failure of empathy, each impact the boundaries of the therapist, who responds prereflectively at least to some extent.

In the case of the overidentification or counter-identification (Fliess 1953), the therapist does not immediately perceive the true danger to ego integrity of relating so closely to the patient, and thus her boundaries are too open. The therapist's inner boundary has been loosened to allow unconscious fantasy similar to the patient's into the ego. The therapist becomes unable to differentiate her own feelings from those of the client. The possibility of the complementary identification occurring due to this openness is the result of the sudden need to close the inner boundary when identification has become a threat to ego integrity. The therapist prereflectively recognizes her momentary loss of self, and closes the inner boundary so quickly that she will only be comfortable in responding to the client in a complementary manner (such as taking care of the patient or judging the patient), which helps bolster the boundaries by way of differentiating the self from the other. That is, closing oneself off from further discomfort while denying the concordant identification and taking the complementary position works to relieve discomfort in the therapist, but fails therapeutically. Although this particular complementary position is similar to Racker's complementary identification, in this position the therapist often remains within the acceptable range of behavior from the perspective of the projecting client as in the case of "loss of control of empathy" (clients are not typically aware of the problematic aspects involved in the therapist being on their side or helping them), but judgmental or other negative complementary reactions (more typical countertransference problems) of the therapist also become possible.

The typical complementary identification works to stir up complementary unconscious fantasy more directly, and is more readily identified by the patient as nontherapeutic. The therapist's boundaries in this situation are also open to the patient, who casts the therapist in the complementary role. The therapist takes on that role in a prereflective manner because at that moment he is open to becoming part of the patient's view of things—that is, that the client is helpless or, conversely, dominant, and so on. On the other hand, it is likely that many therapists react prereflectively to strong projections by shutting down the outer boundary before the projection can have any interpersonal effect. If the boundary is shut before a projective identification is initiated because of the level of discomfort it might cause, then empathy will be blocked as in Greenson's (1960) "inhibition of empathy," or Tansey and Burke's (1985) "blocking of empathic response."

The therapist must be able to accurately perceive the level of threat or relative importance of the client to himself. If he needs the client to love him or think he's a good therapist, or conversely, if he is unduly afraid of the client, he will react prereflectively in anti-therapeutic ways. He will be either too open or too closed to the patient. With self-reflection, the prereflective nature of boundaries is intentionally overcome by the therapist so that he can be open to projective identification and avoid closing boundaries where there is no real threat. Thus, self-reflection allows for the intentional use of countertransference. Still, to the extent that the therapist's boundaries and structuralization of experience are prereflectively healthy, the unintentional use of countertransference, which is always present no matter how self-reflective the therapist might be, is beneficial.

Identification is not always bad, of course. Parents and children go through this cycle constantly throughout a child's growth. But just as the parent must be healthy if the child's identifications are going to be healthy, the therapist's health is essential. In fact, when someone's projections are especially toxic, the healthy prereflective reaction may be to close boundaries before identification even occurs, thus not allowing that person to do harm. In the therapeutic situation, however, the intentional use of countertransference adds a new dimension. The therapist who uses countertransference intentionally must be able to allow the patient's projective identification to take hold in him. Then, instead of reactively closing boundaries, the therapist must self-reflect, allowing the identification to remain intact and at the same time differentiating himself from the identification so that its function within the relationship can be understood. And when the therapist does act out, self-reflection can be used to formulate an intervention that grasps the interactional process developing between therapist and patient. Such an intervention is especially fruitful because it parallels the patient's experience in the world of activity. Due to the typical activity level, this interactive intervention is the most likely intentional use of countertransference in family therapy.

The relational systems perspective hinges on the application of the clinical concepts presented in this chapter to larger systems like the therapist–family system. The level of activity used in family therapy makes the acknowledgment of self-disclosure, even if not intentional, an integral part of family therapy. The therapist uses countertransference prereflectively, which implies self-disclosure in and of itself, and self-reflection is used in making the best possible interventions. The therapist's identity integration is essential when the extent to which she creates process with the family is acknowledged. Although self-reflection allows the therapist to maintain open boundaries when the prereflective tendency would be to become less open, the therapist's character cannot be hidden and her ability to process (hold, contain, metabolize) the family's projective identifications will always involve her own singular characteristics. Thus, as a subsystem within the therapist–family system, although the therapist may use her training to create empathic responses out of complementary identifications, her interpersonal influence will always be a central factor in understanding the system as a whole. With that understanding the therapist can harness the dynamics of the therapist–family system, and forge keys that unlock the ongoing dysfunctional processes within the family.

5

Intrapsychic and Interpersonal Systems in Groups and Families

In this chapter I look to the conflict-laden arguments between different schools of thought, as well as the arguments that integrate those schools. My emphasis is to demonstrate that where conflict has been discussed and viewpoints have been considered contradictory, integration is also possible. In pursuing that emphasis, I will begin by reviewing family therapy views on empathy, a quality which, as has been discussed, is a thoroughly interpersonal one. I will follow that discussion by turning to psychodynamic group therapies to see how that work can help bring a psychodynamic viewpoint to family therapy. In concluding this chapter, I will review the extent to which family functioning has already been understood by psychodynamic thinkers. I will also review some prototypical systems concepts that are clarified by a psychoanalytic perspective.

EMPATHY AND FAMILY THERAPY

Systems theorists do not often consider empathy as a primary factor in therapy, but its use is often implicit within the writings of many family systems therapists. When discussed by family therapists, empathy is often not accompanied by the use of self-reflection. As found in the psychoanalytic literature, however, self-reflection is an essential ingredient in using empathy. For that reason the level of self-reflection implied by various therapists will be assessed in this brief overview of what has been said about empathy within the family therapy literature. I will begin with authors who have used psychodynamic family-therapy techniques and move through experiential authors to the structural and strategic schools.

Nathan Ackerman

Family therapy authors who use psychodynamic approaches think of empathy as central. This is true of Ackerman (1966) who, in discussing the therapist's responsibilities stated: "His primary responsibility is to mobilize a useful quality of empathy and communication, to arouse and enhance a live and meaningful emotional language" (p. 92). The second half of the statement above is revealing about Ackerman's work in general. Connected to the empathy that he prized so much is the way that he used his own personality. The essential "live and meaningful emotional language" of his therapy could not exist without the use of empathy. Ackerman's use of empathy included self-reflection, which he employed in working with all types of countertransference reactions.

Ivan Boszormenyi-Nagy

Boszormenyi-Nagy (Boszormenyi-Nagy and Krasner 1986), another family therapist who uses psychodynamic principles in his work, also considers empathy central. He describes empathy as an aspect of "partiality," a word he uses to describe his commitment toward helping everyone in the "relational world" of his client who is likely to be affected by therapeutic intervention. In describing empathy, Boszormenyi-Nagy states:

> Empathy is an aspect of partiality, that is, a therapist's openness to imagining the feeling mode of each family member as he or she proceeds to describe personal perspectives and conflicted interests. The therapist's own natural feelings and reactions towards particular

family members are reined in by his efforts to be partial. One family member may evoke resentment in him, another may evoke contempt . . . At the very least a therapist has to find room in his feelings to imagine how the offending person has himself suffered as a childhood victim. [p. 302]

Perhaps Boszormenyi-Nagy is using "efforts to be partial" in this statement in the same way that self-reflection is discussed by Greenson (1960) as that part of empathy that prevents the therapist's ego from becoming overly invested.

In this same book, Boszormenyi-Nagy (Boszormenyi-Nagy and Krasner 1986) describes empathic ability as part of what makes a good contextual therapist. He also indicates that empathy is essential within any kind of therapy, including family therapy. In referring to the client's or family's "unconscious, emotionally significant configurations," he emphasizes that "the lack of consciousness over these configurations is the most significant stumbling block in a client's maturation" (p. 397). And he asserts that it is essential for the therapist to pay attention to these emotional cues through empathy.

David Scharff

Empathy is implicit to the work of object relations family therapists. In discussing interpretation, D. Scharff (1991) implies that an empathic response on the part of the therapist is the goal of some interventions. "Through interpretation, we reach to the core of the family experience. An accurate empathic interpretation is an ideal toward which we work by trial and error through clarifying comments" (p. 431). Such a statement is in keeping with the idea that empathy is the ultimate result of an intentional use of countertransference.

Deborah Anna Luepnitz

Luepnitz (1988), an author who uses some object relations principles within her psychodynamic feminist approach, considers empathy and nurturance to be indispensable factors in family therapy (as well as to a connection to feminist theory). "Many of the master family therapists have had little to say about the role of care and empathy in the therapeutic relationship. The fact that object-relations theory not only insists on such care and empathy but also uses the metaphor of mothering—what mothers do— as the essence of healing has clear potential for feminist translation" (p. 23). She criticizes the field of family therapy for not considering empathy more seriously. "It is striking that so *little* [italics in original] interest is given in other theories of therapy to activities that have to do with empathy and care. Many conventional family therapies even disparage such notions ('That's touchy-feely social work stuff'). Most feminists would agree, in contrast, that problems of healing are problems of understanding, and that, in essence, the cure is 'through love' " (p. 189).

Luepnitz discusses the work of Satir as exemplary with respect to empathy, and clearly demonstrates the importance of empathy in Satir's experiential approach. Satir (1987) used herself in a way that Luepnitz (1988) believes leads to growth in families. "Satir's work is not only accessible, it accessibly discusses *nurturance* [italics in original], a matter so taboo under patriarchy that it must always be disguised as 'unconditional positive regard' or 'positive countertransference' or 'multidirectional partiality.' Satir, undaunted by the taboo, writes unapologetically about the uses of care, trust, and even affection in the psychotherapeutic situation" (p. 52).

Virginia Satir

Although it is difficult to find a theoretical discussion of empathy in Satir's writings, her views on the subject are clear. In her work, "The therapist is clearly identified as a self interacting with another self. Within this context the therapist's use of self is the main tool for change. Using self, the therapist builds trust and rapport so more risks can be taken. Use of the self by the therapist is an integral part of the therapeutic process and it should be used consciously for treatment purposes" (Satir 1987, p. 23). Certainly if nurturance requires empathy, then Satir makes empathy a central part of her work. Also, it appears that her "use of self" at times requires self-reflection. In the excerpt above Satir specifically refers to the "conscious" use of the self, which brings to mind the differentiation in the psychoanalytic literature of intuitive empathy from empathy based on internal processing (Tansey and Burke 1989). However, it also appears that the empathy that is discussed by Luepnitz and Satir often overlaps with what might simply be called "holding capacity."

Shirley Luthman

Similar to Satir in her approach to families is Luthman (1974). Again, the word empathy is not often mentioned, but its use seems clear. In describing her use of self in therapy, Luthman describes a process similar to what Greenson (1960) describes as a good use of empathy. In this next example Luthman describes what the therapist does when experiencing emotions during the therapy hour.

> He tunes into his own experience of sitting in with the family system ... The therapist then checks out of the system and into his insides. He picks up a heavy feeling, a chaotic feeling, and he is also aware that he feels more and more constricted as he sits between the two parents. He offers all of this information to the family; thus intervening back into the system in an attempt to shake it up because all the data indicates that the family is not dealing with the real issues. [pp. 53–54]

This statement is similar to Greenson's understanding of empathy in that the therapist is expected to experience the feelings of the family but also to be able to pull out of the situation in self-reflection. In this excerpt Luthman also suggests that the therapist's feelings, empathic or not, should be shared with the family. She does not suggest, however, that negative reactions require processing before sharing them with the family, as is suggested in some analytic models. Rather, the therapist should not act out when recognizing that feelings are coming from the family, but should inject them, relatively unchanged, back into the family where they originated.

Carl Whitaker

Whitaker's methods with respect to empathy are, in theory, almost identical to those of Luthman. Observation of the work of Satir, Luthman, and Whitaker, however, suggests that Whitaker's work is far more dependent on his eccentric personality than that of the other two. Nevertheless, Whitaker describes a process of "uniting with" and then "distancing" from a family (Whitaker and Keith 1981). He does not make the purpose of this back-and-forth process clear, but he seems to find value in reflecting on what the system is doing and feeling. In general, Whitaker seems to believe empathy is important. "The family therapist must develop a basic empathy with the family. We hope his/her transference feelings will include an identification, a feeling of pain and a sense of the family's desperate efforts to self-heal" (p. 210).

And in their book about Whitaker's methods, Neill and Kniskern (1982) make the point that lack of empathy is a terrible mistake for the therapist. They contend that it is a terrible mistake to be aloof or technical in approaching a family and that, in fact, it is the therapist's empathy that acts as "anesthesia" for the "operating" he must do. Of this empathy, they state "This may be either a positive concern for the family members' pain or a negative response to them within himself, but in either case he is emotionally invested in them and that enables his participation to be authentic" (p. 352). In theory then, Whitaker's approach is very similar to that of Luthman. It can also be deduced that among Whitaker's followers, empathy becomes important, not as a curative factor in itself, but as the emotional connection that makes it possible for the family to bear the therapist "doing whatever he feels right in doing."

Within the systems models that follow, it is not clear if the interventions formulated and used involve any concern about how the family might be emotionally affected. Systems models are primarily concerned with the behavioral change that occurs, and perhaps with the emotional change over the long haul, but not much with the emotions that occur on the way.

Salvador Minuchin

A bridge to the strategic schools of therapy is the approach used by Minuchin in his structural family therapy. Minuchin (Minuchin and Fishman 1982) describes his role as therapist as ever-changing.

> Any technique may be useful, depending on the therapist, the family, and the moment. At times the therapist will want to disengage from the family, prescribing like a Milano expert, perhaps with a hidden agenda to his program. At other times he will take a median position, coaching à la Bowen. At other times he will throw himself into the fray à la Whitaker, taking one member's place in the system, allying strongly with a family underdog, or using whatever tactic fits his therapeutic goal and his reading of the family. [p. 31]

In this statement it is not clear if Minuchin uses empathy. If he does, it is certainly not considered of primary concern. He is interested in getting the job done. If he thought using empathy would be conducive to a positive outcome, and if it fit the therapist's personality, it seems he would recommend using it.

Jay Haley

Haley (1976) also does not consider empathy to be of central importance. Although Haley does not exclude the possibility of using empathy in some capacity, his opinion on the importance of emotion, in general, is made clear in this statement about his treatment model, and the elements of the therapist's role that are important in the training of new therapists: "it assumes that they will improve as therapists only by doing therapy under supervision and improving their skills. Instead of helping students understand their feelings or their transference involvement in a case, the teacher will offer active ways to resolve the difficulties in the case . . . It will be assumed that the student will change with action, not reflection about himself" (p. 201). It is apparent from this excerpt that Haley is not interested in empathy with self-reflection as it is discussed by psychoanalytic therapists.

Kleckner and Associates

An interesting article called "The Myth of the Unfeeling Strategic Thera-pist" (Kleckner et al. 1992) discusses the use of feelings, and even empa-thy, by strategic therapists. With the recognition that the client's feelings are an important reflection of the processes within a family, although per-haps not an accurate reflection of the truth within a family, these authors propose that strategic therapists often use those feelings in many ways. For example, empathy is used in joining: "In order to develop the type of therapeutic relationship that is required for change to occur quickly, the therapist must spend time listening to clients' feelings, acknowledging the feelings, and using those feelings in order to understand situations from their perspectives" (p. 44).

Here we see an interest in using empathy to make interventions go well, as the followers of Whitaker have proposed, but without a parallel emphasis on being genuine. These authors see the end-goal of this use of empathy as getting a strategic understanding of the various family member's "positions" as opposed to truly connecting with the family or developing a deeper understanding of the member's feelings. Kleckner and colleagues (1992) explain it this way: "The joining process in strate-gic therapy may look very familiar to anyone who uses empathic com-munication as a way of building rapport with clients. The difference be-comes more obvious when producing behavioral change in that empathy stresses self-understanding and position stresses cooperation" (p. 47). By stressing cooperation, these authors suggest that the strategic thera-pist's aim in acting empathic is to assess where the members of a family position themselves with respect to a particular issue so that the therapist knows what kind of therapeutic maneuver is most likely to move them. As is suggested by Haley (1976), these authors place the focus of strategic therapy not on feelings but on action. "Although we are not suggesting that strategic therapists use feelings in the same ways that practitioners of other models do, it is our observation that they have their own ways of addressing client feelings, ways that are conducive to the strategic goal of behavioral change" (Kleckner et al. 1992, p. 42). It appears, nevertheless, that something similar to self-reflection occurs in the work of these strategic therapists. The fact that strategic therapists use empathy to understand what is occurring in the family suggests that some mental process must occur that takes their focus out of the family's feelings and back to their own working model of families.

Mary Wilkinson

From the systemic school of family therapy has come an interesting distinction of forms of empathy. In a paper about empathy in systemic therapy, Wilkinson (1992) suggests that "systemic empathy" is quite different than the empathy used in most models of psychotherapy. The distinction she makes is that while doing systemic therapy, empathy for the entire system is of value but empathy with individuals can be destructive. She describes empathy for the entire system as encouraging empathy within the family as opposed to a splitting of family members, which occurs when empathizing with individuals. Some of the tactics she prescribes to ensure that systemic empathy is being used are circular questioning, which keeps family members in touch with each others' differing points of view; neutrality, which ensures that the therapist is not taking sides; and positive connotation, which reframes the behavior of family members as occurring due to deep caring about one another. According to Wilkinson, "The emphasis for the systemic therapist . . . is not so much on the therapeutic relationship, or the therapist's entry into the individual's private world, but on the connections between people, and between their different belief-systems. It is this wider system, or network of relationships, which is the focus, and which provides the context for change. That is so whether the therapist is working with an individual, a couple, or a family group" (p. 203).

Within systemic therapy, as in the strategic school, we see a use of empathy that uses reflection, but not self-reflection. These therapists reflect on the system of family relationships but do not self-reflect upon their own experience. In Wilkinson's (1992) systemic article, however, what is being suggested is that the reflection upon the system, as opposed to any one member, assures the therapist that she will not become overly involved in dangerous empathic situations.

Summary

In this brief overview of family therapy's views of empathy, the concept has been shown to have significance to at least some therapists within most models. Of course the way that empathy is used is very different within the various perspectives. From psychoanalytic and experiential schools we see a use of empathy that requires self-reflection or at least some distance from the family. Psychoanalytic schools seem to emphasize the curative aspects of empathy. Experiential schools might consider empathy as a curative factor, but always consider it an ingredient in the genuineness that provides "anesthesia" (Neill and Kniskern 1982) to the family for the painful work of therapy. Systems and strategic therapists for the most part only consider empathy important to the extent that it helps to get the job of behavior change done. When they do use reflection it is upon the system of relationships as opposed to the self-reflection discussed in analytic models.

GROUP ANALYSIS AND COUNTERTRANSFERENCE

There have been numerous efforts among psychoanalytic thinkers to discuss the intrapsychic as well as interpersonal processes inherent in group dynamics. According to Bion (1959b), one of the most influential group analysts, Freud is known for his opinion that "individual and group psychology cannot be absolutely differentiated because the psychology of the individual is itself a function of the relationship between one person and another" (p. 168). Bion also credits Freud with stating that "The individual is, and always has been, a member of a group, even if his membership of it consists of behaving in such a way that reality is given to an idea that he does not belong to a group at all" (p. 168). Thus, although Freud did not research the group, he did leave a legacy pointing to the group as an important subject for study. The clinical theory, including analytic theory, that has been developed in studying group processes is helpful in developing a deeper understanding of how countertransference works in family therapy.

Families, like groups, are aggregates of individuals. Of course, there might be limitations in applying group theory to families. A crucial difference between these two kinds of groups lies in the fact that a family comes to therapy already having deep connections to one another, whereas a group must develop connections over time. This caveat seems to have special validity with regard to countertransference, because countertransference due to projective identification depends on the intrapsychic expectations of clients. Transferences and projective identifications are likely to be far stronger within the family, especially at first, than toward the therapist. But in group therapy, such expectations are stronger toward the therapist than toward any other member.

On the other hand, the strength of the emotions within a family is likely to be far greater than in a group. After all, the group will only become like the family in each member's perception after members have gotten to know one another. (It was suggested by Freud (1921) that the strength of emotion that will lead to the group's cohesion originally developed as a result of each member being in a family.) Bion (1959b) stated "There is ample evidence for Freud's idea that the family group provides the basic pattern for all groups" (p. 187). In that vein it seems the strength of emotion within the family would clearly have a great impact on the countertransference of the therapist. But also, the therapist's countertransference experience in groups is likely to be similar to the family therapist's countertransference experience simply because the conglomerate group is likely to mimic some kind of family constellation.

In the following section I review contributions to understanding countertransference made by several psychoanalytic group therapists. Because the therapist's countertransference can be understood as his or her experience of being in a system with either the group or the family, the contributions of group therapists about systems theory in groups are also examined.

Origins in the Work of Wilfred Bion

Bion is the most commonly referenced therapist in psychoanalytic group therapy. His work with groups (1959b) is best explained starting with his distinction between "work groups" and "basic-assumptions groups." This distinction applies to two different purposes of a group. A group is in work group mode when it is working toward its stated goal. For example, a group assembled for the purpose of developing a new design for a car is a work group to the extent that it concentrates on that task. A group is in basic-assumptions group mode when its work-group task is affected by its intra-psychic defenses and interpersonal expectations. For example, a group assembled for the purpose of developing a new design for a car is a basic-assumptions group to the extent that individuals' intrapsychic defenses and interpersonal expectations interfere with the ability to concentrate on that task. Of course it is not possible for a group to be exclusively of the "work" type or the "basic-assumptions" type. Given these broad definitions every group has characteristics of both. In the therapy group, the task is for treatment or growth, making the basic- assumptions group important as part of the task. An important distinction related to the therapy group is that the therapist is always the leader in the work group. The leader of the basic-assumptions group, however, will be determined by the particular needs of the group and by which one of its members, including the therapist, best fits those needs.

Bion described three different basic-assumptions groups. These three might best be thought of as modes of operation that dominate group process at different times. These modes among basic-assumptions groups are the dependency group, the fight-flight group, and the pairing group. A group can fluctuate between these three several times within an hour or remain primarily in one of the three modes for several months. Each of the three groups requires a different kind of leader. The dependency group requires a leader who the group perceives as nurturing. The fight-flight group requires a leader who the group perceives as strong. The pairing group's leader is the imagined progeny of a group sexual fantasy who represents hope (perhaps best thought of as a leader created by the group to represent some hoped-for group identity).

It is important here to understand how Bion viewed these groups generally. The specifics of each are less important to the topic of countertransference. The two most important ideas related to basic-assumptions groups in relation to countertransference are: first, that they represent a psychotic level of communication, and second, that the therapist is as likely to be affected by these basic assumptions as the other group members.

Bion described a psychotic level of group process that he considered a normal part of group functioning. He also believed this psychotic level of group functioning to be necessary for a positive therapeutic effect to occur. But he was clear in stating that he did not consider the existence of these processes indicative of severe sickness within the group. In fact Bion believed no real therapy could occur unless these psychotic processes unfolded. Groups differ, however, with respect to when such processes will become manifest, some requiring more work before they become discernable. Bion states, some "groups resemble the analytic patient who appears much more ill after many months of analysis than he did before he had had any analysis at all" (p. 181).

By psychotic level functioning Bion meant that a great proportion of group process occurs at a nonverbal level and reflects very primitive anxiety. He described the group itself as representing primitive fantasies about the mother's body and the basic assumptions as related to a "more bizarre" version of the primal scene in which the "breast or the mother's body, contains amongst other objects a part of the father" (p. 164). The therapist's attempt to bring these fantasies to the awareness of group members evokes primitive anxiety. Bion stated that the defense mechanisms for dealing with these fears are characteristic of the paranoid-schizoid position (Klein 1946). The group switches its basic assumptions because of increasingly intolerable levels of this primitive anxiety, which is stirred up due to the possibility of primitive fantasies coming to conscious awareness. " . . . the basic assumptions now emerge as formations secondary to an extremely early primal scene worked out on a level of part objects, and associated with psychotic anxiety and mechanisms of splitting and projective identification such as Melanie Klein has described as characteristic of the paranoid-schizoid and depressive positions" (p. 164). The group switches its basic assumption out of fear and does so through splitting and projective identification.

Bion thought of the therapist as no less affected by the basic assumptions of the group than the other members. In fact, many of his descriptions make it clear that he believed the therapist was even more affected by the basic assumptions than other group members. Group members are likely to have greater expectations of the therapist than of each other. For example, Bion believed that one particular kind of basic-assumptions group, the dependency group, would look to the word of the therapist almost like that of a "deity." The theme of this dependency group would be the need for nurturance from a leader as well as the fear of losing that leader. The group under this basic assumption would look to one of its members, other than the therapist, as the leader if their needs were under the influence of the dependency basic assumption and the therapist did not meet their expectations. At times, any effort to discredit the chosen leader would lead to the canonization of that leader's word, which Bion referred to as "Bible making." The effect on the leader, often the therapist of course, could be a dramatic pull toward action.

Bion is well known for using the term projective identification in discussing interpersonal dynamics. He used the term sparingly in discussing groups but it is clear that he intended its application to group as well as to individual therapy. This next excerpt is representative of Bion's view that the leader is affected by group processes as much as other group members and that projective identification is a regular part of group functioning.

> [T]o me the leader is as much the creature of the basic assumption as any other member of the group, and this, I think, is to be expected if we envisage identification of the individual with the leader as depending not on introjection alone but on a simultaneous process of projective identification (Melanie Klein 1946) as well. The leader, on the basic-assumption level, does not create the group by virtue of his fanatical adherence to an idea, but is rather an individual whose personality renders him peculiarly susceptible to the obliteration of individuality by the basic-assumption group's leadership requirements. [p. 177]

Although in this particular instance Bion referred to a leader who is affected by the projective identification of one individual, it is clear that he intended that term to refer to the influence of the group as a whole. The "susceptibility" of the leader is also an interesting aspect of Bion's approach, and one that is connected to his concept of "valency." Although valency was discussed briefly earlier, in the section on projective identification, I will provide a fuller examination here.

Valency

Bion (1959b) described valency as a readiness for certain types of projections that occur in relation to a group's basic assumptions. Bion had this to say about valency: "I mean to indicate, by its use, the individual's readiness to enter into combination with the group in making and acting on the basic assumptions; if his capacity for a combination is great, I shall speak of a high valency, if small, of a low valency; he can have, in my view, *no* [italics in original] valency only by ceasing to be, as far as mental function is concerned, human" (p. 116). Bion also explained that valency is part of the basic assumptions group in the same way that cooperation is part of the work group: "A group acting on basic assumption would need neither organization nor a capacity for co-operation. The counterpart of co-operation in the basic-assumption group is valency—a spontaneous, unconscious function of the gregarious quality in the personality of man" (p. 170). This last statement rounds out his collective statements on valency: "By it I mean the capacity of the individual for instantaneous combination with other individuals in an established pattern of behaviour—the basic assumptions" (p. 175).

When these statements about valency are put together with Bion's ideas about the psychotic level of communication, especially projective identification, it becomes clear how he felt groups function. The members of a group, including the therapist, each have a certain valency for the three basic assumptions. When enough primitive anxiety is aroused in the group, the pressure from projective identification within the group interacts with each of the members' valency for the basic assumptions. Under siege of such anxiety the primary need is for the basic assumption to change. The new basic assumption that emerges is formed by the collective valencies within the group and is also reflected in the aims of the predominating form of projective identification. The therapist, as part of this group, feels the influence of its primitive functioning and attempts to make the group conscious of whatever basic assumption is currently at work. But short of becoming consciously aware of the pressures on him, the therapist has a natural tendency to identify with certain projective identifications. The leader of any basic-assumption group is someone who is "susceptible" to that particular role. To the extent that the therapist plays out the required role, he has responded from a valency for that role as well as to projective identification from the group.

The Analyst in the Group

Countertransference becomes important in the therapist's function as a work-group leader. Bion offered the "contention" that many of the most important interventions are based in the analyst's emotional reactions that occur because the therapist is the recipient of projective identification. When the analyst feels he is being "manipulated" into playing a role in someone else's "fantasy," or when he has a sense of "being a particular kind of person in a particular emotional situation," if he is able to pull himself out of it, "he is in a position to give what . . . is the correct interpretation" (pp. 149–150). Bion's use of countertransference in groups was integral to his work. He seemed to think of projective identification and valency as the glue that holds the group members together and leads them through their basic assumptions. The group therapist's job is to make the group's anxiety-provoking fantasies conscious. Bion thought that the therapist's experience of projective identification from one patient, or the group as a whole, was often the best way to reach the correct interpretation.

The Contributions of Other Group Analysts

Other group analysts have written on the group as a system and about its effects on the therapist, and all of them appear to owe a great deal to the work of Bion. His contribution will be clearly seen throughout the remainder of this section. Ernest Masler discusses the interpretation of projective identification as it develops between group members. Leonard Horwitz, drawing heavily from Bion's work, describes three "group dynamisms" that are "energized by projective identification." Most recently, Ramon Ganzarain has specifically described the way in which groups are systems made up of many kinds of identifications. Ashbach and Schermer have provided an extensive and comprehensive integration of systems and object relations thinking. Finally, I will present material from a paper written by Helen Durkin in 1974 that specifically calls for a reconciliation between systems and analytic methods in group therapy.

Ernest Masler

In 1969 Masler published a paper entitled "The Interpretation of Projective Identification in Group Psychotherapy." In this short paper he addresses the importance of interpreting the function of projective identification as he observed it in groups. Interestingly, Masler did not discuss the effect projective identification has on the therapist. Nevertheless, his contribution is important in describing how projective identification in groups can be seen as an integral building block.

Masler's primary aim is to demonstrate the kind of interpretation that is useful in resolving the defensive use of projective identification. Simply put, he recommends that the therapist interpret the group's reaction to projective identification among its members. By making the group's collective reaction conscious he hopes the group will de-identify with the projective identification. The effect of this de-identification is that the group members' reactions become less intense. Masler believes the individual using projective identification will begin to introject a modified version of what had been projected based on the change that occurs in the group members' reactions.

Masler's (1969) contribution is in his observation that projective identification can be interpreted between members of a group even if the therapist has not fully experienced its effects himself. As shown above, Bion (1959b) discussed similar views on projective identification, but added the concept of valency. Masler's view of the therapist's role, however, is somewhat different than Bion's, for two reasons. First, his work unfortunately takes the therapist out of the influence of the group; he does not mention an interpretation of projective identification that does affect the therapist. The second difference, however, is an addition to Bion's work. Masler's specific interpretation of projective identification between group members is not done for the purpose of bringing group members in touch with primitive anxiety. Rather, Masler's belief seems to be that the effect of the group members' modifying their reaction to one member's projective identification can lead to a working through of that individual's transference. This aspect of projective identification may be implied, but is not specifically discussed, in Bion's work.

Leonard Horwitz

Horwitz (1983) describes three different ways in which projective identification is manifested in group therapy: "there is little doubt that three significant and interrelated group dynamisms are energized by projective identification, particularly its interpersonal aspect. I am referring here to (1) the phenomenon of role-suction, (2) the use of a member as spokesman, and (3) the pervasive occurrence of scapegoating" (p. 270). Horwitz describes "role-suction" as occurring due to the functional necessity of certain roles within a group. The member who is unconsciously deemed most appropriate for a particular role will be induced by powerful pressure within the group to take up that role. That member will then become the repository of any projections that are associated with that role. These roles are not necessarily leadership roles, however. Leadership roles are more specifically related to "the use of a member as spokesman."

Horwitz's description of the use of a group member as a spokesmen is much like Bion's suggestion that each basic-assumptions group has a particular kind of leader. Spokesmen are those members who take up the leadership for particular kinds of issues. Horwitz explains that groups quickly learn which members best express anger, deal with closeness and attraction, or can be dependent with minimal conflict. Bion's influence can be detected here where Horwitz's three kinds of spokesmen correspond in some ways to the three kinds of basic-assumptions groups.

Both of these concepts, role-suction and the use of a spokesman, require the interplay between projective identification and a person's susceptibility for certain kinds of behaviors. Horwitz (1983) states that in both role-suction and the use of a spokesman "there is always a collusion between the person's conflicts and character style on the one hand and the group's dominant needs on the other" (p. 270). It seems clear that "the person's conflicts and character style" could easily be translated into valency within this particular context, again demonstrating the influence of Bion.

The third dynamic, scapegoating, could be described as often resulting from the other two. There are uncomfortable thoughts for which the group finds a spokesman. The member who represents these thoughts often ends up being castigated for his or her views. Likewise certain roles are required within groups for the purpose of containing the worst thoughts, feelings, and fantasies of the other group members. In another form of scapegoating, aggressive or libidinal impulses toward the therapist are displaced onto a less threatening group member.

One last refinement to the understanding of projective identification in groups offered by Horwitz is the inclusion of the definitions of projective identification given by Ogden (1979) and Malin and Grotstein (1966). Following from the work of these authors, Horwitz also discusses the importance of the therapist using her experience of projective identification within herself, not just for her interpretation of its effects within the group process. This addition is in contrast to Masler's (1969) paper, discussed above. Horwitz demonstrates the growing acceptance of applying these concepts within group therapy. His differentiation of the several ways in which projective identification manifests within groups is important in comparing these ideas to family therapy. That is, similar patterns can be discussed within families. Avoidance of "suction" has been discussed by Palazzoli and colleagues (1978) and "scapegoating" by Vogel and Bell (1960).

Ramon Ganzarain

In 1989 Ganzarain published a book entitled *Object Relations Group Psychotherapy* in which he contributed extensively to an understanding of the way object relations work within and between groups. One of those contributions is his combination of general systems theory with object relations thinking which he had previously outlined in 1977. Ganzarain sees systems theory as a useful skeleton on which object relations theory can be the flesh. He writes, "[T]he systems viewpoint needs to be supplemented with other more specific perspectives because it is too abstract. Only a skeleton, it needs to be filled with specific descriptions of the concrete subject matter that is being studied" (p. 455). He proposes that the general structure of systems theory can be reinforced with "psychoanalytic views on object-relations and groups" (p. 455). Specifically, Ganzarain offers a dialectic understanding of the paranoid-schizoid and depressive positions as described by Klein (1935) and Fairbairn (1941, 1943, 1946). The paranoid-schizoid and depressive positions will be more fully discussed in Chapter 6. Here, it will be sufficient to describe them as developmental positions, the first (the paranoid-schizoid position) representing a desperate need to remain intact through interaction with others, and the latter (the depressive position) representing a desperate need to remain attached and related to others. Ganzarain describes these two levels of functioning as part of a general "decider" subsystem, calling each a "decider sub-subsystem." He describes each the individual person and the group as a whole as whole systems.

Ganzarain's (1977) most distinctive contribution is the boundary sub-system. As a part either of the group as a whole system, or of the person as a whole system, the boundary subsystem has three functions. The functions are "(1) holding together the components; (2) protecting them from the environment; and (3) controlling the permeability through permitting entry or excluding information and matter-energy exchanges" (p. 446). Ganzarain's view can be seen as adding to what has already been discussed concerning ego boundaries. His specific addition is in looking toward paranoid-schizoid and depressive developmental levels in explaining how boundaries function. Like Bion (1959b), he thinks of groups as functioning primarily at primitive levels. He likens "holding together the components" to the schizoid aspect of the personality. The fear of being unable to hold together certain aspects of the system is connected to the possibility of splitting the self and losing some of its parts. "Those are the schizoid anxieties of impoverishment of the self, based upon defensive mechanisms of splitting" (p. 446). "Protecting them from the environment" is akin to the paranoid part of one's personality, according to Ganzarain. In the paranoid-schizoid position, the external world is perceived as dangerous. "Controlling the permeability . . . " can be viewed as the workings of projection, projective identification, and introjection. Unwanted parts, or parts of the self that are in danger, are at times split off and extruded, either through projection or projective identification. Those aspects are also brought back in through introjection, along with the unwanted or dangerous parts of the other, when the paranoid-schizoid "decider sub-subsystem" (p. 455) indicates that it is safe to do so. The paranoid-schizoid decider sub-subsystem itself responds to the world in a way that corresponds to its developmental level.

But these three functions also have depressive position analogs. Bion (1959b) did not elaborate on this aspect of primitive functioning. When the depressive position is worked through, the individual or group must be able to hold onto the internalized good object and protect it. That the individual's or group's rage or destructive impulses could destroy the good object is the anxiety of the depressive position as opposed to the anxiety based on danger to one's own existence in the paranoid-schizoid position. In the depressive position introjection and projection continue to mediate the permeability of the system. If the depressive position is thoroughly worked through, however, the internal object, connected to a self or group cohesiveness, is safe enough to allow for permeability without the fear of damage. This working through occurs only if the individual or group has failed to destroy the object with rage and if the object has allowed for reparation so that the individual or group develops concern (Winnicott 1965b, cited by Ganzarain). But since such working through is never complete, healthy control of boundaries is never complete.

Ganzarain emphasizes that control of boundaries is not generally well-planned or rational. Early anxieties at a paranoid or depressive level determine the reflexive functioning of defense mechanisms without higher functioning rationality available to intervene in the process. Ganzarain writes, "Anxieties connected with holding together the components that make up the system or with threats perceived as being 'out there' in the environment may trigger these primitive defense mechanisms" (p. 448). Groups operating at these primitive levels are Ganzarain's primary concern.

Ganzarain's perspective is that treatment involves the group working through these levels of functioning so that each member begins to view the world more realistically. He describes both the process between group members and, through fantasy, the processes between the group and outgroups. In considering the group as a "whole" system, Ganzarain sees individuals and subgroupings as "components." Introjection and projection are frequently used within this system and lead to identifications that form the "glue which cements the components of the group" (p. 447). Ganzarain indicates that boundaries between members become highly permeable in a therapeutic group as each member casts other members into roles of objects that were important in his past. Projective identification comes into play as each member manipulates other members into fitting those pre-existing patterns that he has come to expect from others. Insofar as the group becomes a cohesive unit, its internal processing will form a boundary between the ingroup and the outgroup. Ganzarain believes that including the outgroup as a fourth transference target has many advantages. The other three transference targets are the therapist, the other group members, and the group as a whole. Since manifestations of projection and introjection in the first three targets are elaborated quite clearly by other authors, Ganzarain's focus on the outgroup will be discussed here.

Frequently, Ganzarain states, projection takes the form of "the 'we/they' paranoid lines of splitting, visualizing the outgroup as the container of all the primitive, undesirable, unacceptable impulses and characteristics" (p. 449). One example he gives is the interaction across the boundary between the group and the marital couples formed by its members. The projection of the group on a group member's partner can hold many of the group anxieties. The influence that partner has on the group can take many forms. The group might respond to a member's stating that his wife does not want him to continue in the group. In a depressive defense, the members might attack the wife with no conscious awareness of their fear of losing an important part of the group system due to their own inadequacies. In a paranoid-schizoid defense, if the wife's complaint is that the group has no efficacy, members might project their own anxiety on her, not accepting their own doubts about the group's efficacy. Ganzarain allows these projections to develop, making an interpretation only later. He suggests that from a general systems point of view, interactions with a wife, as they are discussed within the group, are actually an extension of the group that has occurred through projection. He also points out that, through the patient's introjection of his wife, she is, figuratively speaking, a part of the group. The group therapist, from this point of view, must prevent the group members from excluding important aspects of their own systemic functioning. The therapist does this by including the analysis of projections onto outgroups.

Ganzarain (1977), in referring to the example given above, discusses how this kind of intervention is helpful.

> The group decider "old" sub-subsystem—under the influence of paranoid anxieties—was closing its boundaries so that the expulsion of such "bad" contents could be made definitive. The therapist acted as a "new" and higher decider sub-subsystem, making the group boundaries permeable to the "recycling" of such contents by dealing with them as a new input rather than a finalized output. A vicious circle was thus overcome and a "virtuous" cycle begun. [p. 455]

The "virtuous" cycle to which Ganzarain refers in this case was that the group member developed a new decider sub-subsystem that could analyze situations with a different approach. The group member "began conceiving of a new, more assertive self-representation and thought of possible interaction between himself and his wife, with himself being stronger and less fearful" (p. 454). The group member stayed in the group, facing the risk of divorce, and did get divorced later on.

Like Bion, Ganzarain believes that the therapist can use projective identification, and thus countertransference, to make empathic interventions. But his unique contribution, since Bion had already discussed the use of countertransference, is his integration of systems with psychoanalytic object-relations thinking. The understanding of groups as skeletal systems with object relations flesh, and introjection, projection, and projective identification as the glue between group members, is a valuable way to envision the family group as well. His idea that the safety of the individual's or the group's integrity is dependent on boundaries that determine which identifications will be introjected or held within and which will be expelled via projection or projective identification is a helpful bridge to systems thinking from object relations thinking. As will be seen in Chapter 6, Ganzarain's views on the paranoid-schizoid and depressive functions of boundaries are instrumental to my own integration of analytic and systems thought.

Charles Ashbach and Victor Schermer

The work of Ashbach and Schermer integrates systems and object relations thinking in a different way. Their book, *Object Relations, the Self, and the Group* (1987) is quite comprehensive in its scope, discussing several of the most important concepts integral to this study. They describe the group as a system made up of a space with boundaries containing the object relations of its members. Using an approach similar to Ganzarain's to explain the phenomenon of the group, these authors see the group as containing three dynamic subsystems, each functioning within this space.

Ashbach and Schermer differentiate intrapsychic space, including object relations, from interactive space, that includes communications forming a network that connects personal, intrapsychic space to group space. Thus, they make the essential connection between intrapsychic processes and interpersonal processes. The "interactive space of transactions" (p. 112) consists of general communication as well as projective and introjective identification. The group itself, as well as every combination of relationships held within it, provides various forms of containment for the members' projections. "Each subsystem as well as the group-as-a-whole become containers of meaning, parts of the self, projective-introjective processes, and object relations" (p. 121). It is clear that Ashbach and Schermer envision systems and object relations as integral in explaining the complexity of groups. The group system holds within it the individual dynamics of each member, and the way in which those dynamics interact determines "the group structure, process, and content at a given point" in the group's "evolution" (p. 112).

As part of the individual dynamics they describe, Ashbach and Schermer (1987) view drive theory as complementary to object relations theory. Drive theory, they state, characterizes the individual personality as a "closed system" of "mental representations" connected to "biological tensions" (p. 26). Object relations theory, on the other hand, represents an "interactive social model" (p. 26) that emphasizes the interconnectedness between the person, his environment, and his various group affiliations. They go on to say that the drive model is derived from an epistemology that views the observer and the observed as separate entities, while the object relations model is a product of the view that observer and observed make one unit. This "transactional" method, they argue, "brings psychoanalysis ever closer to group dynamics and a 'multi-body' psychology" (p. 26). Ashbach and Schermer's work is exceptionally integrative. Their description of drive theory and its intrapsychic processes allows for the understanding of one person's drives and individual psychology. Although they do not discuss this topic in detail, their description here demonstrates that they believe some aspects of that model retain validity. Their description of interpersonal object relations, which is their primary focus, allows for openings in the closed system of the person through interpersonal interaction.

In describing the group evolution, Ashbach and Schermer explore various levels of projective identification. The paranoid-schizoid position is more representative of group dynamics at earlier stages and the depressive position is more characteristic of later stages. These authors also make use of the concept "cohesion" to describe the movement into the depressive position of group functioning and then toward better integration of each member beyond the depressive position. Their description of projective identification allows for its use through all of the group's stages. They argue that it is a normal and adaptive response as well as a defense mechanism.

"It has explanatory value for group dynamics because *it points to the ongoing developmental relationship among inner mentation, interpersonal communication and interaction, and the group system as a container which is modified by the content that is projected into it* [italics in original]" (p. 42). This view invokes the definition of projective identification given by Malin and Grotstein (1966).

According to Ashbach and Schermer, the use of projective identification throughout the life of the group can have either paranoid-schizoid or depressive characteristics. However, the group should naturally evolve, at first toward higher-level uses of projective identification, and then to less use of projective identification in general as the group members become better differentiated. In the beginning of a group, when its unknown aspects evoke primitive anxiety, projective identification is often described in this way:

> In group, the paranoid-schizoid position may manifest itself as a pervasive group culture, in interpersonal relations, or in individual valences. Split-off or repressed parts of the self are projectively identified into the group matrix and experienced in a location in the group rather than in the self. The group-as-a-whole (like the responsive mother) changes to accommodate the projected elements. Thus, projective identification plays an important part in group regression, role differentiation, cohesion, and leadership. Each of these dynamics reflects a process through which inner states promote or inhibit group organization in particular ways, and vice-versa. Projective identification is so fundamental to group psychology that it, in a sense, creates the group as a distinctive, coherent experience. [p. 42]

As the group develops, the depressive level of projective identification becomes more dominant in group process. Ashbach and Schermer indicate that the ushering in of the depressive position within the group is marked by overactivity, false hopefulness, and exaggerated or false optimism. These behaviors suggest that issues of "termination, separation, and guilt are emerging" which can only be resolved by confronting the defended against "group-wide disillusionment and depression which is the precursor to accurate consensual validation" (p. 43). Depressive anxiety, the authors state, is the fear of harm to the object as opposed to fear of harm to the self. In the group, depressive anxiety occurs as a result of a threat to group cohesion. When the group develops the "capacity for concern" (Winnicott 1963b), members are able to fear either loss of each other or the group as a whole. The group and its members have become perceived more as whole objects since they have been perceived as constant even when the most destructive or pathetic aspects of individuals have been projected.

Ashbach and Schermer (1987) then describe the relationship of cohesion to the evolution toward mental health. They describe a transformation *"whereby functions previously performed by individuals are assimilated into the group structure itself* [italics in original] (p. 193). Instead of one member absorbing the projective identifications of another, with cohesion the group structure begins to contain the problems of individuals or subgroupings. If development proceeds normally to a "closely knit and coordinated organizational frame" (p. 194), then the group progresses from primitive part-object relations to predominantly mature whole object relationships. Leading up to mature cohesion, the group becomes, at first, like an extended family, and then more like a nuclear family. "The group as it evolves into separation and individuation begins to manifest kinship relationships within a predominantly maternal orbit, the type of grouping analogous to a tribe or extended family. In its further development, a more distinct family constellation, characterized by the Oedipal triad, may emerge" (p. 127).

Finally, when the group has become mature, it controls its own destiny, which is to perform the "work group" function in a way that is consistent with the integration and differentiation of the members. "Upon the resolution of these various conflicts, one can begin to speak of the group as a mature, non-transference object . . . The group is now a creation of the membership, whereas earlier the members had been a creation of the group, that is, of their own projective identifications" (Ashbach and Schermer 1987, p. 128). The description of what it means to have reached relative mental health is refreshing in this work. It seems that often when health is discussed in clinical literature it is typically more abstract and more difficult to understand than when it is described by Ashbach and Schermer.

This clarity is also refreshing when these authors discuss the therapist's experience of projective identification and how it can be handled. Like other authors already discussed, Ashbach and Schermer believe that projective identification affects all members of the group, including the therapist. Their description of that process, however, is far more direct. They use projective identification in exactly the same way it would be used in a one-on-one psychotherapy. The application to groups, however, makes it unique. They state that when the therapist has contained the projective identification, he must tolerate the emotions and derive meaning from them, interpreting them back to the patient or group in a way that is safe and tolerable so that the patient or group can allow private, unconscious impulses to coexist with social identity. Their descriptions of working with projective identification are very similar to that described in the work of Langs (1976a,b) whom these authors often cite. It also fits with the work of Ogden (1979), who emphasizes the necessity of allowing the projection to repose (Bion 1959a) in the therapist, sometimes for many sessions, before interpreting it. In discussing how Langs works with projective identification these authors go even further.

They apply the deliberate processing of projective identifications, as described by Langs (1976a,b), to groups. After observing a "distorted interaction in the group" (p. 242), the therapist first examines his countertransference feelings and tries to understand what effect his reactions have had on the therapeutic frame. This exploration allows group members to investigate their own unconscious responses to these events. Secondly, the therapist attempts to clarify the role that each member, including himself, had on the projective identification that occurred. In providing an integrative experience for group members, they then explore the way in which the interaction relates to individual object relations and the significance of the event for the group as a whole. The work of these authors represents the most advanced development of the use of countertransference among the group analysts.

With its various levels of projective identification and its movement toward mature cohesion, Ashbach and Schermer's discussion of group evolution is the most complete model for integrating object relations and systems thinking thus far discussed. Their work is encouraging in its complex integration of many different aspects of group functioning. The authors' willingness to include the therapist's reactions in a group as part of the group material is atypical. The direct demonstration of the use of countertransference reactions within the complex processes that make up a group is completely unique.

Helen Durkin

The idea that object relations are a part of every human system is not a new one. In 1972 Durkin wrote a brief paper entitled "Analytic Group Therapy and General Systems Theory" in which she described how psychoanalytic and systems thinking are not incompatible. Durkin uses the definition of systems given by Hall and Fagan (1956). Those authors defined systems as a "set of objects together with the relationships between the objects and between their attributes. The objects are the component parts of the system, the attributes are the properties of objects, and the relationships tie the system together" (p. 18). According to Durkin, most analytically oriented group therapists recognize that definition as compatible with their experiences of groups. But she also states that this compatibility is hotly debated. In her view, the debate is based on views similar to those of von Bertalanffy (1968) and Watzlawick and colleagues (1967).

Von Bertalanffy's (1968) objection to psychoanalytic thinking is its reliance on linear causality. Durkin, however, cites Freud's work on groups (1921), in which Freud conceived of man as a bio-psychosocial being and the group as the reciprocal influence among its members. Freud's work seems much more in line with circular causality than is usually thought. Durkin (1972) then cites the ego psychology work of Hartmann (1964) in which mental health was formulated in terms of the equilibrium that exists among the structures of the personality on the one hand and those of the environment on the other. Within that framework, Durkin says, the group can be envisioned as a system that follows the same laws of organization as the personality. She states that analytic group therapy contributed to the modernization of psychoanalytic theory in that it maintained the tenets of ego psychology. Both analytic group therapy and ego psychology focus on "function, relationship, and dynamic interaction" (p. 13). From Durkin's point of view then, the interactive focus of ego psychology was partially brought about due to the work of analytic group therapists. She does not see systems and psychoanalytic thinking as incompatible as did von Bertalanffy.

Durkin states that Watzlawick and colleagues (Watzlawick et al. 1967) consider psychoanalysis and systems thinking to be incompatible because psychoanalysis employs the concept of energy, as opposed to information, as a unit of exchange. She sees this argument as related to the psychoanalytic focus on development of the individual rather than the interaction between group members within the here and now. Because interaction in the here and now is observable, and does not rely on inference regarding unconscious infantile motivations, systems theorists prefer the concept of information over that of energy. Systems theorists see analytic thinking as reflective of closed systems that are not truly influenced from the outside (by other people). But analytic therapists do concentrate on exchanges in the here and now, events at the interface between systems. Durkin argues that systems theorists miss the point. The fact that analytic therapists view the interaction as occurring between intrapsychic attributes of the people within the group does not suggest that those intrapsychic attributes are not translated into communicated behavior. Although analytic therapists see the exchange between members of a group as reflective of development, they also believe that attention brought to those interactions can bring about change in the system as well as the individual. As she says, "it is a mistake to regard the interaction of intrapsychic components as a closed system" (p. 14).

Durkin believes that a delineation of the psychoanalytic concept of transference refutes all arguments against the compatibility of systems and psychoanalytic thinking. She lists the necessary attributes of transference as seen from a systems point of view as: (1) it is clinically observable as manifest distortions in perception, (2) it is a here-and-now phenomenon, (3) it is derived from infantile conflicts that can be verified through the individual's associations, (4) translating it into interpretations effects changes in communication between group members which validates it both as a "theoretical concept and as a change agent" (p. 15).

Durkin thus sees transference as an exceptional explanatory tool for systems functioning. In the next excerpt, Durkin puts the meaning of transference into a context of interpretation within a system. According to Durkin, transference can be perceived as a behavioral manifestation of

personality organization which constitutes a reactivation of the caretakers of childhood. It originates during the process of individuation, and serves the special function of avoiding repeated pain. Over a period of time, the transference emulates other specialized functions in that it tends to become mechanized to varying degrees. Concurrently, there is a loss of spontaneity in the affected areas. In cases of severe conflict, it may dominate the individual's behavior, in which event it regularly interferes with valid communication. Thus the whole thrust of the interpretation of transference phenomena is aimed at breaking through this mechanization and restoring spontaneity. [p. 15]

Durkin believes, however, that group interaction cannot be completely explained by unconscious infantile emotions. "The individual's input is also derived from physiological and complex current psychological needs" (p. 15). She ends her paper by hoping that, in the future, "when the need for defensiveness has died down," those aspects of systems theory that are complementary to psychoanalytic theory, and vice versa, will be further explored.

Analytic Group Theory and the Relational Systems Perspective

The use of countertransference, or the use of self, as described by the authors above, could be employed in family therapy. However, no complete explanation of relational systems has yet been discussed within the family therapy literature. Features of the discussion above that are essential to family therapy include the following. First, and originating in Bion's work, is the idea that projective identification occurs within groups and should be recognized and used to salutary effect. Masler's work also discussed this issue. Beyond projective identification, Bion's work offers other valuable ideas. Family modes of operation can be viewed as basic-assumptions groups that are governed by projective identification. For example, the dependency group might be suspected when one member of the therapist–family system seems to be identified as the nurturing one, the fight-flight group when one member seems to be identified as the strong one, the pairing group when one member is thought of as the special person in the therapist–family system. Recognizing these patterns might help the therapist track process in the family from one basic assumption to the next, thus allowing for deeper understanding of current family functioning.

Horwitz introduces similar group concepts that can be applied to family therapy. The role-suction concept and the use of a group member as a spokesman, along with the scapegoat concept, all have much in common with Bion's views of the basic-assumptions group leader. But Horwitz adds to the basic-assumptions group concept with explanations of how negative roles might come about in response to the need to disavow unwanted attitudes that continue to seek a voice. The term "scapegoat," originating from Vogel and Bell (1960), has become popularized in family therapy, but is not often so lucidly discussed as in Horwitz's paper, in terms of projective identification.

Ganzarain's (1977) paper, and Ashbach and Schermer's (1987) book, are useful in more fully understanding how intrapsychic and interpersonal processes complement one another in group systems. By extension, the family group can be understood as a system in which the components are individuals, themselves made up of intrapsychic subsystems. Ganzarain's description of boundaries structured by paranoid-schizoid and depressive functioning with projection, projective identification, and introjection governing boundary permeability is particularly useful, and will be central to my discussion of boundary formation in Chapter 6. Ganzarain's approach is also unique for the inclusion of outside targets of transference, an addition that reminds us that the group system intersects with many other systems. Ashbach and Schermer help to explain individual growth by maintaining drive theory as a complement to object relations. Their focus on the evolution of the group toward health is instructive with regard to family growth as well, as are their detailed accounts of how the therapist uses projective identification in the group setting, which can be used as a guide for such use of countertransference in the family therapy setting. Ashbach and Schermer as well as Ganzarain, highlight one of the most crucial reasons for combining systems and psychoanalytic thinking, which is to address the fact that systems therapy typically denies the importance of the intrapsychic system.

In that same vein, Durkin's work is important in pointing out the unnecessary shift away from analytic thinking found in systems theory, a shift based on the false assumption that analytic thinking relies on libido theory and therefore presumes linear causality. Analytic thinking has clearly transcended libido theory (Ashbach and Schermer provide the best example) and now encompasses both linear and circular causality in describing human systems. However, a few analytic therapists have begun to describe family systems in terms of object relations theory. Their work is the focus of the next section.

OBJECT RELATIONS SYSTEMS AND FAMILY THEORY

Within family therapy, as in group therapy, several attempts have been made to integrate psychodynamic thinking. Object relations theorists have been able to delineate intrapsychic as well as interpersonal aspects of communication that are very useful in understanding family interaction. Some of the ways these therapists propose that countertransference may be used have already been discussed. However, in this section the description of the family as a system of object relations is emphasized and this emphasis, as found in the work of some object relations group therapists, leads to a perspective that includes the therapist as part of a system with the family.

This section begins with a review of the work done by John Zinner and Roger Shapiro in the 1960s and early 1970s at the National Institute for Mental Health. These authors applied what they called an analytic, group-interpretive approach to family therapy (Shapiro 1979), which expanded on the work of Bion. Their work is especially valuable to this study for its description of the family group as a single psychic entity held together by object relations (Zinner and Shapiro 1974). Scharff and Scharff (1987), in their popular work on object relations family therapy, use many of the conclusions reached by these authors in defining their own approach. After discussing the implications of Zinner and Shapiro's work, I will review the work of Scharff and Scharff. Slipp (1984, 1988) is also a major contributor to this area. Slipp's work is useful here in two ways. First, Slipp describes family interaction as made up of transference and countertransference reactions of family members to each other. Although these terms are usually used in relation to a therapist, his application of them to family members simplifies a discussion of how projective identification functions within the family. Second, Slipp details some of the assumptions made in family systems therapy that he sees as better explained through object relations therapy. In fact, he sees his own formulations as being in better keeping with the tenets of systems theory as it is described by such principals of that philosophy as von Bertalanffy (1968), Gregory Bateson (1962, 1972, 1979), and Norbert Weiner (1954), than the methods employed by dedicated systems therapists.

John Zinner and Roger Shapiro

The work of Zinner and Shapiro (1972, 1974) with families of adolescents is the earliest attempt to apply to families what is commonly referred to as British object relations theory. Zinner and Shapiro rely most heavily on the extension to groups of the work initiated by Bion (1959b). In making the transition from Bion's work on groups to their work with families, these authors (Shapiro 1979) postulate that both mature and primitive aspects of family functioning exist in every family, just as they do in every group and every individual. They argue that the same shift that Bion (1959b) made from individuals to groups must also be made from individuals to families.

They explain that families differ from groups in very important ways, including shared developmental background; specific role relationships; and shared assumptions, motivations, and defenses that do not exist in a randomly organized therapy group. Because of these differences, they believe family processes are more similar to individual psychodynamics than they are to group processes. According to these authors, within the family, internal processes become external processes. Because there is a shared developmental history in families, what is projected by one member is very close to being the reality of the other member who has, through his or her development in that family, internalized those projections. From this point of view, each member of a family becomes one part of a larger personality that is the family system. One important difference between the functioning of an individual and the functioning of the family, however, is that many of the processes that would be internal within the individual are external within the family. Thus those processes are made available for observation and then intervention. The family system functions in such a way as to allow for inference about the intrapsychic systems within each of its members.

In their discussion of families, Zinner and Shapiro concentrate on work-group versus basic-assumptions group functioning and on the common use of projective identification in families. Their formulation of projective identification is very useful because they describe it as detectable through observable behavior. Zinner and Shapiro (1972) describe their view of the family in very accessible language with their use of a concept they call "delineation."

> Included within the realm of parental behavior are acts and statements that communicate to the adolescent his parents' image of him. We have referred to these behaviors as *delineations* [italics in original]. As observers of the family, we make inferences, based upon an accumulation of delineating statements, about the composite object representation of the adolescent residing within the parental psychic structure. [p. 111]

Zinner and Shapiro explain that some delineations are more dependent on defensive functioning within the parents than others. "Defensive delineations" constitute perceptions of the adolescent within the parents that help the parents avoid some conflict between them or in one of them. Since these perceptions are part of the defensive personality organization within the parents, they are tenaciously sustained. As one behavioral aspect of projective identification, delineations express a need within the parents, and have a powerful influence on the adolescent within the family. These perceptions are so tenaciously sustained through delineating comments and attitudes that they lead to behavior within the child that is congruent with the parental perception.

But projective identification is not always considered unhealthy by Zinner and Shapiro. They also refer to delineations that are healthy. For example, the idea that the adolescent can be responsible for himself is likely not a defensive one on the parents' part, and results in parental behavior that allows for the adolescent to develop in a healthy way. In describing the way in which psychopathology is transferred from one generation to the next, Zinner and Shapiro (1972) emphasize the "content of the projected material, the capacity of the parent to differentiate himself from the child, and the intensity of the parental defensive requirements" (p. 117). They report that, depending upon these factors, projective identification can be healthy and beneficial or, on the other hand, bind the child into the defensive psychopathology of the parents.

Thus their perspective on projective identification is close to that of Malin and Grotstein (1966) presented earlier. Although they do not specifically advocate any one theorist's view of projective identification, they do cite

Malin and Grotstein, as well as Racker (1957) and Searles (1963) in describing their view. Like these therapists, Zinner and Shapiro see projective identification as part of a natural process between people. Since their work is dedicated to determining the role of family process in psychopathology, however, the reader will notice their emphasis on the problematic aspects of family process.

Interestingly, they do not discuss Bion's concept of "valency," even though that concept is consistent with many aspects of their approach. For example, they credit Anna Freud (1936) with implicitly suggesting the "willingness, unconscious or not, of the recipient of the projections to collude in providing vicarious gratification on behalf of the other" (Zinner and Shapiro 1972, p.113). They say that this next statement is an extrapolation from Malin and Grotstein (1966): "In the absence of this collusive process the defense fails, or the projection is 'lost'" (p. 113). It is clear that Zinner and Shapiro intend to describe something very similar to valency as instrumental in family process.

They suggest that the adolescent also takes part in the process of becoming what the parents have projected. They account for the adolescent's collusion in fulfilling the expectations of parental delineations by citing a variety of motivations and influences. Among these, Zinner and Shapiro include impulse gratification, feelings of power associated with taking part in determining the parent's self-experience, parental compliance with the child's defensive needs, and parental reinforcement of those behaviors that are consistent with parental projections. However, they indicate that the most important influence on the adolescent is the possibility of losing parental love if she does not behave consistently with parental defenses. They state, "If we view our disturbed adolescents as walking a fine line between fulfillment of their own strivings for an autonomous identity and conformity with a parental delineation serving parental defense, we are deeply impressed with the power that parental anxiety holds in tipping the balance" (p. 118).

The behaviors these authors refer to as delineations are a key to understanding how the family system functions and is sustained. They use these delineations to understand intrapsychic processes within each group member. They also see delineations as applying a great force on the recipient of projective identification. Shapiro (1979) explains that "the power of these projections, with their accompanying unconscious identifications, may push the individual into more extreme role behavior and into feelings that are very powerful and may be experienced as unreal and bizarre" (p. 239). The extent of regression mentioned here is more fully explained by Shapiro and Zinner (1979) in their work on boundaries between subsystems within the family as a larger system.

Like the authors in the section above on group systems, Shapiro and Zinner (1979) describe boundaries as an essential aspect of the family system. They also (Zinner and Shapiro 1974) describe a dysfunctional family system as a single psychic entity with individuals who are incomplete without the whole. "Taken as a whole, the family appears to constitute a single, relatively complete, psychic entity; taken alone, each individual seems to be psychologically incomplete and overrepresentative of one mental structure. Consequently, internal psychological conflict within members is transmuted into interpersonal conflict *between* [italics in original] those who have come to represent the agencies of impulse and superego" (p. 187).

Within that system are subsystems. Boundaries between various subsystems, and the boundaries between the whole family system and the larger community, are important in describing the functioning of the family. Shapiro and Zinner (1979) put it this way: "We assume that there is an important correspondence in the structure of the personality system and its subsystems and the structure of external reality—especially the social system and its subsystems—that impinge on that personality (Edelson, 1970)" (p. 204). Starting with the developing adolescent, these authors describe how boundaries are involved in explaining the correspondence between the individual personality and other systems.

The adolescent's development can be conceptualized as a remodeling of psychic structure and an increase in the secondary autonomy of the ego (they cite Jacobson [1964]). According to Shapiro and Zinner (1979), increased strength develops in the boundary between independent action and ego functioning on one side and functioning limited by childhood anxiety and conflict. Likewise increased strength and definition develop in the boundary between the adolescent and his objects. The familial and societal response to the adolescent's growing autonomy facilitates or interferes with the development of self boundaries. When either childhood conflict or the impingements of the adolescent's current environment interferes with developing ego organization or ego autonomy, the adolescent's self boundaries become "chaotic."

Zinner and Shapiro (1979) refer to the work of Miller and Rice (Miller and Rice 1963, Rice 1967, 1969) in explaining how the subsystem of the adolescent might interact with other subsystems within a family. Rice's basic propositions are that every interaction—whether it be between individuals, within groups, or between groups—is an intergroup interaction, and that the effectiveness of any intergroup relationship is determined by the extent to which the groups involved have to defend themselves against uncertainty about the integrity of their boundaries. Thus the adolescent who is just developing her self boundaries is less certain of those boundaries and is thus less likely to have effective relationships. This is even more likely to be the case where either childhood internalizations or ongoing relationships with others are not conducive to boundary formation.

Shapiro and Zinner (1979) explain that Rice's formulations point to a relationship between the integrity of boundaries within systems and the integrity of the boundary between systems. Integrity of the boundary between systems implies that each system has a clear sense of differentiation from other systems. Differentiation within a system is dependent on "internal authority for integrated functioning" (p. 209) or the ability within that system "to be self-regulating, and to control task implementation, including intergroup transactions" (p. 209). Shapiro and Zinner (1979), applying this thinking to an interaction between two systems, state that the boundary between two systems is defined by the understanding within each system of the intergroup task. If these understandings are different, or if there is a change in one of the two systems that requires the intergroup task to change, then "each system is strained, with anxiety arising over the possibility of breakdown in authority in each system" (p. 209). A breakdown in system functioning occurs if there is unclear role differentiation, if either subsystem is too fragile to play its part, or if authority within one subsystem is too inflexible to handle changing situations. Under these circumstances, either abrupt separation from the group, or a breakdown of boundaries with ensuing chaos, occurs. When individuals are thought of as systems, it becomes clear that ego autonomy, identity integration, and self boundaries are essential in the effective functioning of interaction.

"Definitions" within the family system and its subsystems can be thought of as parallel to the basic assumptions as described by Bion. The basic assumptions that become prominent in a family at any one time reflect the overriding defensive functions of the parents. Shapiro and Zinner (Shapiro

1979) describe family regression as interaction dominated by projective identification that results from a breakdown in the ego differentiation and self boundaries within the family. Thus family regression, chaos, or separation occurs as a result of a combination of inadequate self and other definitions as well as inadequate self integration and inflexibility within the family's members. The expression of that regression can be viewed as the dominant basic assumption at that time. This next excerpt captures their point of view:

> In family regression, there is rapid reduction in usual ego discriminations. Dissociation and projection are increased, with confusion over the ownership of personal characteristics that are easily attributed to other family members. When one individual assumes a role compatible with the attributions of others in the family at the regressed level, he quickly becomes the recipient of projections which tend to fix him in that role. [p. 239]

In persons who have less well-developed ego autonomy and self boundaries, whether they be children, adolescents, victims of trauma, or adults with unresolved childhood conflicts, projective identification is likely to become operative with more powerful induction.

Shapiro and Zinner (1979) discuss the breakdown in the family as resulting from parents who have not been able to tolerate their own anxiety well enough to avoid projecting aspects of themselves into their children. The functioning of these parents falls far short of "good-enough." The "good-enough" mother, as described by Winnicott (1960a), is able to tolerate the infant's intolerable affects as they are projected into her. The parents described by Shapiro and Zinner have, over an expanse of time, been unable to tolerate the difficult, though developmentally normal, affects of their children. And beyond this inability to tolerate their children's affects, they have also been unable to tolerate their own anxiety without projecting it into their children.

Zinner and Shapiro (Shapiro 1979) see the family's development at the point where a child reaches adolescence as especially anxiety provoking for parents and thus very likely to bring on basic assumptions group functioning within the family. The family's effective work-group functioning toward normal growth and daily functions is interrupted. According to

Shapiro (1979): "Family group behavior now appears dominated by assumptions that particular meanings of childhood and adolescent individuation represent a danger to family requirements, cohesiveness, and even survival" (p. 236). Shapiro and Zinner (1979) give examples of family regression or the operation of basic assumptions within the family. They observe that family behavior appears to be determined more by fantasy than by reality; work failure is evident in the emergence of confused, distorted thinking, and failure of understanding and communication; it becomes impossible to maintain discussion in which family members respond realistically to their problems. The family's behavior at these times is indicative of primitive communication via projective identification. These authors go on to say, following the work of Klein (as described by Segal 1973) that the family's anxieties are evoked by issues at the depressive level that cause defense at the paranoid-schizoid level of communication. This kind of defending they describe as the essence of Bion's application of Klein's work: work-group level functioning is interfered with by depressive anxiety, which then sends the group into primitive, paranoid-schizoid level functioning marked by group defenses at the basic-assumptions level.

Shapiro and Zinner (1979) specifically describe transactions at the boundary between the patient and the therapist as well as between the adolescent and the family. Unfortunately their discussion is limited, for the most part, to the boundary between the individual adolescent patient and the therapist. Their only comment on the boundary between the family and the therapist (or therapists) is that "the transference issues in this situation are complex and must be approached with the recognition that family therapy is an intergroup meeting with a number of subgroups present" (pp. 213–214).

One caveat to the work of these authors exists and is highlighted by them. The sensitivity demonstrated above about the complexity of the family system with its many subgroups suggests that their descriptions of family functioning are, by necessity, oversimplified (The many subgroups they describe are similar, perhaps, to the Minuchin and Fishman [1982] formulation of the family as being made up of many different "holons"). Zinner and Shapiro (1972) criticize their own oversimplification of family dynamics by stating that their reductive analysis may highlight specific phenomena while obscuring the more fluid complementarity of behavioral sequencing within family process. They are specific in criticizing their lack of differentiation among siblings. They state that a general style of parenting is not what determines each child's personality, but rather that each child becomes influenced by different parental delineations depending on what particular purpose that child serves or what role he plays in the family. Even this criticism seems oversimplified in that it does not consider the delineations reverberating throughout the family from various family subsystems and other influences. But the formulations of Zinner and Shapiro generally provide an adequate theoretical picture of family functioning.

If one views the influence of delineations coming from all persons and subsystems of the family system, rather than just one way, from the parents into the child, this family picture is quite complete. Refreshing within the work of Zinner and Shapiro is the clarity with which they use boundaries in describing the workings of the family system and its subsystems. In reading their work, one can readily understand why and when projective identification is likely to become forceful in the family. They explain the developing individual in the family system, her function with respect to other parts of the family system, the functioning of the system as a whole, and the functioning of the family system in contact with other systems. Although not specifically discussed by Zinner and Shapiro, the developing valency within each member of the family adds to this picture. Zinner and Shapiro's work provides so much clarity in the application of object relations to families that it has been widely cited by authors who now advocate an object relations approach to family therapy (Scharff and Scharff 1987, Slipp 1984, 1988).

The importance of countertransference and its use is, however, a notable omission from Zinner and Shapiro's work. They do remark that transference to the therapist might be of use. Given their discussion of boundaries, it might be assumed that therapists are able to detect transference toward them in the "strain" (or countertransference) that is caused by the family having an incorrect "definition" (transference) of their function. Also, the increased likelihood that family members' defenses would include strong behavioral influences when their systemic integrity is threatened, which occurs in the family regression these authors describe, would seem to indicate that the boundary between the therapist and the family would often be projectively breached. Thus, although not directly discussed by them, it would seem that their views on family functioning would naturally lead to the use of countertransference in family therapy.

Jill and David Scharff

The Scharffs also use the work of Bion in applying object relations to families. However, they advocate three important additions. The first is a use of countertransference in family therapy, as already discussed. Second, Scharff and Scharff (1987) discuss the effects of projective identification on family members in a broad way; they look at its effects throughout the development of the family. Zinner and Shapiro, of course, limit their discussion to working with the adolescent period and, by their own admission, fail to assess the different effects of projective identification on different children within the family. Third, Scharff and Scharff elaborate on the basic assumptions functioning within families and believe it is important to add a fourth basic assumption when working with families. To Bion's dependency, fight-flight, and pairing basic-assumptions groups, they add the dimension of "fission/fusion." This concept is important in describing families that fall into the dimension of enmeshed or disengaged, a concept popularized by Bowen (1978) and Minuchin (1974).

The addition of family development is important in making an understanding of family object relations clinically useful. Understanding the effects of parental projective identification is greatly enhanced when these are looked at as having certain consistent attributes with respect to each child from birth. Also, genetic interpretations can be seen as focusing on the buildup through introjection of the projective identification that has occurred in the family. Like Zinner and Shapiro, Scharff and Scharff (1987) emphasize that projective identification can be used at a healthy as well as a regressed level. Either way, the buildup over many years results in very strong identifications within the child that constitute, to a large extent, the child's personality. In the Scharffs' view, a child's current behavior and personality are the result of genetic endowment, temperament, and experience, including the buildup of projective identifications and introjection within the family. They view projective identification as essential, in empathy as well as pathology, from the beginning of life and even before birth, as can be seen in this next excerpt:

> The mother, who is in constant physical relationship to the fetus inside her, learns about the fetus's rhythms of stillness and movement, fantasizes about who it will look like and whose qualities it will have,

and, while physically meeting its needs, automatically prepares for responding to its needs after birth. In attending closely to her inner experience, she picks up physical clues and, putting herself in the baby's place, imagines its feeling state . . . Unconscious fantasies may not [however] promote empathic understanding of the baby. Instead, the baby may be used as a repository of unwanted or secret parts of the selves of the parents. Then the couple does battle with what it finds in fantasy in its child, rather than struggling within the couple relationship. [pp. 93–94]

Thus, beginning even before birth, parental projection is at work. After birth, projective identification begins to form in the parents' interactions with the child. Their expectations and projections are, of course, influencing the development of the child, who learns who she is through the parents' eyes (See Ogden [1989], Chapters 5 and 6, for a comparable viewpoint). The parents may be using projective identification in a healthy way. For example, they may feel confident that their child will be intelligent, capable, and strong. Through his introjection of the parents' perceptions, the child begins to think that way about himself, and act that way with others.

It is also possible to see various developmental milestones as impinging on particular aspects of parental personalities. Pathological types of projective identification are more likely to become an issue when a child is going through phases of her life that are particularly problematic for the parents. The parents might not have worked through some aspect of their sexuality, which is more of an issue when the child reaches puberty. Thus some form of sexual acting out might be expected. Or, a parent might not have a well-developed capacity for empathy, a quality that is so important in holding a newborn. Thus the inadequacy the parent feels is projected into the child, causing relentless crying in the child and causing the parent to perceive the child as difficult.

Scharff and Scharff (1987) differentiate "pathological projective identification" from healthier kinds. Like Zinner and Shapiro (1972), Scharff and Scharff (1987) consider projective identification as ranging from mature and healthy to pathological. Also like Zinner and Shapiro, they focus primarily on pathological aspects of projective identification. With their developmental perspective, however, they expand the implications of projective identification to include its influence over many years as well as to the special significance it might have when the family is going through particular life stages. Thus their approach allows for intervention at the genetic level, the developmental level, and the here-and-now level. In other words, they are able to make an interpretation that involves the current influence of behavior, its meaning with respect to life stages, its buildup over time as reflective of parental needs, and the genetic background of those parental needs. Their hope is that such a complete interpretation allows for near total empathic understanding.

Scharff and Scharff (1987) elaborate briefly on the manifestation of the three basic-assumptions groups posited by Bion. Interestingly, they believe that basic-assumption processes within the family can sometimes support work-group functions, but can at other times interfere with a child's current developmental phase. For example, they note that dependency assumption behavior, meaning the need for a nurturing leader, helps to support a family through a crisis, whereas fight/flight behavior, which requires a leader ready to do battle or plan an escape, supports separation and individuation within, and can defend against attack from outside the family. On the other hand, dependency behavior at a time when separation and individuation are necessary is regressive, as is fight/flight behavior when a family needs to pull together. The idea that basic-assumptions–level interaction can be healthy fits with the idea that projective identification is a natural part of family functioning. It appears that sometimes these authors are equating basic-assumptions functioning with normal defenses and at other times with primitive defenses.

Scharff and Scharff's inclusion of a "fission/fusion" basic assumptions group for families is very interesting in that it accounts, in their view, for psychotic-level functioning in the family. The next excerpt demonstrates their view of this fission/fusion basic-assumptions group.

The threatened family regresses to primitive merging (fusion) or splintering (fission) in order to remain safe. In either case, understanding and progress are blocked. In fusion, merging substitutes for understanding and conflict resolution, whereas in fission, conflict attacks linking and murders understanding. These processes predominate, sometimes in alternation, in psychotic families in response to fear that an integrated experience will lead to annihilation of the self, of the other, and of the family. [p. 134]

Scharff and Scharff (1987) believe that the four categories they use for basic assumptions roughly follow traditional steps in psychosocial functioning. These four basic assumptions follow development from "an early fused stage (fusion) with paranoid-schizoid anxiety (fission) through oral (dependent), anal (fight/flight), and genital (pairing) to oedipal (cooperative work) stages" (p. 135). Therapy aims to bring awareness to these obstacles so that underlying fears can be addressed and work-group functioning can be resumed.

It is not clear how this view of basic assumptions fits with other views. For example, Bion, working with groups, and Zinner and Shapiro, working with families, both employed a Kleinian model where paranoid-schizoid level functioning was equated with the basic assumptions. In the model suggested by Zinner and Shapiro, such primitive-level functioning was the result of overwhelming depressive-level anxieties. Although the fission/fusion category for basic assumptions is a welcome addition, equating each basic assumption with traditional developmental steps does not seem compatible with the original meaning of basic-assumptions groups as discussed by Bion.

Compatibility would require a different meaning for "paranoid-schizoid" than that used in the above excerpt. Perhaps by considering depressive-level functioning as oedipal/cooperative, and all four basic assumptions as paranoid-schizoid levels of functioning, a useful compromise can be reached. It would still be possible, given this scheme, to consider the four basic assumptions as reflective of the traditional psychosocial stages.

The ambiguity raised by the descriptions of Freudian/Ericksonian psychosexual/psychosocial stages and the Kleinian stages has long been debated. Klein's model pushed back the oedipal stage by describing a very similar phenomenon, the depressive position, as developing at the end of the first year of life. The work of Margaret Mahler bearing on this subject has become widely accepted. Her work posits that the sine qua non of entering both the depressive position and the oedipal stage, object constancy, generally occurs around the age of $2^{1}/_{2}$ years. Nevertheless, Klein's (1946, 1948b) model is useful in describing a dichotomy between generally healthy functioning and relatively unhealthy functioning. The traditional psychoanalytic model is also useful in describing particular kinds of fixation. Therefore, an integration of the two is desirable for comprehensive description.

The work of Scharff and Scharff provides a useful extension of previous applications of object relations theory to families. After reading the views of Zinner and Shapiro, one might naturally have wondered about the extension of their views throughout the development of the family. Scharff and Scharff address that issue. Adding to their developmental perspective, and fitting the work of Bion to the family, Scharff and Scharff also develop a new construct, the fusion/fission basic-assumptions group. The addition of the fission/fusion dimension of basic assumptions makes for a much better fit of Bion's theories to family therapy. Authors such as Bowen (1978) and Minuchin (1974) have used constructs like enmeshment and disengagement to describe similar states observed in their work. It is interesting that Scharff and Scharff have attributed this level of functioning to "psychotic" families. Much of the family systems literature developed out of work with schizophrenic families. But the original basic-assumptions groups as envisioned by Bion accounted for a primitive level of functioning among otherwise neurotic group members. It is not clear if Scharff and Scharff are making a similar claim, or if they are referring strictly to very sick families. Certainly the way the terms enmeshment and disengagement are used within family therapy does not always indicate psychotic-level processes. It seems the fusion/fission basic-assumptions group, like other basic-assumptions groups, could be found in otherwise neurotic families. Thus the basic-assumptions concept is useful in understanding family behavior in a way that is compatible with other family theories (like the extended-systems notions of Bowen or the structural ideas of Minuchin).

Samuel Slipp

Slipp has worked toward the integration of family systems with individual psychodynamic therapy since the publication in 1980 of his paper "Interactions Between the Interpersonal in Families and Individual Intrapsychic Dynamics." This effort toward integration is unique among the object relations family therapists. Two essential aspects of Slipp's work will be highlighted here. First, his description of the concept of countertransference is different from that found in other authors' work in that he seems to define it simply as the effect of projective identification on the recipient. In this view, the person experiencing countertransference feelings is not necessarily the therapist, as in most descriptions of that concept. Thus, a transference–countertransference system exists inside the family. Second, Slipp discusses many systems concepts through the framework of object relations theory, making them understandable at intrapsychic as well as interpersonal levels.

Instead of restricting the use of the term countertransference to the therapist, Slipp (1984, 1988) regularly refers to it as it is evoked in any recipient of projective identification. A good example of this can be found in Slipp's (1984) description of the often-used family-therapy concept of triangulation (Bowen 1978). According to Slipp, triangulation occurs through splitting and projective identification, as one person induces a second to act out the all-bad part, and a third to act out the all-good part, of an internalized object. In this way, symptoms within one patient in a family can be seen as the "countertransference reaction" induced by strong projective identification originating within another family member. By applying the word countertransference to any member of a family who has been induced by projective identification to think or behave in a certain way, Slipp becomes able to describe family dynamics using object relations theory in a simpler way than is typical. Instead of using phrases like "the induced behavior in the recipient via projective identification," for example, he is able to say simply "the induced countertransference reaction." This latter phrase implies that projective identification is involved.

Slipp sees family dynamics as largely constructed from projective identification. In his discussion of triangulation, for example, Slipp (1984) describes the family as one entity and compares the results of projective identification to other popular concepts in the field such as "the undifferentiated family ego mass" (Bowen 1978), pseudomutuality (Wynne et al. 1958), and enmeshment (Minuchin 1974). This viewpoint is similar to that of Shapiro and Zinner (1979) as well as to Scharff and Scharff (1987).

But Slipp turns away from those views by defining projective identification in a different way. Slipp (1984) specifically states that his use of projective identification is different than that of Malin and Grotstein (1966) and also of Grotstein (1981). He believes Malin and Grotstein do not differentiate projective identification from projection. In pure projection, however, Slipp asserts that firm ego boundaries are maintained and the interactional influence of projective identification is not included. While in projection the other is "perceived and experienced only in terms of the inner feelings and images that are transferred," with projective identification, he argues, "ego boundaries of the patient must be fluid . . . and pressure is exerted to induce the other to think, feel, or behave in a manner that is congruent with the internalized self or object" (p. 57). Slipp also specifies that "a close, continuing relationship" (p. 57) must exist between the projector and the recipient for projective identification to take place.

As discussed, Slipp defines countertransference in a very liberal way. But his definition of projective identification is very conservative. With the liberal use of the term "countertransference" and the conservative view of the term "projective identification," Slipp clearly defines the patient as projector and the therapist as the recipient of forcefully projected identifications. Although it is difficult to fit Slipp's views on projective identification into the relational systems perspective, his flexible use of the terms *transference* and *countertransference* works nicely in describing family systems.

Slipp's work is also useful in facilitating the application of many psychodynamic concepts in family systems therapy. In his 1984 book, Slipp offers a comprehensive argument for the application of psychodynamic thinking to families. His approach to using countertransference becomes clearer as his general application of psychodynamic concepts is reviewed.

Slipp discusses the move away from psychodynamic thinking in family systems therapy in his critique of the work of Jackson and his followers. According to Slipp (1984), Jackson's move away from psychodynamic thinking, after many years of training as an analyst, is likely to be the result of some animosity. He states: "There undoubtedly were strong feelings involved in this move, because none of his subsequent work contains theoretical constructs derived from psychoanalysis" (p. 33).

At a theoretical level, however, the move away from psychoanalytic thinking was based on the erroneous assumption that psychoanalytic thinking could be equated with libido theory. According to Slipp (1984), Jackson and his colleagues (Watzlawick et al. 1967) believed that Freud's libido theory was mechanistic, representative of linear causality, and constituted a closed system. In other words, according to their view of libido theory, if human energy is regulated through defenses, and ineffective defense mechanisms can only be adjusted by working through early trauma, then ongoing actions and reactions in the here and now are relatively unimportant. Jackson and his followers wanted to intervene in the here and now by exclusively using observable behavior to inform their formulations. They used inductive reasoning (formulations based on observation) as opposed to the deductive reasoning used by Freud to infer the causes of current behavior in past trauma. They wanted to adhere to the notion of circular causality, which takes into account action and reaction in the here and now, as opposed to the linear causality (emphasis on past trauma) they saw in Freud's work.

But Slipp points out that with the development of the repetition compulsion in "Beyond the Pleasure Principle" (1920), Freud's libido theory was much changed. According to Slipp, Freud's concepts of the death instinct and repetition compulsion, which are theoretically conceived as responsible for the perpetuation of psychopathology, can be equated with negative feedback as it is described by Jackson and his colleagues. That is, the death instinct, as the trend toward maintaining the status quo resulting from the fear of change, and the repetition compulsion, as the reliving of past trauma without change, are related to perceiving the environment as negative feedback (through projection or projective identification). A person continuously perceives his environment based on past experience, acts as though the environment cannot change, and thus simultaneously creates new experience that confirms old perceptions and reads new experience as if it were the same as old experience. There is an unconscious desire to confirm old expectations so that life's challenges can be perceived as already mastered, even though the repetition occurs so that unmastered difficulties can be mastered. These concepts can thus be used to describe the often-discussed family systems concept of homeostasis in analytic terms. Families perceive change as threatening even though their difficulties signal that they are basically dysfunctional.

Since Jackson and his colleagues (Watzlawick et al. 1967) looked for a circular, open-systems way of intervening with families, it makes sense that they wanted to drop libido theory. After all, if libido theory were correct, here-and-now interventions would only be effective to the extent that they involved the reworking of old trauma. However, by distancing themselves from psychodynamic thinking, these writers failed to recognize the changes taking place within the psychodynamic literature. Jackson and colleagues, according to Slipp (1984), thus gave up individual development in their formulations. They viewed pathology as existing exclusively in relationships, and especially in the family. Any utility to psychoanalysis was completely denied. He states, "The part played by the patient was also ignored. It was as if the patient were a black box or victim of pathogenic family interaction" (p. 32). However, many of the changes that have occurred in psychoanalytic theory since Freud's introduction of the repetition compulsion in 1920 have moved toward the circularly maintained aspects of psychopathology while retaining individual aspects of the earlier theory.

In referring to the development away from the individual within psychoanalytic thinking, Slipp cites the work of several neo-Freudians and object relations therapists. He points to Adler's (1917) stress on the competitive nature of society and the evolution of the individual's personality out of relationships, Jung's (1927) emphasis on social patterns in culture that influence personality development, and Horney's (1937) idea that cultural forces could corrupt and bury the spontaneous real self of the individual. Slipp (1984) states that Harry Stack Sullivan (1953a) abandoned the linear, mechanistic libido theory and viewed the personality as developing out of interpersonal relations with parents, peers, and the culture. He points out that "some of the theoretical underpinnings of this perspective can be found in general systems theory, cybernetics, communications theory, game theory, field theories, and the behavioral sciences in general" (p. 31). Thus, many psychoanalytic theorists had begun to see the here and now of relationships as an integral component of psychopathology. However, those psychoanalytic theorists who recognize the interpersonal aspect of personality functioning continue to view the development of the personality over time as significant in current relationships and in psychotherapy.

The essential new development for therapy is the belief that a person's current personality functioning can change through a change in current relationships. Object relations theory, and the therapy that goes with it, works from this perspective. Slipp advocates this view and cites the work of Ferenczi, Klein, Bion, Fairbairn, Winnicott, Kohut, and Mahler in supporting it. It is the work of these authors, and the neo-Freudians, that Slipp believes the family therapy movement has largely ignored.

Slipp also remarks on a contradiction inherent in family systems work.

According to Slipp, systems therapists advocate working with families from an open-systems point of view but employ a linear approach in their actual work with families. Jackson's work was largely influenced by Bateson, with whom he founded the Mental Research Institute, where many central family systems concepts were generated. Bateson and Jackson were interested in the work of Whitehead and Russell (1910) on logical types, and that of Wiener (1954) on cybernetics and von Bertalanffy on general systems (1968).

However, while Jackson's description of family functioning was completely consistent with these theories, some of his methods as a therapist contradicted them. For example, Jackson devised interventions with families to create either deviation-amplifying or deviation-correcting feedback. Based on cybernetics, these interventions recognize the family as a system that is either too static or too unstable. Thus the system requires some of the opposite kind of feedback to either help it grow and change or stabilize. Given cybernetic theory the logic is sound, but Jackson's method of bringing about these changes in the family system is epistemologically incorrect. According to Slipp (1984), "In devising these techniques . . . Jackson fell into a linear and dualistic distortion of the use of cybernetics. He viewed the observer as outside the system and considered the observer thus able to manipulate and control the system. According to cybernetics and other modern epistemologies, the observer is part of the system and is affected by its part–whole constraints" (p. 36).

Bateson is known to have criticized the work developed by Jackson and his colleagues, and others like Haley (1976), because that work depends on manipulation as well as power and control. Haley was influenced by the directive approach of Milton Erickson (Erickson and Rossi 1983) who viewed therapy as a power struggle for control by patient and therapist. According to Slipp, Bateson opposed this kind of therapy, especially if it sought legitimacy in modern epistemology. Bateson (1979) considered issues of power as arising from linear epistemology and not from cybernetics. Although the use of influence from within the therapist–family system could be seen as epistemologically correct (from a systemic view), Slipp feels that such interventions rely on pathological behavior similar to that which is already found in the family and that such interventions cannot effect therapeutic change in the long run.

In his 1988 book, Slipp expresses much concern about the way strategic therapists use their position with families. Strategic therapy relies on distrust and control for its paradoxical interventions to work. He likens this position to the dependency basic-assumptions group described by Bion (1959b). In this dependency basic-assumptions group, the family looks to the therapist as the absolute authority on which they depend for a cure. But there is a split-off persecutory perception of the therapist as well. The resultant effect is that the family members both feel that they need the therapist and that they are being forced to do what the therapist demands. The family then often becomes angry at the therapist rather than at the family scapegoat. Sometimes they rebel. As Slipp (1988) puts it, "The very same type of disturbed object relations in the family that contributes to psychopathology is replicated in the treatment situation. In more seriously ill families, dependence on an idealized good maternal object is maintained, while rage is split off, repressed, and displaced onto the patient or spouse, who is demeaned and scapegoated" (p. 154). Thus, although Slipp views strategic therapy as at times effective, he also sees it as worse than failing to help the family.

After discussing the failure of systems theorists to recognize those aspects of psychoanalytic theory that could complement their own work, Slipp describes several family therapy concepts in terms of object relations theory. His most important concept is the "symbiotic survival pattern" (1984). Slipp describes the symbiotic survival pattern in dysfunctional families of all kinds as part of his description of homeostasis. This pattern involves the maintenance of "narcissistic equilibrium" in patients "who have not internalized the mothering function during the separation-individuation phase of early development" (p. 68). Such a person finds others with whom they can become symbiotic, either excessively depending upon them or controlling them, in an effort to sustain emotional balance, self-esteem, or self-cohesion.

Homeostasis is a result of this symbiotic survival pattern. Slipp continues to explain homeostasis, describing its beginnings in the relationship between two parents who rely on primitive defense mechanisms that fit together. When two people meet, they transfer their internal object relations onto one another, each according to his own symbiotic survival pattern, each attempting to reach a state of internal equilibrium through a relationship with the other. Unresolved developmental arrests are not worked through within the coupling, however. Rather, a homeostatic pattern or defensive equilibrium is reached between the pair that, in some compromised fashion, meets the symbiotic needs related to the developmental arrest of each member. "Family homeostasis thus can be explained by the mutual transference–countertransference balance that becomes permanently established between spouses. A form of unconscious collusion occurs that serves as a negative feedback cycle to perpetuate pathological functioning" (p. 69).

Jackson's (1957) views on family homeostasis were derived from the cybernetic theory of Wiener (1954). Wiener's concentration on feedback mechanisms in explaining how behavior was governed by various kinds of communication was a major focus of family systems theory for many years. Applying this theme to families, Jackson viewed them as resisting any change to already existing patterns of communication by way of negative feedback. Negative feedback occurred within the family whenever there was a chance that a change might occur. Scheflen (1968) has even provided a detailed examination of the behavioral cues within families that regulate the intimacy, direction, and speed of interaction. Scheflen used the term "monitoring" to describe behavior that served to warn family members of deviation from rule-governed family action.

Jackson (1957) believed that these concepts, when applied to the family, could explain family pathology. The "identified patient" would become the only bearer of symptoms, which allowed the rest of the family to function relatively easily. While deviation-amplifying techniques could be applied to help the family change its general homeostatic pattern, deviation-correcting techniques could be used to help the family change the function of the identified patient within the family. That is, since this one member of the family helped to maintain homeostasis through problematic behavior, his behavior required the deviation-correcting intervention. The deviation-correction of this one member would serve to amplify deviation away from homeostasis, or the deviation-amplification with the whole family could serve to correct problematic behavior in the one member.

Slipp (1984) discusses triangulation as a particular kind of homeostatic mechanism or symbiotic survival pattern. Triangulation can refer to the identified patient. Slipp believes one of family therapy's most useful contributions is recognition of the movement of attention away from the triangulated family member.

Perhaps the greatest contribution of family therapy has been to re-move focus away from the symptomatology of the identified patient, thereby altering the pathological processes of splitting and projec-tive identification. The patient is only the container for the family pathology, or the manifest expression of more widespread pathology in the family system of interaction. This shift away from the patient, which is in direct opposition to the medical model, tends to neutral-ize the splitting and projective identification, instead of reinforcing these defenses. When the patient is taken out of the role of scapegoat in the family, the countertransference of the patient is profoundly diluted. [p. 71]

Thus, simply by viewing the family system (rather than a single family member) as the container of pathology, the therapist helps the family to-ward intrapsychic as well as interpersonal growth.

Slipp states that the paradoxical intervention furthers this process. By reframing the patient's behavior as positive and necessary, the whole equi-librium or homeostasis set up through projective identification is turned on its head. The paradoxical intervention can even reveal the projective identification. For example, consider a family in which a child is accused of being a lazy irritant by a father who is depressed and angry. It is no-ticed that, if not for the battles waged between them as an outlet for the father's anger, the father either would have to confront his employer and his wife with his complaints or become completely emotionally isolated in his angry depression. In this case, if the son is asked to continue being as lazy and irritating as possible so that the father will not have to become more depressed or have fights with the mother or the employer, the inter-vention reveals the father's projective identification. The son contains the intolerable parts the father projects, and thus allows the father to maintain self-esteem. As Slipp explains, "Once this pathological interaction is re-vealed, it is difficult for the father not to own this aspect of himself. In addition, the patient's self-definition is changed from a negative to a posi-tive one, resulting in enhancement of the patient's self-esteem" (p. 71). Slipp clearly shows how a concept like the paradoxical intervention, which is typically thought of in descriptive terms or in terms of power and con-trol, can be viewed, when seen through the object-relations lens, as re-vealing of intrapsychic as well as interpersonal dynamics.

The Double Bind

Finally, Slipp discusses the double bind, broadening the concept beyond its direct link with schizophrenia. As is true of the other concepts thus far covered, he sees the double bind generally as a manifestation of projective identification. What occurs in the double bind is that one person passes on feelings to another by putting another in an impossible situation. An impossible situation is the essence of the double bind, which has as its main components two contradictory messages, one verbal and one nonverbal (two different logical types). Both of these messages, if not complied with, will result in negative consequences. It is also necessary that the person receiving these messages can neither leave nor comment, actions that might otherwise resolve the paradox she has been put in. In a family situation, the inability to leave or comment is present until the child becomes much older. It is also possible that with projective identification one person attempts to create a situation in which the other person is extremely limited in his responses. The response to which the recipient is limited is congruent with a split-off aspect of the projector (an explanation of the double bind as it relates to projective identification will be more fully considered in Chapter 6).

Slipp (1984) states that the double-bind theory resembles in many respects the theory of the schizophrenogenic mother as described by Fromm-Reichmann (1948). Both of these concepts, of course, developed out of attempts to understand the etiology or maintenance of schizophrenia within the family, with Fromm-Reichmann's formulation of the rejecting mother opposed to Bateson and colleagues' (1956) formulation of the double-binding mother. Perhaps rejection is one possible kind of punishment that could be involved in the double bind. In Slipp's broadened version of the double bind, the application of the term goes beyond schizophrenia. The double bind occurs in families with borderline, narcissistic, hysterical, and depressed members. Slipp's clearest application of the double bind to nonschizophrenic families occurs in some cases of depression. He believes a common theme in these families is the "double bind on achievement" (p. 115).

The double bind on achievement occurs in families in which the child learns that she must achieve to gain approval while at the same time the parents never recognize any of the child's achievements. One example of this type of double bind results in what Slipp (1984) calls the "help-rejecting complainer" (p. 66).

> The help-rejecting complainer comes from a family where he or she was exposed to a "double bind on achievement" during childhood. The patient attempts to satisfy the narcissistic demands of a parent, yet any action taken is not rewarded and is insufficient. As an adult, the patient repeats this process with others, demanding others do something, but what is done is never enough. [p. 66]

The double bind on achievement can be viewed as less severe than what has been said to occur in schizophrenic families, yet the same component parts of the double bind are present.

Projective Identification as the Key to Systems Concepts and the Work of Samuel Slipp

Slipp's work is more integrative than that of other object relations family therapists, and is especially useful in reformulating systems concepts into psychoanalytic language. The key concept in understanding systems theory from the relational systems perspective is projective identification. When projective identification is defined as it has been in this study, to include as essential the recognition of valency in the recipient, it is possible to arrive at a clearer idea of Slipp's specific views on systems concepts.

Slipps' Work and the Therapist in the System

Slipp's combination of a liberal use of the term countertransference and a conservative view of the term projective identification makes for an interesting mixture that is difficult to understand. He advocates a use of countertransference by the therapist, but by definition shelters the therapist from being fully influenced by projective identification. He defines the prerequisites of projective identification as involving a close, continuing relationship as well as fluidity of ego boundaries, although neither is necessarily descriptive of the therapist. The therapist's relationships with family members cannot possibly be as close as their relationships with each other, and the therapist's ego boundaries, although flexible, should not be fluid. Also, Slipp clearly does not consider the concept of valency essential, a position that limits the therapist's role as part of the therapist–family system. In reading his work, one finds that the therapist's part in the therapist–family system seems to be decentralized, and therefore the use of countertransference in his work, although essential, is nevertheless less pervasive than the relational systems perspective would support.

Systems therapists have not fully appreciated the extent to which the therapist becomes part of a system with the family, and that fact makes the introduction of the concept of countertransference essential in bridging the gap between psychoanalytic and systems approaches. Using countertransference requires that the therapist see his part in a system with the family, and makes the fact that he is part of that system useful. No matter what approach a therapist uses, he is affected by the family. The unconscious influence of the family can be intentionally or unintentionally (prereflectively) used by the therapist, and also can become part of the therapist's own countertransference acting out.

Systems work, including structural, strategic, and solution-oriented approaches, would seem to make the therapist especially vulnerable to countertransference acting out owing to the fact that the therapist is not required to observe her own actions or to self-reflect. Although the therapist's prereflective activity can, at times, be either benign or even helpful to the client-family, an awareness and intentional use of countertransference can prevent acting out and harness the power of the therapist's personality to maximum effect.

An intentional use of countertransference requires the therapist to recognize her part in the dynamics of an observer–observed system. Interventions that recognize the therapist–client system would be advocated by theorists like Bateson who believe that the observer cannot be separated from the observed. Because using countertransference can take into account the therapist's part in an observer–observed system, it is a better fit with modern epistemologies (like general systems and cybernetics) than the systems approaches so far devised.

But it would seem wrong to assume that it is epistemologically incorrect for the therapist, as part of a system with the family, to use strategic approaches that require the use of power. Perhaps the important distinction is that one might use perceived power in the perceived battle for control. To the extent that people view the world according to those principles, interventions that depend on them can be effective. The work of Haley, Erikson, and Jackson, as well as many others, has proven effectiveness that can be attributed to an intentional use of influence within systems where influence is very important.

An analysis of such systems methods would show that behaviors that bear great similarity to projective identification are used. However, the influence of these techniques should not be attributed to defensive functioning in the therapist. Rather, the therapist recognizes patterns of projective identification in the family and uses those patterns to formulate interventions that might be efficacious in changing the family. In other words, in strategic therapies the therapist intentionally uses methods that are similar to projective identification.

But such a use of projective identification, as Slipp (1988) points out, relies on the same pathological mechanisms that cause family problems and thus cannot work in the long term with more pathological families. For these methods to work, families with a high level of pathology are likely to rely on the therapist's maintaining a part in the family system. The essential point here, however, is that if the therapist using these techniques connects them to his countertransference reactions, then strategic approaches could be considered an intentional use of countertransference.

In thinking about systemic approaches as involving a use of countertransference, however, it is important to recognize that the therapist who uses these methods is likely to have a valency for power and control or for being the leader of a dependency group. If the therapist were to intentionally use countertransference, he would have to be aware of the way he is pulled into this position as well as of his having the tendency to be pulled in this direction. Of course, strategic therapists do not consider their interventions to be related to countertransference so such awareness is not discussed in the strategic literature.

Slipp's Work and Projective Identification as the Key to Integrating Dynamic and Systems Theories

Just as projective identification can be identified as part of the process of strategic intervention, in the same way it is apparent in Slipp's work (although not specifically stated) that projective identification is the key to understanding systemic concepts in object relations terms. Systems concepts typically describe behavioral phenomena and ignore intrapsychic factors. Projective identification becomes unifying when applied to family therapy concepts because it helps explain observable interpersonal phenomena by connecting them to intrapsychic mechanisms and human emotions. Triangulation and the double bind are two examples of systems concepts that are well explained by the concept of projective identification, and both are identified by Slipp as integrally involved in family homeostasis.

For example, in Slipp's "double bind on achievement," the projective identification involves putting worthlessness into the child by limiting her possible responses. The parent feels as though he must be the greatest to be of any worth at all since his own parents (the grandparents of the child) demanded this. The parent's own lack of parental recognition as a child results in feelings of worthlessness that must be warded off by putting the child in the same situation the parent was in as a child. Like the parent, the child must try to achieve for emotional sustenance, but finds that no achievement is great enough. The child becomes a depressed failure from learning that effort has no efficacy. The parent has been successful in splitting off this bad part and putting it into the child. While the parent has achieved some psychic equilibrium from warding off this bad self-image, he continues to put the child in the double bind because he nevertheless continues to find this part of his self, even when in the child, intolerable.

The child might eventually, maybe not until adulthood, succeed in creating a self-image of success. Yet even this self-image will be false because it will grow out of the same need to please the unpleasable parent and will likely involve the splitting off of the bad self into someone else, which was not an option as a child. Such success does not represent true individuated achievement, which grows from an increasingly differentiated sense of what one likes for oneself. Thus, as an adult, the child is likely to repeat the cycle. The depressed child becomes a success-oriented parent and splits off feelings of worthlessness, finding a home for them in the new family.

It becomes clear in examples like this one that projective identification can, in many respects, be considered a type of double bind and that its recipient is often triangulated as a way of maintaining homeostasis. But if projective identification does constitute a double bind, then therapists who use countertransference should recognize how their countertransference reaction has involved them in becoming the target of a double bind with their clients. The rules of the double bind make this clear. The therapist must be given two different messages, both of which must be complied with if the therapist wants to avoid negative consequences. The therapist must also be viewed as initially unable to leave or comment. But in reality, the component parts of the double-bind situation must take place only in fantasy since the therapist does not truly need to worry about consequences and can leave and can comment. I believe the way therapists do resolve the double bind of projective identification is to comment. Yet the pressure has already been felt. The pressure, when self-reflected upon, informs the comment that will release the therapist from the double bind of projective identification.

And of course it is also essential for therapists to recognize their sensitivity as part of the reason they notice such communication, because the double bind can only take effect when the therapist cares enough about the family or its members to momentarily perceive herself as trapped. The therapist is, by definition, open to helping the client, and thus is very sensitive to what the client communicates as her needs. Moreover, where other people resolve the double bind by leaving, or by acting out in compliance with the limited number of options that are available, the therapist's job is to stay and help, without acting out in deleterious ways. It is both the therapeutic situation and the sensitivity of the therapist that allow for the transmission of projective identification in the therapeutic situation.

Translations from systems theory to object relations theory are common in Slipp's work and are essential in the relational systems perspective. A sharp contrast between Slipp's work and the synthesis I am attempting here, however, can be seen in the definition of projective identification. In Slipp's (1984, 1988) work, the definition of projective identification is very definitely limited. I believe he prefers a narrow definition because it clearly focuses the weight of an interaction on one person, the projector. Thus, in his formulation of transference–countertransference systems among family members, it is always clear who is projecting and who is the recipient. His view of projective identification in the family, while helpful in bridging systems theory and object relations theory, limits the use of countertransference by the therapist because no concept like valency is used to emphasize the extent to which the therapist is part of the projective system. Slipp's emphasis is clearly on not acting out one's feelings toward the family. He believes the pull to do so can be strong but that the therapist should resist that pull. His statements about using countertransference require that the patient be completely responsible for the feelings involved in projective identification. Thus, the interactive nature of a transference–countertransference system, although particularly well discussed by Slipp in reference to relationships between family members, is lost in reference to the relationship between therapist and patient.

SUMMARY : INTRAPSYCHIC
AND INTERPERSONAL SYSTEMS

In this chapter I have presented material pertinent to an integration of psychoanalytic and systems theory. This material is essential to the use of countertransference in family therapy. The importance of empathy within the family therapy movement was reviewed in order to demonstrate that concepts that are closely related to the use of countertransference have been highly valued within the family therapy movement. The section on analytic group therapy covered the work of several authors, from Bion's views on object relations in group therapy through other authors who have described groups as object relations systems. The presentation of object relations family systems led to a discussion of projective identification and its part in families and in family systems concepts.

In the section on analytic group therapy, Bion's work was demonstrated as integral to all current approaches. Bion's (1959b) contributions on projective identification, valency, and the therapist's ability to make use of these interpersonal phenomena through countertransference, were revolutionary concepts for group therapy, and have been elaborated on by other authors. Projective identification has become accepted as a regular part of group process by many authors, who have described it as representing primitive levels of communication that occur even in relatively mentally healthy clients (Ashbach and Schermer 1987, Ganzarain 1977, 1992, Horwitz 1983, Masler 1969). It was also suggested that object relations can be viewed as providing flesh for the systems-approach skeleton (Ganzarain 1977), that boundaries can be described as functioning at various primitive and healthy levels based on developmental personality growth

(Ashbach and Schermer 1987, Ganzarain 1977), and that successful therapy groups evolve into healthier, better-functioning cohesive systems (Ashbach and Schermer 1987). All the authors reviewed contribute to an understanding of how countertransference might be used in family therapy, in which another kind of group, the family group, is influenced by similar properties.

In the section on object relations family systems, Zinner and Shapiro's (1972) concept of delineations was described. Parents use delineations (the behavioral part of projective identification) based on their own pathology or health, thus determining what kind of identifications children will take on. Boundaries between systems were then explained as involving the integrity and role clarity of each system (Shapiro and Zinner 1979). When integrity is not intact, or when role clarity is lacking, boundaries break down and excessive projective identification is more likely to occur. This actuality was shown to be inadequately assessed as applied to the boundary between therapist and family, thus placing a limit on the extent to which boundary concepts have been applied in the use of countertransference. Bion's basic assumptions were also applied to families and were explained as descriptive of progressive developmental levels within the family that are subject to regression under stress (Scharff and Scharff 1987). A transference–countertransference system was discussed as occurring wherever projective identification is successfully used as a defense (Slipp 1984). However, according to that view, the therapist does not necessarily have to be the person who experiences countertransference.

Finally, many systems concepts that grew out of the family therapy literature were explained as being the result of projective identification. I have suggested, based on the writing of Slipp (1984), that projective identification itself could be viewed as a double bind with special circumstances that are not as stringent as the original double-bind theory. That is, with some forms of projective identification, the possible behavioral responses available to the recipient may seem as limited as the recipient's ability to leave or comment. Yet as more behavioral responses become clearly available, or as self-reflection helps to separate the recipient from the projector, projective identification can be used to understand the projector. This relational systems viewpoint requires that the therapist recognize his own valency as part of the projective identification and double-bind phenomenon. Whether or not one perceives that one's options are limited by this double bind depends upon one's valency or desire to be of help in the therapy situation.

6

The Relational Systems Model

INTRODUCTION

The relational systems model is a unified intrapsychic/interpersonal theory of the human mind that combines family systems and psychoanalytic theory in a way that fits the relational systems perspective. Family systems theory has integrated biological and cybernetic models of interpersonal functioning in describing observed behavior in families, but has not explained the intrapsychic system. Psychoanalytic theory, with its offshoots into object relations as well as intersubjective and relational approaches, has provided a detailed, but complicated and diffuse understanding of the intrapsychic system. The relational systems model emphasizes the most relational of the psychoanalytic theories, including object relations and interpersonal approaches, in the attempt to establish a more parsimonious model of intrapsychic functioning that is fully compatible with systems theory. The end result is a systematic theory of intrapsychic and interpersonal functioning that accounts for clinical findings in behavioral and experiential therapies, as well as psychoanalytic and family systems approaches.

From the relational systems perspective, countertransference can only be fully utilized if interpersonal interaction is viewed as a function of groups of intrapsychic systems that impinge upon one another in creating a larger system. What becomes clear in discussing the pertinent psychoanalytic literature, however, is that although there is a presumption that psychoanalytic intrapsychic theory has been systematic enough to be combined with systems theory, that combination has never been clarified. In fact, psychoanalytic theories have not been systematic enough to be integrated with systems theories. The best effort yet, as I have indicated in Chapter 5, is that of Ashbach and Schermer within the realm of group psychotherapy. But even this effort ultimately fails in many respects because it does not address the central difficulties that such integration poses. The model described in this chapter is far more systematic because it does address these difficulties. Special emphasis is placed on the direct connection between intrapsychic and interpersonal equilibrium, but the model also provides a more complete, step-by-step, explanation of how the intrapsychic system fits within interpersonal systems. Within the realm of relational theory, Paul Wachtel (1997) has called for a seamless integration of behavioral and analytic theories. The relational systems model describes a comprehensive latticework for a theory that seamlessly integrates intrapsychic and interpersonal systems.

Intrapsychic and systems models are integrated within the relational systems model by combining the concept of drives from psychoanalysis with the concept of equilibrium from systems theories. The central proposition in the relational systems model is that *emotional life exists as tension and balance*. Intrapsychic tensions result from the individual's effort to live within a community. These tensions cause drivenness and must be balanced so that the individual can maintain intrapsychic equilibrium within the equilibrium of that community. At the surface, the tension that exists between individual and community is clear. For example, laws and rules governing conduct are established to balance the tension between the interests of the individual and those of the community. It is perhaps less obvious that this same tension is integral to the individual personality. Plainly stated, there is no meaning in being an individual without the existence of others to impinge or reflect upon. That we are by default born into a relational world is central to every personality. In other words, not only does life exist in constant tension and balance between individual growth and the community in which the individual lives, but so does its representation within the human psyche. This tension and its balance are so central to the individual personality that they become the very stuff of emotional experience.

In this chapter the relational systems model will be presented as a new perspective on the way tension and balance between individual and community impact the intrapsychic system. This presentation begins with processes of interpersonal influence, explained from a psychoanalytic perspective, and then seeks intrapsychic explanation for such influence. After developing an understanding of the intrapsychic system that is compatible with patterns of interpersonal influence, a diagnostic system revealed by the model will be detailed. Finally, the relational systems model will be placed within family systems theory, thus bringing this presentation full circle to a holistic picture of human interaction.

VALENCY, PROJECTIVE IDENTIFICATION, AND EXTRACTIVE INTROJECTION

If an intrapsychic theory is to be compatible with an interpersonal systems model, then the way the intrapsychic and interpersonal levels of the system interact must be made clear. All of the major relational models for psychotherapy, including Wachtel's (1997) cyclical psychodynamics, Greenberg and Mitchell's (1983, Mitchell 1988) relational-conflict model, and Sullivan's (1953) interpersonal theory, hinge upon the relationship between intrapsychic and interpersonal. Family systems theory, although not focusing on the intrapsychic, has been interested in the pressures behind interpersonal phenomena, and has even demonstrated observable behaviors that appear to have influence (Scheflen 1968, Watzlawick et al. 1967). However, clear connections between intrapsychic processes or forces and the interpersonal forces that are their counterparts have not been emphasized. In this section analytic concepts that describe interpersonal processes will be discussed and the need for an intrapsychic theory that adequately explains these processes will be demonstrated.

Projective Identification

The process involved in projective identification was detailed in Chapter 3. It is so central to the development of the relational systems model that its most important components will be reviewed again here. It was first described by Melanie Klein (1946), and has been described by Ogden

(1979) as "a group of fantasies and accompanying object relations having to do with the ridding of the self of unwanted aspects of the self; the depositing of those unwanted 'parts' into another person; and finally, with the 'recovery' of a modified version of what was extruded" (p. 357). Ogden goes on to explain that "the depositing of those unwanted 'parts' into another person" involves behaving in a way that evokes feelings in the recipient that are similar to those unwanted parts. He also explains that because the recipient as a separate person cannot have the exact same experience as the projector, the depositing of those unwanted parts always results in a modification of what has been projected within the recipient's reaction.

Another way to describe projective identification is as an interpersonal process in which one person, the projector, uncomfortable with experiencing the self in a particular way, behaves in a way that evokes emotions and experience in another. The emotions and experience of the other, the recipient, are similar to those unwanted and uncomfortable emotions avoided by the projector through the interpersonal process. Thus, the projector is allowed to experience the self as relatively free of those emotions, and is able to observe the effects of those emotions on the recipient.

For example, it could be said of the playground bully that he is uncomfortable with feeling extremely vulnerable. The way he avoids that feeling is by intimidating other children. These other children, in turn, do feel intimidated and vulnerable. Their reaction is observed by the bully, who can learn ways of dealing with vulnerability or, as the need may be, continue to use projective identification to avoid the experience.

Although the causal link between behavioral influence and intrapsychic pressures has been presented in a somewhat mystifying manner in the analytic literature, Ogden (1979) has considered it. The first step in projective identification, according to Ogden, "must be understood in terms of wishes to rid oneself of a part of the self either because that part threatens to destroy the self from within, or because one feels that the part is in danger of attack by other aspects of the self and must be safeguarded by being held inside a protective person" (p. 358). According to Ogden then, projective identification occurs because there is an unbearable threat perceived within the self that is associated with a wish to protect parts of the self by projecting threatening or nurturing aspects of the self into others via behavioral pressure. Ogden does not further differentiate the nature of threat to the self that leads to projective identification, and thus the causal link from internal threat to external pressure remains general.

Extractive Introjection

Bollas (1987) has discussed a concept called "extractive introjection," which can be thought of as a subset of projective identification. Extractive introjection is a phenomenon in which a person actively introjects self-representations from others.

> I believe there is a process that can be as destructive as projective identification in its violation of the spirit of mutual relating. Indeed, I am thinking of an intersubjective procedure that is almost exactly its reverse, a process that I propose to call **extractive introjection** [bold lettering in original]. Extractive introjection occurs when one person steals for a certain period of time (from a few seconds or minutes, to a lifetime) an element of another individual's psychic life. Such an intersubjective violence takes place when the violator (henceforth A) automatically assumes that the violated (henceforth B) has no internal experience of the psychic element that A represents. At the moment of this assumption, an act of theft takes place, and B may be temporarily anaesthetized and unable to "gain back" the stolen part of the self. [p. 158]

Bollas goes on to give examples of this phenomenon, which can include the theft of mental content, affective process, mental structure, and theft of self.

Imagine a father who feels inadequate as a man and sets out to work on construction projects in his home with his teenage son. The father gives instructions often, sometimes grabs tools out of his son's hands, and orders his son to fetch things or to make lunch. The teenage son starts feeling inadequate and as though he cannot be trusted to figure out any part of the job. Over time he may even specifically feel that he is inadequate as a man. The father, meanwhile, enjoys working with his teenage son because he feels strong and manly as he demonstrates powerful, manly skills. In this case the father's inadequacies result in the extractive introjection of strength and manliness from his son.

Extractive introjection, like projective identification, involves soothing some threat within the self. Because extractive introjection involves behavior that induces the relinquishment of a part of self, it can be thought of as a subset of projective identification. With extractive introjection, however, the primary goal is to introject, or gain something, rather than to project, or get rid of something. As can be seen in the example above, in many instances, the loss of a part of the self experienced by the victim of extractive introjection leaves the victim with a feeling similar to the one that required soothing in the introjector. Thus extractive introjection and projective identification are similar and complementary processes, and the motivating factor behind both is originally to soothe some uncomfortable feeling. Again, as in the work of Ogden, Bollas does not differentiate the specific threatening experiences within the introjector that lead to the inductive behavioral pressure of extractive introjection.

Valency

Other authors have emphasized an individual's sensitivity or willingness to take on projective identifications, an idea that is equally applicable to an individual allowing others to extract introjections. Bion (1959b) used the term projective identification as it is described by Ogden above, and amplified his description by introducing the term "valency" to suggest the tendency of a person to engage in certain levels of communication, verbal or nonverbal, that have particular kinds of content and emotional qualities. He described valency as the "unconscious function of the gregarious quality in the personality of man" (p. 170). In his view, a person can have "*no* [italics in original] valency only by ceasing to be, as far as mental function is concerned, human" (p. 116).

Bion's use of this term suggests more or less valency in people for specific emotions and behaviors being evoked by specific emotions and behaviors of others. Projective identification and extractive introjection have typically been thought of as extremes of interpersonal influence that suggest a tendency to act in particular ways with others who have some level of valency for engaging in a complementary fashion. But all interpersonal communications involve some level of valency and some level of influence. Not only does the concept of valency include projective identification and extractive introjection, but also the unconscious aspect of every communication. The concept of valency is consistent with this statement made by Sullivan (1962): "No two people have ever talked together in entire freedom of either one from effects of interaction of the other" (pp. 292–293).

The concepts of projective identification and extractive introjection would be considered by most analytic theorists to denote fairly strong behavioral inducements occurring mostly among persons with fairly severe personality pathology. The concepts of projection, introjection, and introjective identification, which are considered far less pathological, also have some level of behavioral inducement associated with them. Malin and Grotstein (1966), however, have suggested that there is always some element of projective identification in every projection or introjection. It has also become not too uncommon for projective identification to be associated with the interpersonal communication of relatively healthy individuals. Bion (1959a,b, 1970) described a "normal" amount of projective identification. Langs (1978) even attributed the use of projective identification to the analyst. Kernberg (1965) described a continuum with regard to the effect of projective identification that suggests greater behavioral inducement associated with worse psychopathology, but that includes some level of inducement even at relatively healthy levels. It could be said that valency of any type or strength, within any interaction, involves some level of both projective identification and extractive introjection as part of the influence of communication.

Although the concepts of projective identification and extractive introjection might often be considered to be related only to severe psychopathology, it is important to note that such emotional communication occurs between all kinds of people, even if little behavioral inducement is involved. Every communication has a set of valences that involve some level of projective identification and extractive introjection. For an intrapsychic theory to be consistent with interpersonal systems theory, it must explain these valences and the pressures behind them. Thus a clear understanding of the causes of valency, projective identification, and extractive introjection must be rendered.

TENSIONS, DRIVES, AFFECTS, AND ATTACHMENTS

The intrapsychic forces that produce valency are accounted for within the relational systems model by the tension between individual growth and the community. This tension is represented within the intrapsychic system in various states of drivenness that are experienced as affects or emotions. Unlike other analytic theories that propose inborn intrapsychic energy sources, the relational systems model does not subscribe to any predisposition within the intrapsychic system for aggressive or libidinal forces. Rather, in the relational systems model, intrapsychic forces are created to the extent that the child is unable to negotiate a state of equilibrium for optimal growth through attachments with others in the community. These forces become stronger, and less well balanced, to the extent that the environment does not provide empathic nurturance of unbalanced states. Emotional understanding allows for rebalancing toward equilibrium, the ideal intrapsychic state for growth.

Some theorists, who also reject the theoretical necessity for inborn intrapsychic sources of energy, have suggested that there is no need to postulate how drivenness is created because all psychic phenomena can be explained by the internalization of interpersonal patterns (Mitchell 1988, Summers 1994). These forces, however, even if not inborn, must be explained if the process of interpersonal influence, or valency, is to be understood in a systematic way. Without such an explanation, it is difficult to deduce how valency is created or where it comes from. If the internalization of interpersonal patterns is to explain valency, then some elucidation of the process by which such interpersonal patterns lead to tension states must be given.

Essential to understanding the force behind valency is the fact that all forms of life grow within a context that variably facilitates or hinders that growth. Winnicott (1965b) has emphasized a similar process, which he called the balance between the "maturational process" and the "facilitating environment." As discussed above, personality growth is one pole in the bipolar system of human life in which the other pole is community. In the relational systems model, the push to grow is recognized as being connected to, and entangled with, community by attachment to others. The newborn infant does not survive without others. He depends on attachments to others for ensuring sustenance and safety. And because of this dependency on attachments for the most basic physiological requirements, the emotions related to attachments quickly become interpreted in terms of sustenance and self-protection. That is, emotions experienced toward others are experienced as various levels of aggression, fear, emptiness, and fullness.

Tension

Experiential tension within the intrapsychic system is a function of the balance maintained between individual growth and community, which is mediated through attachments. When an interpersonal hunger is experienced it creates the need for some kind of social contact. When an interpersonal threat is perceived it creates a need for withdrawal from, or attack on, social contacts. The tension created in this way can be seen as the primary energy source for drivenness within the individual system. Emotional drivenness is the tension created by individual need states as they are experienced within, and specifically concern, the community environment. Interpersonal behavior is the result of the attempt by the intrapsychic system to balance these tensions or need states.

Drives and Affects

By postulating that affects are specifically the result of tension states related to sustenance and self-protection, the relational systems model presents a far more experience-near theory than has previously been offered. The view that the relational world is, at first, interpreted in terms of sustenance and self-protection in the form of affects or emotions (hungers, fears, rages) is quite similar to Kernberg's (1976) view of drives as built from instinctual derivatives themselves built up through self-affect-object connections. However, Kernberg retains the Freudian drives of aggression and libido, a position that makes all human behavior so derivative that it is almost unrecognizable as being related to common experience.

In contrast, the relational systems model associates drivenness with the most commonly experienced motivational states, and recognizes these motivational states as primary components of emotion. Sustenance and self-protection, although physiological necessities, have parallel qualities at a psychological level, where feelings about others have occurred within a context of the objects of attachment who cared for the maintenance of such physiological needs. Affects related to others have a quality that mimics physiological growth needs (sustenance and self-protection) because physiological needs are satisfied within a context of attachment.

It is important to understand that from this view attachment is a drive as strong as the physical needs for sustenance and self-protection. Bowlby's work (1969, 1973, 1975) is absolutely convincing in demonstrating that attachment is as primary as any other physiological force. The child needs the mother for much more than simply sustenance and self-protection. And, in fact, psychological growth, as opposed to physiological growth, is *forever* tied to attachments.

Attachments

Although attachment is just as strong a force as are sustenance and self-protection, in early infancy at a psychological level it is secondary; sustenance and self-protection maintain highest priority because they are most necessary at a physiological level. That is, emotional sustenance fed by affection, and emotional safety maintained by withdrawal or aggression, become primary over the other aspects of attachment. Thus inborn proclivities toward others, such as orientation to the human face, differential treatment of human and nonhuman objects (Lichtenberg 1983, Stern 1985), and interruption of feeding to view visual stimuli without any other tension reduction (White 1963), are not only important by themselves, but also become interpreted, interpersonally, in their relation to getting enough (or too much) of loved ones, and being able to assert the self and be protected within the environment. Nevertheless, emotional experiences of drivenness toward sustenance and self-protection are no less an expression of attachment than these subtle indicators. In fact, it could be said that emotional equivalents of the physiologically experienced need for sustenance and self-protection are the first, and strongest, ways that the drive toward attachment expresses itself.

As issues of psychological sustenance and self-protection become less powerful, that is, as a child gains more confidence that such psychological needs will be met, attachment pushes further into developing relatedness (a more mature attachment) with others. The strength of relatedness, however, is limited by the extent to which the individual infant's perception of self-confidence is developed with respect to the earlier psychological needs of sustenance and self-protection. One can think about the importance of emotional sustenance and self-protection as being the psychic equivalent of their physiological analogs. The inability to maintain confidence in psychological sustenance and self-protection is perceived as having life-or-death consequences at an emotional level, just as physiological sustenance and self-protection truly do have life-or-death consequences at the physical level.

When there is confidence that psychological sustenance and self-protection will be maintained, however, the individual becomes better able to tolerate more complicated concerns, such as the needs of others. Certainly when an individual has confidence that physiological sustenance and self-protection will be maintained, the kinds of activities which can be engaged in become more varied. Similarly, the same confidence at a psychological level makes interpersonal possibilities more varied, richer, and deeper.

The Optimal Growth Pattern

Ultimately, the outcome of the negotiation of growth needs through attachments is an optimal growth pattern, given systemic circumstances that include genetic endowment (physiological capacities and requirements) and community standards, capacities, and requirements (with the community here connoting parental, sibling, or larger groups within the larger community of the world). An individual develops more or less confidence that psychological sustenance and self-protection will be maintained, and more or less maturity in interpersonal functioning based on that confidence. Style or personality represents the self that has been negotiated, beginning with genetic endowment and then as shaped by the necessities of growth within the given environment. This optimal growth pattern, is most influenced by early relationships, however, because those relationships are part of a context in which the individual is completely dependent, and is only slowly able to grow more independently.

By its very nature this optimal growth pattern continues to function in new relationships as though they were similar to the relationships in which it was originally developed. The pattern develops for the purpose of growing within a particular kind of environment. To the extent that the ongoing environment is perceived as similar to the environment from which the individual originated, the individual can be confident that sustenance and safety will be maintained by the same behaviors, thoughts, and feelings that maintained him within the original environment.

Dysfunctional patterns and symptoms that eventually necessitate therapeutic intervention are thus caused by an early adaptation to an environment that no longer exists, but continues, in many respects, to be projected upon the world because the individual knows how to deal with that particular kind of environment. In other words, patterns of motivation, or drivenness, emotional hungers, and patterns of consumption, as well as aspects of the patterns in the interpersonal environment that anger or frighten, are all part of an optimal growth pattern developed for the specific purpose of maximal growth of an individual infant with a specific genetic endowment born into a particular environment. As that environment changes, however, and because the personality was largely developed within a stage of dependence when psychological sustenance and self-protection were fundamentally attached to their physiological counterparts, the optimal growth pattern does not change accordingly. The threat of experiencing emotional pain (seemingly equal to the threat of death) while in this infantile state of dependence is so great that the original optimal growth pattern is very resistant to new perceptions and new behaviors. New ways seem to signal a vulnerability to those emotions for which the optimal growth pattern has provided needed defenses.

THE THREE CONTINUA

The tensions between individual growth and the community are expressed within the personality in three primary ways, only the first two of which were emphasized in the section above. The first two are, as discussed above, sustenance and self-protection. The third is relatedness, a quality that develops as greater and greater confidence in sustenance and self-protection can be maintained. These three kinds of tension can be conceptualized as three intersecting continua (see Figure 6–1). The x and y axes in Figure 6–1 represent the Sustenance and Self-protection continua, considered in the relational systems model to be the first two issues through which attachment expresses itself most forcefully. These continua are represented

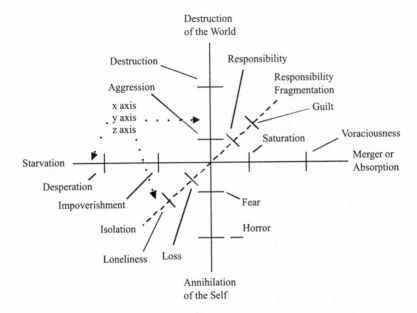

Figure 6-1.
A three-dimensional rendering of the three continua intersecting. Paranoid-schizoid mechanisms deal with issues related to the x (Sustenance) and y (Self-protection) axes, while the z (Relatedness) axis deals with issues of the depressive position. The extent to which x and y are worked through is what determines the extent to which relatedness can develop in a healthy way and the extent to which repression, as opposed to splitting, is used as a defense. Repression is the defense most prominent in protecting the self from the perception of danger to relatedness as opposed to danger to existence. The center intersection of the three continua represents emotional confidence. On the x axis such confidence, or balance, is characterized by satiation, on the y axis calm focus, and on the z axis relational interdependence.

as orthogonal for the purpose of demonstrating their separation from each other as separate factors of growth, and because it is useful in discussing the balance of the three continua in relation to each other. Additionally, as will be seen in the section entitled Diagnostics (page 328), presenting the axes in this way also elucidates the diagnosis of personality functioning. The three axes will be discussed separately at first, and then in relationship to each other.

The x axis, representing Sustenance, reveals the commonly experienced emotions that correspond to the extreme of hunger and its opposite, voracious consumption. As can be seen, desperation, impoverishment, saturation, and voraciousness are plotted on the x axis between starvation and merger/absorption, all of which represent various levels of need or maintenance of sustenance. The concept that fits the Sustenance continuum at its center is satiation. Sustenance in life is clearly necessary for growth, and the theory postulates that these physiological states are symbolized in psychophysiological states that are affects or emotions experienced as levels of emotional hunger and emotional consumption. Hunger and consumption are at all times in a state of tension that is variably well-balanced, depending upon the individual's ability to get these needs met within a particular environment.

The y axis, representing Self-protection, reveals the commonly experienced affects from the extreme of aggression to its opposite, extreme fear (more commonly referred to as "fight or flight"). As can be seen, horror, anxiety, aggression, and destruction are planted between annihilation of the self and destruction of the world. These concepts are seen as representing varyingly powerful degrees of the fight-or-flight phenomenon. At the center of the y axis is calm focus. Self-protection in life, like the need for sustenance, is also clearly necessary for growth. The theory postulates that these physiological states are symbolized psychophysiologically as the emotions anger and fear. Just as hunger and consumption are in a constant state of tension, the relational systems model postulates that anger and fear, too, are constantly in a state of tension that is variably well-balanced.

The z axis is postulated by the theory to be relatively undeveloped in its nascent state. At that point it represents only attachment. It develops into Relatedness as the issues of the other two axes become better resolved. At birth, the z axis, representing relatedness, is experienced as life or death, in that lack of attachment literally would result in death, while attachment holds the promise of life. Only with attachment are self-protection and sustenance possible at birth, and thus, although the issues of those two axes separate themselves from the general push toward growth, that push is by necessity permanently linked to attachment. Since the development of the continuum from attachment into relatedness requires that the issues of sustenance and self-protection be relatively resolved, full discussion of the z axis will be delayed until the workings of the x and y axes can be more fully examined. However, as with the x and y axes, the z axis is a continuum of affective experiences. It is bounded by isolation at one end and responsibility fragmentation at the other. Loneliness, loss, responsibility, and guilt fall between the extremes; a balanced state, represented by the concept of relational interdependence (the ability to be both independent and related simultaneously) is at the center of the continuum.

As Figure 6–1 suggests, within the relational systems model the tension between individual and community is manifested in every part of the personality, thus indicating that there can be no meaningful way of differentiating whether social context or individual endowment (drive, instinct, temperament, and so on) is most important in understanding intrapsychic psychological functioning. Community and individual are inescapably intertwined within the deepest and most central parts of the psyche. That connection is so central that the original connection between death and physiological sustenance or self-protection is, at the extremes, connected to psychological sustenance and self-protection. The threats to sustenance and self-protection at the psychological level, however, are not life-or-death threats to existence but are, rather, threats to interpersonal existence.

At the ends of the x and y axes, these threats to interpersonal existence drive the emotional states corresponding to issues of sustenance and self-protection. Starvation represents starvation from others. Merger or absorption represents the complete enmeshment of the individual due to extreme consumption that causes such an obliteration of boundaries that the self no longer exists as a separate entity. Annihilation of self, resulting from extreme fear and avoidance of others, at its extreme threatens the self with complete disappearance from existence. Destruction of the world resulting from extremes of aggression ultimately threatens an end to a world within which to exist. All of these extremes, at the emotional level, involve the experience of the individual's existence among others.

These kinds of threats have been described within psychoanalytic object relations theory since its inception. Melanie Klein (1935, 1948b) believed an aggressive drive gave rise to "annihilation" and "persecutory anxiety." Kohut (1971, 1984) described "disintegration anxiety" arising from his "principle of the primacy of self-preservation," which is that protection of the self has the greatest motivational power and threats to the self will result in extreme reactions. Winnicott believed all anxiety is experienced as "annihilation anxiety" when the child's lack of a self makes anxiety completely unmanageable and the sense of existence uncertain. Schafer (1978) described a "devouring engulfment" or "annihilation" that occurs in relation to the caretaking of the powerful mother. Fairbairn (1941) and Guntrip (1969) described the fear of destroying the mother with one's hunger.

All of these theorists described such threats as motivating particular orientations to others. But these threats have never been differentiated in a way that adequately describes the many facets of the intrapsychic system. In the relational systems model, issues of merger and absorption and their opposite, which is sustained emotional starvation (consistent with the theories of Fairbairn and Guntrip), are separated from issues of destruction of others and their opposite, which is annihilation of the self (more consistent with the Kleinian model). By separating these issues, the relational systems model becomes descriptive of all kinds of pathology that combine the two issues to varying extents. The model also captures a more comprehensive understanding of the human psyche.

As suggested above, it is the normal need states, as represented on the x and y axes, that create interpersonal drivenness. The push to "consume" another, or "desire," which leads to sustenance of emotional growth, is created by the threat of emotional starvation. The push toward aggression, for the purpose of protecting growth, is created by the threat of annihilation. Thus what is called "drive" in the Freudian model is further elaborated in the relational systems model. That is, in the Freudian model drives are considered innate, while in the relational systems model what is considered innate is the push toward growth and attachment to others. Psychological emotions are part and parcel of physiological needs and both require connection to others. Because that push is threatened by the threat to social existence, energy is created in the form of tension. That tension can be relieved by driven behavior that sustains and protects emotional growth and equilibrium.

The three continua in Figure 6–1 represent the three primary ways in which the tension between individual growth and the interpersonal community manifests itself. Each continuum itself represents a kind of tension. These tensions combine in various ways to create interpersonal drivenness in which desires are sated and fears are avenged. Emotional growth occurs chiefly in balanced states. When the three continua are more balanced—that is, when the emotional state of an individual falls somewhere toward the middle of them—equilibrium leads to the ideal state for emotional growth.

THE OPPOSITION OF SPLITTING AND EQUILIBRIUM

The concept of splitting is used in many ways in analytic theory. Originally it described a process by which negative or bad parts of the self or bad identifications with others are kept separate from good parts of the self or identifications with others (Klein 1935, 1948b, Fairbairn 1941, 1943, 1946). In other words, splitting was originally a concept that described how the personality attempted to maintain self-esteem. In the Kleinian version, goodness within could be attacked by badness within, or the aggressive drive. In Fairbairn's version, goodness within could be attacked by bad identifications from without. Splitting resulted within the personality for the purpose of protecting the integrity of the self. As a consequence of splitting, aspects of self would be projected upon the world, either to safeguard good parts in someone else or to rid the self of bad parts. That is the process known as projective identification. Extractive introjection could also be thought of as serving these purposes.

The concept of splitting has been extrapolated to very observable behavioral processes. One example is the cycling from idealization to devaluation in relationships, a process that some people utilize to boost self worth and then to de-emphasize the importance of another when that other no longer supplies needed reassurance. Another example is the interpersonal process in which personality triangles are created by the projection of good qualities into one person and bad qualities into another, thus externalizing a conflict between positive and negative parts within the projector's personality. A final example is the observed tendency within the personality to protect against fears by manifesting the opposite qualities at the surface, a process by which those fears are reduced and others in the environment are more likely to experience them (as with the bully who masks feelings of vulnerability with aggressiveness). It is clear from clinical observation that splitting does occur within the personality. That is, people are often unaware of aspects of themselves that seem to have a strong influence on their personalities and their behavior.

Although the fact that splitting occurs within the personality is quite clear, the causes of splitting are not so clear. The relational systems model is very different from other relational theories in its view of splitting. For example, in the relational systems model, there is no "good object" that is threatened by "bad objects." In the Kleinian model (1935, 1948b), the positive force of libido, or the "good object" is not initially strong enough to compensate for the destructiveness of the aggressive drive (or death instinct), both of which exist within the child. According to that model, when the "good object" is threatened by "bad objects" (parts of the self accreted from aggressive drive derivatives), "splitting" occurs so that threatening objects will not damage the "good object." Although Fairbairn did not believe bad objects originated from within the personality he nevertheless believed splitting occurred so that bad object identifications could be separated from the positive forces of libido. Klein believed the "good object" had to be built up through good experience and, similarly, Fairbairn viewed positive experience as the key to healthy development. When this buildup is accomplished, splitting (and thus projective identification, which is initiated in splitting) is no longer necessary. This line of reasoning, that splitting is necessary to separate the "good object" from "bad objects" or bad experience, is common in object relations theory (where the good object within connotes a feeling of self-worth and self identity built up over time). The relational systems model also recognizes, and even emphasizes, that splitting occurs within the personality, but differs in its view of why splitting occurs.

Splitting in the Relational Systems Model

In the relational systems model, the concept of "splitting" is used to describe what happens within the individual psyche when it cannot tolerate an extreme affect or perceived threat to interpersonal existence. When a person is threatened by the experiential extremes of any of the continua described above, that threat must be split off and projected while other elements of the environment are extracted to bolster a sense that the threat is not so great. For example, if a person's anger is so immense that she wants to destroy her interpersonal world, the consequent threat to her interpersonal existence will cause a split in the personality. Destructiveness will be split off and projected upon others, or onto the environment, and her feeling state will be mostly fearful and possibly paranoid. To some extent others in the environment will feel the projection of destructiveness and may act upon it while at the same time their own fears and paranoia will likely be projected into the paranoid person. Again, these are the processes of valency, projective identification, and extractive introjection as described above. The initial stage of these processes is a splitting of experience caused by the perception of extreme threat within the personality. This process resembles the way projective identification is initiated in other models but is quite different with respect to the rationale for it.

Other theories have difficulty explaining interpersonal processes due to a focus on the intrapsychic level of functioning without proper regard to interpersonal influences. That interpersonal phenomena lead to the maintenance of personality problems in the individual and the passing on of further personality problems in offspring is accepted in analytic theory. However, no clear language exists within analytic theory for the way these interpersonal processes occur. The "good object" within the individual, and its vicissitudes, do not clearly explain the process by which protection of the good object leads to various kinds of personality formation within others. The need for intrapsychic and interpersonal equilibrium, a concept more in keeping with systems theory, does explain this phenomenon. Although most object relations thinkers believe their theory explains interpersonal phenomena, connections are rarely made, and when they are, they are cumbersome.

The problem posed by the intrapsychic system, as seen from the perspective of the relational systems model, is that the outcome of the processes of valency—that is, splitting and the projective processes it requires—leads to interpersonal equilibrium and the perception of intrapsychic equilibrium, but not to balance or true equilibrium within the intrapsychic system. When an individual splits off a threatening aspect of experience he in effect balances some exaggerated aspect of intrapsychic experience by limiting his experience to only oppositely exaggerated experiences. He interacts with his environment in such a way that interpersonal equilibrium is accomplished. Between him and his environment destructiveness finds fear, or starvation finds voraciousness, and there is

a kind of interpersonal order. But all individuals so involved are unbalanced at an intrapsychic level. They feel balanced, but this sensation
only occurs as a result of the interpersonal interaction. The intrapsychic
system thus requires the interpersonal system for maintenance of equilibrium and growth. Without others with whom to balance the self, an individual who happens to require an extreme amount of projective
and introjective processes cannot function. This person will always
seek out relationships that allow for the sensation of balance. Others
will be engaged who react in the most complementary ways, with their
own projections and needs for introjection. At an intrapsychic level,
these others will be equally as needy and as unbalanced as the projector.
These interpersonal patterns become the optimal growth pattern of the personality, created for the specific purpose of adaptation to a particular social environment, even though they do not lead to optimal intrapsychic
growth.

Equilibrium and Intrapsychic Growth

In the relational systems model, intrapsychic growth is most suited to intrapsychic equilibrium. The closer an experience comes to supporting
growth and equilibrium the more likely it will be sought and will be pleasurable. Equilibrium is sought in sexuality, which in an emotional sense
involves all three continua: sustenance or desire and merger, self-protection or aggressiveness and masochism, and relatedness or issues of intimacy. It takes the form of "effectance" (one of Greenberg's [1991] drives)
in that the hunger for an activity or an accomplishment requires assertion
and is satisfying, but when the activity no longer satisfies the individual,
and is pushed upon him, it can interfere with growth. Equilibrium as the
primary expression and requirement of growth is also consistent with the
approach to pleasurable experience and the avoidance of painful experience, in that pleasurable activities are perceived as supporting growth and
balance whereas painful experiences are perceived as detracting from
growth and pushing the individual away from equilibrium.

In the relational systems model splitting does not occur to protect the "good object," but because threats to interpersonal existence (the opposite of growth and equilibrium) require drastic measures at the level of affect. Where absorption or merger is threatened, an inner starvation, with associated disconnection from emotion, is sustained in an effort to maintain intrapsychic balance. Where starvation or abandonment is threatened an inner voraciousness or controlling nature is sustained for the sake of equilibrium. Likewise, with respect to the self-protection continuum, where annihilation or death is threatened, a desire to destroy is sustained for equilibrium, and where the possibility of destroying others is threatened a fearful or masochistic tendency is sustained. In the relational systems model, splitting occurs as a way of protecting a sense of equilibrium in an interpersonal world that is perceived to be out of balance, due to lack of balance at the intrapsychic level. The part of the self that leads the individual to feel threatened is driven out of experience to avoid destruction, absorption, annihilation, or starvation, which threaten equilibrium. Likewise there is an attempt to extract from the environment those experiences that will soothe these threats to interpersonal existence.

But in this splitting process, interpersonal relations that would reaffirm the safety of the self are not allowed into experience. When a threatening aspect of self has been split off and projected, it is unlikely that soothing aspects of the environment will be perceived, since the intrapsychic threat requires immediate proof that the threat is not within the self. Such proof can only come in the form of seeing that threat within the environment. Others must be seen as depleted to confirm that the self is full, and only others who recognize fullness in the individual will be recognized as having worth. Situations cannot be experienced as merely good but must be great to compensate for feelings of emptiness. Fear seems to require immediate aggression, and makes fear an emotion that exclusively exists in others. One cannot view the self as having some influence on an outcome but must experience complete control. There can be no delayed gratification but only immediate elimination of threats or satisfaction of urges. When others behave in ways that would suggest anything other than what has been projected, that behavior is not noticed or is misconstrued because the need to confirm what has been projected is so strong.

The Role of Defenses

Such defenses tend to create a self-fulfilling prophecy as others tend to react against strong tendencies. For example, if a person controls others because the fear of being abandoned or starved is too great, the other who is being controlled will eventually need to leave for the sake of maintaining her self-identity, or will hide so much of her personality from the controller that the control being applied is rendered useless. A person who tries to avoid aggression behaves fearfully and is targeted as a victim for aggression or through paranoia accuses others so much that they do begin to think negatively and thus confirm the paranoid's suspicions. Persons who behave responsibly at all times for fear of becoming isolated from others become so wrapped up in doing the right thing and being perfect that they become unable to become close to anyone. Exaggerated responses seem necessary to regain some semblance of equilibrium within the human personality system, but bring only ephemeral relief, exclusively at the interpersonal level, while exacerbating long-term threats to intrapsychic growth and equilibrium. By projecting what threatens the self, the individual avoids the pain associated with recognizing his own tendencies but also misses the opportunity to integrate, or adapt to, that aspect of the self, making its projection all the more necessary.

When the threats to existence that are portrayed by the ends of the Sustenance and Self-protection continua are tempered, as in the relatively healthy personality that is typically near a state of equilibrium, some level of psychological drivenness is nevertheless created. When a person feels the need or hunger for interpersonal contact, that contact is sought. When another person feels crowded by others she might become actively self-sufficient. When one person feels afraid, he might avoid the feared other. When he feels angry, aggressive behavior might be expected. However, when an individual's experience approaches the extremes of these affects, either extreme discomfort must be sustained within, and the person must introject an aspect of the environment that seems to reduce the threat, or the person must rid herself of the unwanted discomfort. Splitting and its consequent projective and introjective processes, or interpersonal communications, are caused by these threats to existence.

Communication and Equilibrium

It is interesting that although the splitting caused by threats to interpersonal existence produces communication that only briefly leads to states of equilibrium, such communication also provides the only clue to what is needed by the intrapsychic system to reach more fruitful states of equilibrium. When threatening affects are projected and soothing affects introjected, others will experience the state that is so uncomfortable that it requires such drastic measures. As mentioned above, others typically respond to such feelings with defensiveness that leads the projector to confirm by observation that what he has projected truly exists in reality. The projector need not recognize the projected feelings within the self.

A healthier equilibrium, however, can occur when others act with understanding of the projected feelings or need for introjection. Communication that recognizes such discomfort within the projector and attempts to soothe that discomfort while reifying interpersonal existence can make the projector less in need of splitting and more likely to enact a more balanced state of equilibrium. In the case of the paranoid, for example, if he can be in the presence of someone with whom it is okay to have destructive feelings, someone whose concern for him is clearly not destroyed by those destructive feelings, then it becomes possible for the paranoid's existence to be less threatened by his own destructive wishes. He will be less in need of projecting those wishes upon others and less likely to introject fearfulness. In more healthy situations such a process occurs between parents and their children from birth, thus making splitting less necessary and healthy states of equilibrium more common. When splitting is prominent in the personality of an adult, however, special therapeutic relationships are required to effect such change.

Infantile dependence, in fact, plays a powerful role in personality formation but in such a way that personality becomes particularly attuned to the reality of the infantile environment. Aggression in the environment, for example, leads to an intrapsychic system that is likely to perceive the world as aggressive later in life and thus balance itself in other interpersonal situations in a way that corrects for aggression in the environment. In the Kleinian (1937, 1948b) model, the infant's inborn out-of-balance instincts must be tamed by good experience in the interpersonal world. With such a view, if a patient perceives the world to be aggressive, it could merely be the projection of his own aggression that was never tamed. In a Fairbairnian model, aggression results from introjection of "bad objects," and there is no explanation of drivenness outside of object-seeking, making for vague explanations for the power behind the projective process. In the relational systems model, the infant's tenuous connection to interpersonal existence and its balance therein must be made secure. From this perspective, if a patient perceives the world to be aggressive, then somewhere in the past his connection to interpersonal existence was either threatened by aggression or by the inability of the environment to make him secure despite his reaction to fear with destructive behavior.

With respect to the issues of splitting and equilibrium, the important difference between the relational systems model and other relational theories is the extent to which intrapsychic balance is determined by, or depends upon, interpersonal systems. In the relational systems model, equilibrium of the intrapsychic system is always connected to interpersonal systems or to the individual's perception of them. Accordingly, when interpersonal existence is threatened to a significant degree, so that intrapsychic equilibrium is lost and the consequent emotional experience is intolerable, splitting occurs to reinforce intrapsychic equilibrium within a perceived interpersonal environment that has its own patterns of equilibrium, and not to protect one aspect of self from another. Splitting, although seemingly at odds with intrapsychic equilibrium, actually gets its power from the need to maintain intrapsychic equilibrium within a larger system that is perceived by the intrapsychic system to be out of balance.

AFFECT CONTINUA AND REPRESENTATIONS

In the past sections I have discussed a new model for understanding intrapsychic functioning. However, the original goal, to provide an explanation of the way unconscious influences are created by the intrapsychic system, requires further understanding of intrapsychic phenomena before the projective and introjective processes can be fully understood at the behavioral level. Although the intrapsychic pressures that lead to projective and introjective processes have been identified, both the way those pressures are expressed, and the way their expression leads to influence of others must be elucidated. Clarification of this process will require a discussion of (1) the manner in which emotions are stored in the mind, (2) the discrete periods of interpersonal development that determine emotional growth, and (3) the way interpersonal boundaries are developed in order to define which environmental phenomena are identified as threatening.

Affective Role-Representations

In the relational systems model, memory for human relationships is coded within the intrapsychic system in the form of complementary roles between self and others. Affectively charged roles are projected or introjected by an individual in order to soothe threats to existence. These role-representations (the concept of role-responsiveness, a very similar idea, can be attributed to Sandler [1976]; the concepts of object- and self-representations originated in Jacobson [1964]) are connected affectively by the emotional experience that was most prominent at the time of the interaction. This formulation is in basic agreement with Kernberg (1976), who proposed that object relations units consisting of self and object images connected by affects are stored as affective memory. Because emotions are experienced along various continua in the relational systems model, however, it is the continua, as opposed to one single affect as was proposed by Kernberg, that connect roles. (Also, Kernberg would not agree with the use of the word "role" in such a general sense, since he uses that term only when a person has developed the ability to identify with others. The term is used here, however, only to suggest that the self is always in relation to others.)

Projective and introjective identification are utilized to form role-representations of relationships that build up over time, either allowing for balance within the personality (through integration at a point of equilibrium when these processes can be soothed by empathic parenting), or creating a cycle of compensation for threatening affects (making integration difficult). As suggested above, interactions with others are represented within the personality as though there were a pair of roles attached to a continuum of possible and opposing affects, with one of these roles perceived to be part of the self and the opposing one considered to be part of another. Perception of these roles is used by the individual personality to create a sense of relative equilibrium so that one feels emotionally protected from threats perceived outside the self. Sullivan (1954) would have referred to these roles as "illusory me–you patterns." In describing the relational systems model these representations will henceforth be referred to as *affective role-representations.*

Part-Representations

The two roles attached by any particular affective continuum can be referred to as part-self and part-object representations (thus differentiating them from the concept of "role" Kernberg [1976] discusses, which requires identification and thus integration of part-self and part-object). A part-self representation is maintained within and remains as the portion of the affective role-representation that is most comfortable to the individual. A part-object representation is perceived as though it is within another person because to maintain it within the self would be perceived as threatening to the projector's existence.

To the extent that projection of the most threatening role allows the individual to regain a sense of equilibrium, the individual will experience some level of attunement within. It is the projection of very threatening roles and the consequent rebalancing of the projector that has led clinicians to the belief that a good object is protected by projective and introjective processes. In fact, as discussed above, the consequence of splitting and projection is rebalancing, which allows one to feel better by comparison to what one is projecting into others. It is not a good object that is built up within, but rather more and more confidence in one's ability to balance inner affects.

The fact that those roles that are projected are the ones most difficult to maintain within the self should not lead to the misconception that only nonthreatening part-representations are maintained within the personality system. Rather, the most threatening of two threatening affective experiences is perceived as outside the self. The role that is projected might be kindness, for example, if maintaining that role within makes the projector feel vulnerable. The opposing role of harshness or malevolence might make such a person more comfortable and slightly more balanced.

In terms of projective and introjective identification, the most feared affect in an affective role-representation is made part of the role that is projected. For example, when a child experiences a parent as angry and feels scared, a dual role-representation develops with the self-protection continuum covering the range of associated affects. While the child is still young the most threatening affect is anger which, if unleashed, could lead to very real physical consequences from, or a severing of the child's primary attachment to, the angry parent. Thus the child maintains the role of fear while the parent maintains anger.

To the extent that such a relationship was a typical interaction in the child's life, the affective role-representation remains intact. Later, in other circumstances in which fear is the more intolerable affect, fear is projected while anger is maintained. This turnabout can occur when others are perceived to have less potential for damaging the individual, either via the existence of a mutual relationship or through more direct negative action. To the extent that fear becomes intolerable in this individual, aggressive behavior will be expected, and it could be said that such an individual introjects aggressiveness and the role of the aggressor, while projecting fear and the role of victim. Thus, it can be seen that the affective role-representation consists of two roles and a connecting affect. Which of the two roles will be identified with at a particular time depends on which role is more threatening to individual integrity or interpersonal existence.

Although this example is demonstrative of the self-protection continuum, the sustenance and relatedness continua work similarly. Typically, an affective role-representation hinges upon a continuum that is some combination of the three axes, making for a vast array of possible affect continua. Such an affective continuum can be pictured as a line drawn through the center of Figure 6–1, with one end that has x, y, and z coordinates and another end that has -x, -y, and -z coordinates. The nature of the particular combination accounts for what role is projected or introjected based upon which end of the continuum or which affect is most threatening to the experiencing individual. Integration results from there being such a large number of combinations, with most of them reflecting experience that soothed (or failed to corroborate) apparent threats to existence, that a great number of possible role-representations have been developed for every situation.

There tends to be a dominant and stable affective role-representation given an individual's perception of any situation (Greenberg's [1991] view of the wish as the self, an object, and an interactional field has many similarities to this view of the way affective role-representations are evoked). To the degree that all affective role-representations are balanced, however, the individual allows the situation, to ever greater and greater extents as greater integration occurs, to unfold without prejudging. The more integrated the personality, the more accurate is the individual's perception of reality.

It is also important to note that, with maturation, as affects become less threatening, the nature of projective and introjective identification changes along with the nature of affective role-representations. As an individual learns that threats do not lead to annihilation, destruction, starvation, or merger/absorption, the need to rid the self of threats becomes less powerful. The part-selves and part-objects are less exaggerated and can be thought of as closer to the center of whatever affective continuum holds them together. Projective and introjective identification become less powerful at a behavioral level as it becomes less essential to the individual that others in the environment behave exactly according to the individual's needs. The continua that depict healthier and more integrated emotions are then shorter because threats have been soothed and no longer hold as much power within the personality system (existential threats do not reach the level of severity represented at the ends of the continua and states of equilibrium are more likely). This level of maturation will be explored in more detail in sections to come. The process of development from lesser to greater integration of roles can be explained through a discussion of the paranoid-schizoid and depressive positions.

THE PARANOID-SCHIZOID POSITION IN DEVELOPMENT

The description of the paranoid-schizoid and depressive positions found throughout object relations theory, which originates in the work of Klein (1935, 1940, 1946) and R. W. D. Fairbairn (1941, 1943, 1946), provides a brilliant outline for individual development within the relational systems model. A projective-introjective cycle begins in the earliest stages of life. In Klein's view (1948a) this cycle occurs for the purpose of protecting the libidinal "good object" from aggressive, inborn, "bad objects." According to Klein, projection offers the first and most dependable mechanism for such protection. After projection the infant introjects what is perceived as reality. To the extent that reality changes the infant's perception from what was projected, the infant's projections must change. If, over time, what is introjected is in fact less dangerous than what has been projected integration occurs, as inner "bad objects" lose some of their power in comparison with the strengthening of "good objects."

Fairbairn (1941) and Guntrip (1969) discussed a similar cycle that is initiated for different reasons. These authors emphasized the developmental need for connection with others that can take the form of extreme voracious hunger and have a tendency to push the infant into a wish to devour. The basic formulation of these theorists with respect to schizoid tendencies is that the infant can desire to devour his objects so strongly, that is, he can desire to merge with them so much, that he becomes afraid he will destroy them in the process. As Fairbairn (1941) might put it, the dilemma is "how to love without destroying by love" (p. 271). The consequent compensation is to withdraw from objects in order to preserve them, but to leave the self empty and hungry. Such compensation can be decreasingly necessary as through development the child learns that the desire for merger does not, in fact, lead to destruction of the object. These aggressive and merger tendencies, and their associated processes, have become known as the paranoid-schizoid position.

Klein, Fairbairn, Guntrip, and the Relational Systems Model

A central discrepancy between the work of Klein, on one hand, and Fairbairn and Guntrip on the other, is that for Klein the projective-introjective cycle is the result of the need to protect the "good object" from inborn aggressiveness, whereas for Fairbairn and Guntrip this cycle occurs as a way of dealing with fearfully strong libidinal connections to objects (projective-introjective cycles related to aggression are explained in the Fairbairnian system as secondary efforts to deal with frustration of those fearfully strong libidinal needs). The relational systems model works quite differently, even though issues of aggressiveness, fear, hunger, and merger/absorption remain central.

From the relational systems perspective, it is not necessary to differentiate aggressive drives or drivenness from libidinal attachments to objects and needs, because drivenness is conceived to be created from threats to interpersonal existence and equilibrium. In this model, a projective-introjective cycle ensues within the paranoid-schizoid position because threats to interpersonal existence are so central, and the infant is so desperately in need of equilibrium for both individual and interpersonal growth. Equilibrium is sought with such vigor, and existence seems so tenuous, that reactions to environmental failures in empathy are exaggerated in the effort to regain equilibrium.

At the paranoid-schizoid level of development, the individual intrapsychic system regulates emotions by splitting perceptions of the self and/or others and then projecting and/or introjecting emotional aspects of self or others (part-selves or part-objects) to stave off threats to existence. In the relational systems model, the projective-introjective cycle begins with splitting. Splitting occurs for the purpose of separating the experienced self from other aspects of self that, if experienced, would threaten existence and make a state of equilibrium impossible. Projection is an interpersonal part of splitting that completes the separation of threatening aspects from the experienced self. Extractive introjection is an interpersonal aspect of splitting that allows soothing aspects within others to bolster the experienced self.

Splitting always occurs to the extent that any valency exists. Thus when any projective or introjective process occurs, a split has occurred in the personality system. This split results from the inability of the system to tolerate the full range of affective possibilities that lie between all four ends of the paranoid-schizoid level continua (only later, in the depressive position, are the two ends of the relatedness continuum also involved in this split). The more threatening any particular affect, the more likely it is that a split will occur and projective or introjective processes will follow. Whether or not projective and introjective processes occur depends upon the level of threat from the four primary affective states driving the paranoid-schizoid position. These affective states are (refer to Figure 6–1, p. 273): (1) annihilation, or being destroyed; (2) starvation, or impoverishment; (3) destruction of the world, or rage; and finally (4) merger/absorption, or enmeshment. These are the threats represented at the ends of the sustenance and self-protection continua.

The Self-Protection and Sustenance Continua

The processes of the paranoid-schizoid position can be clarified in revisiting the self-protection and sustenance continua. The self-protection continuum extends from annihilation of the self, through anxiety, to calm focus (or confidence), and the destructive attitude, to complete destruction of the environment. The sustenance continuum extends from starvation, through impoverishment, satiation, and voraciousness, to absorption into the environment. The affects close to the center of each continuum represent experience that is only possible when the extremes no longer threaten the individual. The area where the continua intersect, and where equilibrium is found, can be called "confidence." The extent to which an individual's intrapsychic processes can be located around that intersection can be thought of as a three-dimensional confidence interval (it becomes increasingly three-dimensional as the third continuum develops).

In examining the self-protection continuum, for example, it can be seen that a person might feel his destructiveness to be an overwhelming threat. The person feels as though his aggressive traits may destroy all that is known, thus ending his existence within a relational world. The need for emotional equilibrium will then cause this person to split off destructive parts and project them into the environment. The result of such interpersonal action is a sense of equilibrium in which the threat of one's destructiveness is balanced by a view that the world is more dangerous than the self. In such circumstances, the desperate fear of being a threat to the world is nullified.

However, as a consequence, terrible anxiety floods the individual. That anxiety makes others uncomfortable and likely to act out toward the projector in aggressive ways so that the perception of the environment as destructive becomes justified. It could also be said that fear is introjected in this case, because inner destructiveness is so threatening that only the introjection of fear can adequately stave off the perception of the self as destructive. The person who must maintain the self in such a fearful state is, unfortunately, never able to gain experience of the self as strong, since such experience can only come as a result of having aggressiveness understood and soothed, without consequent destruction, within the environment.

Take as another example the opposite case, in which the person feels the environment might annihilate her. Fear is so great that it is split off and projected into the environment. As a reaction to the person's destructive behavior those in the environment now act fearful. Such a person has warded off fear that is part of her personality and justified a less threatening perception of the environment, while also maintaining a more comfortable internal state. Again, the aggressiveness of others could be understood as being introjected in this case because only aggressiveness can allow the individual to be fully split from experiencing herself as fearful. The unfortunate consequence of maintaining the self in an aggressive state is the inability to ever perceive the self as protected by the environment, which can only occur when one is protected while in a fearful state.

At the ends of the sustenance continuum, two other clear examples can be differentiated. Perhaps an individual is threatened by his voraciousness because there is a feared possibility of becoming one with the environment through emotional consumption of others, with a consequent loss of individual identity. This voraciousness is thus split off and projected into the environment. The environment is perceived as voracious and controlling and the individual perceives himself as impoverished and hungry and behaves accordingly. Such behavior brings about further voracious, controlling behavior in others, which leads to the need to maintain the self, ever more strongly, in an impoverished state. In this instance it could also be said that hunger is introjected. This hunger is costly in that it makes connections to others impossible. It also makes exercising control over the environment impossible.

At the other end of the sustenance continuum, an individual is so desperately impoverished that starvation or abandonment appears as the threat. The starving part is split off and projected, while the individual becomes voracious or controlling. The environment is perceived as starved and in need of the individual who attempts to control the environment. In this instance it could be said that self-sufficiency is introjected. However, such self-sufficiency is costly within a person who remains truly starved because nourishment from the environment cannot be accepted.

Fear, destructiveness, impoverishment, and voraciousness have many meanings. On the sustenance continuum the human experience of wanting someone so badly that it hurts can become, through acting upon that pain in desperation, the feeling of being overwhelmed by the other, with a loss of identity. The attempt to soothe the intrapsychic fear of starvation results in voraciousness, and the attempt to soothe the intrapsychic fear of merger/absorption results in desperate impoverishment. On the self-protection continuum, many kinds of fear can become many kinds of aggression, and vice versa, because the affect perceived as most threatening is soothed by defenses that result in their opposite. Furthermore, these two affective continua combine to form many other affective continua that link many different kinds of affective role-representations. At the paranoid-schizoid level of development raw threats to existence tend to cause extreme interpersonal measures. Through interpersonal processes these raw threats are variably well-soothed.

DEVELOPMENT FROM PARANOID-SCHIZOID TO DEPRESSIVE POSITION FUNCTIONING

The paranoid-schizoid position, while it is a part of every person's development, continues to plague those (they become fixated at that level of development) who were required as infants and children to fulfill the needs of others to an exaggerated extent. Adults who meet their excessive needs through relationships with infants and children do so while damaging infant self-growth. Their actions prevent the development of increased ability, self-sustenance, self-protection, self-definition, and confidence because their actions skew the ongoing equilibrium of the child. The paranoid-schizoid position creates exaggerated need states and is associated with external blame due both to the exaggerated response to perceived threats within, and to the resulting projections into the environment. Thus the child born within a family where these mechanisms are prominent is subject to being perceived by others who project into her as having something essentially good that these others need, while at the same time she is blamed for the difficulties these others have. The child perceives a reality-based level of threat to self-protection or sustenance in the environment as she develops. Others in the environment attempt extractive introjection of the perceived nurturance, goodness, purity, or strength within the child and may employ projective identification to the extent that their own never-ending emotional hungers or anxieties frustrate introjection.

Within a healthy environment, developing through the paranoid-schizoid position is a natural developmental process caused by the reality that the child is defenseless and unable to care for itself. The environment can be variably soothing to the needs of the infant but cannot perfectly soothe every need. The extreme dependence and vulnerability of the infant make for a situation in which even the slightest lack of understanding in the environment leads to the threatening points of the sustenance and self-protection continua. As Winnicott put it (1952), in the earliest stages of development the infant lives on the brink of "unthinkable anxiety." The infant is so vulnerable and dependent that the threats of the paranoid-schizoid mode require exaggerated affective responses and associated role-representations no matter how perfectly the environment attempts to meet emotional needs.

Some experience of these threats is inevitable. To some extent these experiences are even necessary for growth. Both Winnicott (1963a) and Kohut (1977) have emphasized the benefit to personality development of momentary breaks with empathy by caretakers. Such breaks with empathy allow for a slow introduction to reality. If the personality can perceive that despite perceived threats, existence remains intact, then resiliency is developed. When this introduction occurs within an environment that, more often than not, allows the infant appropriate levels of self-sufficiency and loving care, the result is special or unique character. The child adapts to his unique environment with whatever unique characteristics he was born with. This is the generally "good-enough" environment that will shield the infant from too much experience of threat, occurring too early, and too much of the time.

When the infant acts destructively, links are not severed because the caretaker understands that the baby does not yet have the ability to control such impulses. The baby also learns that she is not destroyed by the destructiveness of the parent, who has learned to control such impulses. When the infant acts as though starving, links are not severed by starvation, but rather the caretaker recognizes the need for soothing or food. Moreover, the baby learns that she will not be overwhelmed by the caretaker's response because the caretaker is able to empathically understand when the baby is sated or has had enough affection. Empathic caretaking within the environment ensures that the issues of self-protection and sustenance do not reach the point of desperation. The child learns the potential of others as well as the ability to delay gratification. The child born within a prominently paranoid-schizoid environment, on the other hand, never adequately works through this normal developmental period because issues of self-protection and sustenance are constantly played out at immature levels within reality.

The Depressive Position

The depressive position describes an individual's ability to perceive others as both good and bad at the same time (referred to as "whole object relations" within the object relations literature). This ability originates in the experience of maintaining confidence that threatening parts of the self (destructive, fearful, hungry, or voracious) can remain intact within to some extent because the individual can nurture himself and find others who will be nurturing. As one learns to nurture the self, based on the nurturing one has already found in the environment, threatening affects become acceptable because they are no longer so threatening. If a person knows that he will never be starved for affection from nor overwhelmed by another, and if that person knows that he will never be annihilated by or need to destroy another, then it becomes possible to maintain opposing affects simultaneously. When confidence has built up from the recognition that relationships do not necessarily result in pain or threat in one form or another, it becomes possible for the individual to feel afraid yet know that assertiveness will likely result in satisfaction. Likewise, consumption or pursuit of another is likely to resolve hunger or desire for another.

This process is essentially the same as that which Kernberg (1976) refers to as the shift from splitting to self and object integration. Nonthreatening affective role-representations build up over time as an individual experiences others to be understanding or not too rejecting despite the individual's aggression, desperation, fear, or voraciousness. Working through of the paranoid-schizoid position occurs by a process of projective and introjective identification in which outside systems are able to tolerate projective identifications, and lend confidence from within themselves by maintaining empathic connection despite the difficult affects transferred within the interaction. Balance or confidence (again, represented by balance in the center of Figure 6–1) within others is thus transferred to the individual throughout development. Through this process the infant recognizes that the environment is not likely to cause annihilation and is not likely to be destroyed by impulsive aggression. Furthermore, this process allows the infant to recognize that he or she will not starve for affection nor overwhelm others in pursuit of sustenance.

When the issues represented by the ends of the sustenance and self-protection continua within the paranoid-schizoid position are no longer so threatening that they require immediate projection or introjection for alleviation of threat, the depressive position develops. Because those threats are no longer perceived as so imminent, the individual no longer interacts with others out of desperation, forever seeking to stave off a threat to existence. Instead, to a greater and greater extent, as confidence grows, relationships with others are pursued by choice—not for sustenance or self-protection, but for companionship that includes genuine concern.

An essential milestone in the development of the depressive position is in the infant's preconscious understanding that reparation is possible once aggressive and/or voracious impulses have been projected into the environment. As Klein (1935, 1957) views this process, reparative longings arise as the child regrets having hurt the mother with destructive projections. In other words, because the infant can now perceive that the mother who is caring for her is the same mother that moments ago was seen as a threat that needed to be destroyed, the child feels that her own thoughts of moments ago are threatening to this caring mother. The development of the "capacity for concern" (Winnicott 1963b) occurs as the child's impulses meet the reality of disapproval in the caretaker who, however, continues to love and accept the child. Through this process the child learns that both her good and bad characteristics are accepted, even if they do not always meet with approval. The child also learns that she is able to accept bad and good within others. Thus the relatively full working through of the depressive position can be viewed as the road to true empathy. It is also the path to proper limit-setting, which requires the maintenance of love despite feeling disapproval. Respect for the self as well as the other as separate, whole people cannot be achieved without the desire to repair and the capacity for concern. Also, therapeutic behavior, as well as adequate (good-enough) parenting, can be seen as deriving from the integration within the individual of this essential milestone.

In the depressive position the individual will continue to avoid threats to interpersonal existence through relationships to the extent that the powerful affects of the paranoid-schizoid position have not been worked through. But now positive experience and the ability to perceive others in a more balanced way temper these threats. Although paranoid-schizoid affects cannot be completely resolved, and do continue to drive behavior, with concern comes a deeper caring for others. Rather than just using other people out of desperation, others are cared about for who they are, and attachments to them are valued in a more permanent, less mercurial, volatile, or capricious way. Before fully describing how the depressive position allows for development of relatedness (the z axis), however, it is necessary to discuss the way the paranoid-schizoid and depressive positions regulate the needs of the individual so that the results can be described as "boundaries."

PARANOID-SCHIZOID AND DEPRESSIVE POSITION BOUNDARIES AND THE RELATEDNESS CONTINUUM

The use of the word "boundaries" is common in psychoanalytic theory but the term is typically not well explained. As discussed in Chapter 4, Federn (1952), more than any other theoretician, has clarified the meaning of boundaries in analytic theory with his differentiation of an "inner boundary" between unconscious and conscious and an "outer boundary" between the individual and what or who in external reality is given "narcissistic investment." Federn (1952) proposed that an inner boundary maintained separation between the ego and frightening affects, and that an outer boundary governed what or who can affect or be affected by an individual. The work of other authors such as Ganzarain (1977) and Ashbach and Schermer (1987) has also been important. They have demonstrated in what ways the paranoid-schizoid and depressive positions influence boundaries. Ganzarain has suggested that the paranoid-schizoid and the depressive positions account for two boundaries with similar functions to those proposed by Federn. The relational systems model integrates these ideas in the description set out below where the

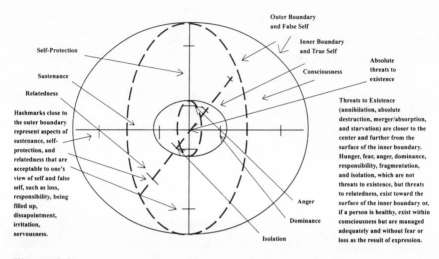

Figure 6–2.
Three-dimensional model of the continua turned inside out. Threats to existence are contained within by the inner paranoid-schizoid boundary while the depressive-level, (outer) boundary determines what or who will be allowed to affect the individual. What is contained within the paranoid-schizoid boundary is often repressed because of its potential for damaging the connections we have with others, as determined by the depressive-level boundary. Repression pushes down the affects of the paranoid-schizoid position and to the extent that repression is successful, splitting need not occur. But with repression comes the development of a true-self–false-self dichotomy. In the hypothetical case of complete working through of the depressive position, the affects or threats of the inner core would be acceptable enough so that a person could spontaneously present the self to cared-for others without fear of loss. As the affects of the inner core become less threatening, the inner boundary approaches the outer boundary, which signifies *confidence* and *authenticity*. This process can also be described as the true self coming up to the surface so that the false self is no longer needed.

"inner boundary" is characterized as regulated by the paranoid-schizoid position and the "outer boundary" by the depressive position. Figure 6–2 turns the relational systems model inside out in demonstrating the inner, paranoid-schizoid position boundary and the outer, depressive position boundary.

As indicated above, the workings of the paranoid-schizoid position can be thought of as representing an inner boundary of the personality. This inner boundary can be inflexibly permeable or impermeable or, with maturation, can be flexible and change in permeability with the needs of the individual. In the case of psychosis, for example, the inner boundary of the prepsychotic individual can be described as inflexibly permeable. This inflexible permeability occurs because practically no development of the inner boundary has been allowed. Early infant experience has been characterized as existence in an interpersonally chaotic world in which the child is unable to differentiate his own need states from what is occurring within his environment. This existence has been described as a symbiotic unit (Mahler et al. 1975), an "environmental-individual setup" (Winnicott 1960a), or the "domain of core relatedness" (Stern 1985). Although these ideas about early infancy are, in many ways, at odds with one another, all of them suggest an extreme dependency upon the environment.

Etiology of Psychosis

Psychosis occurs as a consequence of a particular kind of molding to the environment in which the infant's self must be almost completely denied for the sake of others' needs and fantasies. Thus, the threats of the paranoid-schizoid position can only be staved off with an adaptation to reality that denies individual freedom and self-sufficiency while allowing the environment to control and define how (or who) the infant will be. Rather than learning that the environment can be safe, the infant learns to believe that existence is threatened at all times unless individuality is relinquished. This occurs to such a degree that very little development of the ability to stave off the threats of the paranoid-schizoid position occurs. That is, personality integration is given up for the sake of maintaining safety under the control of others. The caregiver's definition of the infant becomes the definition the infant maintains within, but the maintenance of any experience of equilibrium with that self-definition requires constant feedback from the caregivers who control the definition.

Such an orientation can develop in two ways (or by a combination of the two). The first way occurs when caregivers in the environment have a powerful need for the infant to be a very specific way. In such an environmental setup, the caregivers are typically intent on taking care of the child's every need beyond the true existence of such needs within the child. In other words, the child's need for independence is never fully realized. Nevertheless, and even though in reality the child's caregivers' efforts are motivated more by their own powerful needs than by concern for the child, they demand absolute devotion and loyalty in return for those efforts. The second way such an orientation can develop is that actual threats within the environment can be perceived as so extremely dangerous that only the complete relinquishing of individuality seems to promise relief from them. In other words, it seems to the infant that being what others want him to be makes them behave in ways that are caring and balancing. Either way, the infant's adaptation is so exaggerated that the inner boundary never develops. Instead, the infant orients himself to the outside world with extremely little focus on his own needs, pains, or distress so that those difficulties will be taken care of by others.

The permeability of the inner boundary does not cause problems for the prepsychotic individual until the defining environment changes. If feedback from the original environment or caregivers is not available to define him, the prepsychotic comes too close to experiencing threats to existence. In other words, it is as though the prepsychotic individual has learned to play an intricate game in which following the rules precisely leads to generally safe interactions. The prepsychotic has trouble when the rules change. The inner boundary is inflexibly almost completely permeable and the prepsychotic loses the ability to differentiate the "cold shoulder" from emotional starvation, suggestions offered from absolute commands, pointed conversation from extreme aggression, or avoidance of a topic of conversation from utter horror. Normal discourse becomes a mixture of fantasized threats that cannot be differentiated from reality.

When the environment changes and as the inner boundary fails to hold any contents of the psyche, projection and introjection occur with little or no control, and yet an equilibrium state is still sought. The individual loses all sense of his ability to control threats to social existence and thus severs reality-based social ties while creating in fantasy a world that is less threatening or seemingly more controllable. This severing of social ties and assumption of a fantasy world mark an overdetermined reaction to the threats in the environment. If this now-psychotic state is prolonged, that is, if the individual does not reorganize according to the dictates of a new defining environment, the inner boundary changes, in an all-or-nothing fashion, from inflexibly permeable to inflexibly impermeable. Only very specific perceptions of the environment are allowed so that the desperate state of the psychotic individual can be balanced. Either the environment must be exactly as the psychotic needs it to be, as in a delusional state, or there must be a complete cutoff from the environment as the individual dissociates himself from internal chaos, as in the catatonic state.

Boundaries and Delusional States

In the delusional state, projections onto the environment rule what is perceived. That which is introjected from the environment is essentially the same as that which has been projected. Thus the psychotic's perceptions of the environment are confirmed. For example, paranoid delusions focus all danger outside the self in a fantastical manner so that destructive tendencies within the self do not have to be realized. Essentially, the adaptation to the environment is one in which the environment is perceived to be exactly what will balance inner threats, and reality is given up for that purpose. In the dissociated catatonic state, on the other hand, external reality is simply not perceived as the individual struggles to manage the emotional quagmire that has heretofore been managed by connections with defining others. In both of these prolonged psychotic states the inner boundary is rigidly impermeable, in that projections and introjections allowed across the boundary are extremely limited and specific.

To summarize, in prepsychotics, almost complete permeability of the inner boundary occurs due to a lack of development in cases where the environment interferes excessively with childhood self-definition. When feedback changes, complete permeability of the inner boundary can allow for a chaotic psychotic state as the psychotic person reacts to the chaos of her own emotional state, which had always before been managed within relationships. If the psychotic individual is unable to find a defining environment for a prolonged period, a relatively absolute shift, from inflexible permeability to inflexible impermeability, occurs in the inner boundary as the intrapsychic system for the first time attempts to balance extreme affects without the availability of defining relationships. (It should be noted that the switch to impermeability of the inner boundary is not in agreement with Federn's views. Federn [1952] considered the projection and confirmation of projection in the psychotic to be representative of an extremely permeable inner boundary. In my view, extreme permeability can cause a wild projective process in the beginning phases of a psychotic break. However, the switch to extreme impermeability occurs as extreme threats are dealt with in an exaggerated manner, resulting in prolonged delusional states and catatonia.)

Early phases of the paranoid-schizoid position resemble psychosis as the switch from almost complete permeability of the inner boundary to almost complete impermeability takes place, marking the most immature development of the paranoid-schizoid position. As the developing self begins to experience the reality that others will not always meet needs perfectly and yet these needs do exist, the experience of needs becomes intolerable and creates a sort of desperation about meeting needs. The infant is not well protected by experience and integration, and the possibility of interpersonal threats, such as emotional starvation or abandonment, voracious emotional consumption or enmeshment, destructiveness, and emotional withdrawal or disappearance, creates exaggerated responding to ward off such experience. The boundary system is not well developed, but because threats to individual existence become possible, the system must do something to protect itself. That protection comes in the form of the inner boundary being inflexibly impermeable, allowing only very specific perceptions of the self and the environment. Flexibility develops over time; however, those who remain primarily in the paranoid-schizoid position, although not perceiving life exactly as they need it to be, continue to perceive life according to very narrow definitions.

The Paranoid-Schizoid Position in Adults

In the case of persons caught primarily at the level of the paranoid-schizoid position in adulthood, the inner boundary is inflexibly impermeable to a lesser degree than in the prolonged psychotic state. Threatening affects still come too close to experience, but the person maintains some sense that such feelings can be modulated. Projective and introjective identification are utilized by the intrapsychic system as outside sources or containers are sought to balance a system overwhelmed with concerns of self-protection or sustenance. When there is an extreme threat to existence (annihilation, absolute destruction, starvation, or engulfment), projective and introjective identification go into full operation.

Thus the inner boundary that regulates what is allowed into and out of the core of the individual system remains to a great extent inflexibly impermeable, while the most threatening part-representation is desperately maintained outside the individual system. That is, the boundary is so inflexible at this level of intrapsychic threat that projective and introjective identification work to maintain internal stability with no conscious awareness that existence has been threatened. The inner boundary is imperme-able in that only very specifically defined contents are projected and ex-tracted. Part-selves are thus projected that seek to define the world and to only see the world with that definition. Only part-objects that are specifi-cally enough defined to fit a role that is seen as opposing (or complemen-tary to) the most threatening part-self that was projected are allowed in for extractive introjection. But to the extent that others have appropriately recognized the needs of the individual over time, thus allowing the indi-vidual to experience relational life as less threatening, this inner boundary develops flexibility. With development one can experience the self as some-what hungry but able to consume and be sated, or somewhat anxious but able to assert the self and be secure.

The Depressive Position Boundary

The depressive position can be understood as regulating a boundary that decides whom or what the individual will allow to affect him, as well as whom and what he will feel he affects. This only becomes possible when the capacity for concern has at least partially developed. Once the indi-vidual realizes that he has been destructive toward or has withdrawn from the same person who loves him and who is also needed, anxiety about hurting that person becomes an issue. That anxiety becomes generalized to all others to whom the person makes an emotional connection. The depressive position boundary limits who or what will be allowed to affect a person so that he will perceive himself as only affecting those about whom he really cares. This boundary is necessary because the person cannot maintain concern or be anxious about affecting everyone and everything without becoming fragmented. And also because the possibility of caring about no one, given certain parameters of this boundary, would result in complete isolation (see Figure 6–1 and the z axis, Relatedness continuum).

The depressive position operates its boundary efficiently to the extent that the self-protection and sustenance issues of development are resolved, making it possible for others to have significance as whole objects—per-sons with weaknesses and strengths. Only by being treated as a person with strengths and weaknesses, and who is loved no matter what, can this level of development begin. To the extent that these issues are not resolved, the depressive position boundary will never operate efficiently, and rudimentary depressive-boundary functioning will fluctuate, in an inflexible way (like the paranoid-schizoid boundary), between relatively complete permeability and impermeability. Permeability at this level is understood as the extent to which the individual's understanding of the environment is crystallized. In other words, when the boundary is very permeable, the definition determining who or what will affect the person is very broad, and when the boundary is impermeable, that definition is very specific.

For example, a narcissistic person could be said to be relatively sensitive to issues of self-protection and sustenance and thus be expected to use a constantly impermeable depressive-level boundary (as well as a constantly impermeable inner boundary, as is the case in most character-disordered patients who continue to have difficulty with paranoid-schizoid issues), to ensure that projected threatening parts remain outside the system. Thus, she appears to care only about those things or people that seem to consistently mirror the grandiose sense of self that is needed, in order to stave off fear of dependence and fear of the aggression of others. A dependent personality could be said to have equal sensitivity (an equally impermeable inner boundary), but the depressive-level boundary is extremely permeable in allowing constant projection into and introjection from the environment. Thus this person consciously cares about everyone's opinion, seeking approval to stave off fear of others' discovery of his aggressiveness or voraciousness. Where the narcissist needs to maintain a highly crystallized, malignant view of the environment with an extremely impermeable depressive-position boundary in order to maintain a positive self view, the dependent needs to maintain an amorphous, open view, with an extremely permeable depressive-position boundary, so the self can be defined by the environment. Although these forms of the depressive position boundary can be understood as related to personalities in which self-protection and sustenance continue to be the primary issues, depressive-position boundary development will occur over time if paranoid-schizoid issues are relatively worked through.

To the extent that the depressive position has developed, it pertains to a flexible outer boundary. But to the extent that it has not developed, others in the world are perceived as so essential to self-protection or sustenance, with emotional impoverishment, anxiety, voraciousness, and destructiveness in the environment perceived as so strong, that the outer boundary must remain inflexible and the person can be described as primarily in the paranoid-schizoid position. When primarily in the paranoid-schizoid position there is a tendency to never become intimate with others (inflexibly impermeable outer boundary), or to always put others first (inflexibly permeable outer boundary), or to fluctuate between these two extremes (inflexibly all-or-nothing outer boundary). But it is important to understand that the depressive-position boundary only develops in these all-or-nothing ways when paranoid-schizoid issues are not well worked through. As paranoid-schizoid issues are worked through, the depressive-position outer boundary becomes increasingly flexible. When individuals are limited to these broad boundary fluctuations, however, the personality disorders become the only possible character orientations.

In the paranoid-schizoid mode the individual is affected by everyone and everything, with all elements seen as sources of possible pain or desperation. Defenses work very diligently and in inflexible ways to avoid that pain or desperation by either cutting off the emotional influence of everyone (inflexibly impermeable outer boundary) or pleasing everyone (inflexibly permeable outer boundary). When the depressive position is reached by way of working through the paranoid-schizoid position, the individual is better able to regulate intimacy because others are not so threatening to the internal world. He is able to choose those to whom he wants to become close, and maintain emotional distance from others. Nevertheless, the depressive-position outer boundary does function even when the depressive position has not been reached by way of working through in the paranoid-schizoid position. The extent to which the depressive boundary functions flexibly is determined by the quality of the person's attachments and relatedness, and is limited by the extent to which the paranoid-schizoid position has been worked through.

When the depressive position is reached and paranoid-schizoid functioning is relatively worked through by positive experience, one issue that remains is that the threat of loss of others who have become more intimately related to the individual (as well as of relatedness itself) seems more ominous—that is, loss now has real meaning. To the extent that they have not been worked through, the affects controlled by the inner boundary may now endanger attachments and relatedness. The working through of the paranoid-schizoid position is never complete, but once it reaches a certain level others can be cared about and working through of the depressive position can begin. For the individual, the problem changes from desperately needing to soothe inner threats, to desperately needing to hold onto attachments and relatedness. To the extent that the paranoid-schizoid affects are still dangerous, repression develops so that attachment and relatedness will not be threatened.

ANXIETY, REPRESSION, THE RELATEDNESS CONTINUUM, AND MENTAL HEALTH

Repression is the defense of the depressive-position outer boundary. The feeling that is created by a leak in repressive defenses is what is generally referred to as "anxiety." This anxiety must be differentiated from the "fear of being destroyed," or fear of losing interpersonal existence via withdrawal, of the paranoid-schizoid position. The feeling that is typically referred to as anxiety is the fear of threat to one's attachments and relatedness that strikes one when repression is not fully successful in pushing down destructive, fearful, hungry, and voracious attitudes or affective role-representations. To the extent that the paranoid-schizoid position has been worked through, these affects no longer threaten interpersonal existence. Thus the inner boundary no longer needs to be so inflexibly impermeable as to define with extreme specificity what will be perceived in or understood from the environment. But with development of the capacity for concern and whole object relations (the ability to simultaneously maintain good and bad feelings about oneself or others), the flexibility of permeability that develops in the inner boundary creates a problem. As the paranoid-schizoid boundary becomes more flexible, powerful affects are allowed into consciousness where they threaten relatedness. A different kind of force is employed within the intrapsychic system to protect relatedness from these destructive, fearful, hungry, and voracious affects. Whereas splitting occurs in the paranoid-schizoid position and involves the inner boundary, repression is the defense of the depressive position and the outer boundary.

Defensive Orientations

Repression develops to push these "bad" affects back down and away from consciousness so that they cannot damage relationships. It generally works by operating the outer boundary in defining who or what will be allowed to affect the individual, and what inner affects will be allowed to affect those about whom the individual cares. In other words, by pushing down "bad" affects and determining what and whom the individual will care about, repression allows an individual to be affected only by those who in some way justify the particular way in which the individual manages to deny those "bad" affects. There are two primary defensive orientations that allow inner "badness" to be denied and that reflect incomplete working through of the depressive position. These two orientations can be understood in looking at the relatedness continuum (the z axis, Figures 6–1 and 6–2).

Just as issues of self-protection and sustenance can be thought of as existing along a continuum, so too can issues of loss or threats to relatedness. The relatedness continuum runs from isolation, through loneliness, secure attachment, and guilt, to responsibility fragmentation. To the extent that issues of self-protection and sustenance have been worked through, the depressive position's outer boundary regulates relatedness at levels ranging from loneliness to guilt. Thus the two primary defensive orientations are that (1) the individual can care very little about others, keeping distance despite loneliness, or (2) she can care too much and maintain responsibility for others despite guilt.

The connection between repression, caring, and the relatedness continuum is that concern for others creates a feeling of responsibility for maintaining the connection to others that could be damaged by destructive, fearful, hungry, or voracious affects or impulses. If these affects or impulses threaten relatedness (if the paranoid-schizoid position has not been fully worked through but has been worked through enough for the affects to be allowed into consciousness) the personality system must find a way to protect relatedness. Repression works to protect relatedness by erecting a "false self" (Winnicott 1965a). In determining who and what will affect the individual and will be affected by the individual, the false self protects relatedness through "environmental compliance."

The false self complies with a perception of what will be accepted and prized by others who are allowed to affect the individual. Thus a whole self-image is created. It includes adorning oneself with material objects related to complying with what is important to these others who are allowed to affect the individual. The false self created by repression, or the manner in which the outer boundary defines who or what is important, will not allow others deemed as important to be hurt by the true self, which contains affects that are deemed to be dangerous. Likewise, others who are not allowed to affect the individual, never damage the true self or even touch off its many affects. Unfortunately however, unless the true self, complete with fears and hungers as well as anger and voraciousness, is exposed to others, no true intimacy can develop. This dilemma becomes the primary problem of the depressive position. In the words of Fairbairn (1941), the dilemma is "how to love without destroying by hate" (p. 271). Using terms consistent with the relational systems model, the dilemma is how to be intimate with others, thus allowing others to see the deepest sensitivities, faults, and impulses of the true self, even though there is fear that those aspects of the true self will damage relatedness.

The relatedness continuum represents the two complementary and opposing ways in which the personality system attempts to protect relatedness from those "bad" impulses (bad because one cares about relatedness and these impulses threaten that relatedness). On one side of the z axis is responsibility and guilt and on the other is loss and loneliness. The intrapsychic system can bolster repression (which exists to the extent that bad affects are perceived as threatening relatedness thus causing anxiety) by taking care of, or providing for, others. Or, alternatively, the system can avoid the possibility of badness contaminating relatedness by maintaining some level of emotional distance. On the z axis, taking care of or providing for others, is represented by "responsibility." To the extent that bad affects continue to surface, a person who tends to take responsibility will start to feel guilty. On the z axis, the avoidance of caring for others causes emotional distance which is represented by "loneliness." To the extent that bad affects continue to affect relations despite the attempt to not care deeply, a person who tends to maintain such emotional distance will become lonely or isolated.

The affective role-representations that occur on this continuum work in the same way as those that were described as related to the self-protection and sustenance continua. That is, a person who takes responsibility and becomes guilty most fears isolation, and his guilt is in reaction to the possibility that isolation or loss could occur if others were affected by his bad affects. A person who tends to remain emotionally isolated most fears responsibility fragmentation, and her emotional isolation is in reaction to the possibility that she would be extremely responsible for the damage caused to relationships if her bad affects were perceived by others. The concept of responsibility fragmentation denotes the possibility that one is so responsible for the misfortune of others that the self must be completely divided and forfeited for those others' benefit.

An example of the person who maintains a position of responsibility is the obsessive. The obsessive has worked through the paranoid-schizoid position enough so that the outer boundary corresponding to the depressive position can develop to some extent. Her concern is not with threats to existence but with threats to relatedness if her inner badness were to leak through. She is afraid that she will be shunned for this badness, especially weakness and fear, and thus she fears isolation. The solution is to take care of everyone and to clean up her own messes before anyone else is affected. The fantasy of having control over the fate of others and her relations to them protects the obsessive-compulsive from the immense anxiety about her weakness and badness leaking through and damaging relationships. Her weakness or badness is thus not allowed to hurt others.

An example of the person who maintains a position of emotional loneliness is the hysteric (not to be confused with the *DSM-IV* "histrionic"). Although this personality style is not so obviously lonely, it must be noticed that the hysteric maintains such a different presentation to the world than what is felt inside that others never get close and intimacy never fully develops. Like the obsessive, the hysteric can be understood as a person who has worked through the paranoid-schizoid position enough so that the outer boundary and repression can develop to some extent. Like the obsessive, the hysteric's concern is not that actual existence is threatened but rather that inner badness, especially owing to a perception of the self as better and stronger than others, can leak through and sever ties. The paradox for the hysteric is that he perceives ties to be severed because others view his strength or goodness as threatening, so he often acts as though he were weak. But because he maintains some inner perception of himself as special and strong he is able to handle the kind of emotional isolation that exists on this end of the z axis.

Intrapsychic Systems and the Depressive Position

Intrapsychic systems that have developed into the depressive position are far more complicated than those that remain stuck at the paranoid-schizoid position. Since paranoid-schizoid concerns continue to have an effect to the extent that they are not worked through, both the paranoid-schizoid and the depressive-level functioning of the individual must be examined.

Taking the example of the obsessive described above, it can be seen that the inner badness most shameful to such an individual has to do with feeling weak and dependent. These feelings are closer to the patient's conscious awareness than the extreme aggressiveness and voraciousness that require feelings of weakness and dependency at the paranoid-schizoid level. For the obsessive, feelings of destructiveness and voraciousness are so threatening at the paranoid-schizoid level that she exaggerates her defenses in projecting strength and introjecting weakness. But the weakness and dependence are, in turn, also unpalatable to the obsessive, who must demonstrate strength in taking care of others or face the idea of causing damage to her attachments that would result from not taking good enough care. What is most complex here is that the obsessive needs to be soothed for having dependent and fearful aspects, but at a deeper level needs to be soothed for aggressive and voracious impulses. Because she acts as though she were capable, and asks others to notice this strength, the obsessive can never receive the kind of relationship she needs for maximal growth. Even when feeling guilty, such a patient is taking credit for being strong. It is interesting to note that Guntrip (1969) thought of guilt, which implies strength as a responsible person, as a difficulty that covers for weakness and shame. Shame for weakness and dependency, and ultimately shame for the aggressiveness and voraciousness that weakness and dependency cover for, is the deepest issue of the neurotically obsessive patient. Guilt is merely the first layer to surface when repression initially fails and is thus the first issue that must be addressed before moving to the deeper issues of dependency and weakness, and then, finally, aggressiveness and destructiveness.

The case of the hysteric is of course similar. The badness hidden here is the feeling of being better and more worthy than others, and is closer to consciousness than the more threatening issue of being fearful and dependent. This feeling of being better and more worthy than others is unpalatable in that the hysteric is afraid of being held accountable for the severing of relationships—sometimes in others, like the parents, one of whom may prefer the hysteric to the spouse. The hysteric avoids, often in a controlling way, becoming emotionally attached because attachment brings such accountability into focus. The hysteric holds emotional attachment at bay by presenting a pleasing image that betrays his feelings of specialness. What is most complex in the hysteric's case is that he needs relationships that recognize, at the deepest level, the fear and hunger that drive him to the need to feel strong and better than most. But the presentation of the hysteric makes this impossible, since no one can get emotionally close enough to affect him and because his presentation is one of not caring deeply about things. These patients may surround themselves with many people who reflect only their presentation or false self, and thus they do not appear lonely. They often do not recognize their loneliness as a problem because they have so many others surrounding them. Nevertheless, at a deeper emotional level, they remain isolated and it often becomes clear that they have difficulty with intimacy.

Triangulation and Responsibility

The triangular nature of relationships that occurs when repression is employed within the system is also accounted for in the relational systems model by the notion of "responsibility" and the relatedness continuum. Once the capacity for concern develops, the child begins to be concerned about his effect on the relationships of others. Children learn that the paranoid-schizoid level feelings they have toward any of various significant others can be especially dangerous. A child might desire the attention of one significant other and then must deal with the possible consequences of having that wish fulfilled. In the case of hysterical personalities, paranoid-schizoid–level feelings of fear and hunger threaten to evoke complete withdrawal and emotional starvation from loved ones, which is so intolerable that a counter-feeling of specialness develops to ward them off. In turn, the possibility that his own specialness and strength will be appreciated by a significant other becomes so threatening to the hysteric that he hides his specialness as though it were destructive. It seems to him that his specialness threatens his attachments to significant others (including the other parent, siblings, or other figures) for whom the targeted parent cares, or the attachments between those significant others and the targeted parent, due to the anger and jealousy these significant others may feel. The hysteric avoids all competition for fear of winning. Yet he continues to crave exclusive attention to bolster his specialness and must "unintentionally" draw attention to himself in such a way as to draw others away from their other relations. He typically then finds himself in troubling situations where everyone else is angry and he deals with it by not caring, and by feeling as though he has done nothing to create that situation.

In the case of obsessive personalities, the dynamics are in many ways just the opposite of those found in the hysteric. While the hysteric fears the possibility of winning and hides any specialness, the obsessive fears losing relatedness and becomes perfectionistic and overly responsible as a way of hiding weakness. This state develops out of a two-level triangulation. The obsessive has aggressive feelings toward one significant other while perceiving that she is in competition for the affection of another significant other. These aggressive feelings must be thwarted because they seem to threaten the very existence of the obsessive at the paranoid-schizoid level. The obsessive manages the threat of interpersonal destruction by perceiving herself as weak and bad. However, weak and bad feelings become associated with loss of relatedness at the depressive level as well, because the obsessive finds that expression of badness and/or weakness results in difficulties between significant others. This weakness or badness often leads to one significant other disapproving of how another significant other deals with the weakness or badness. The obsessive is faced with losing the love of one significant other—or perhaps both if their attention turns toward each other within the struggle. Thus weakness and badness within must be denied and responsibility for others and perfectionism are used as a defense against this weakness and badness. Unfortunately, in reality, although the obsessive attempts to maintain relationships through perfectionism and taking responsibility, hiding a part of oneself results in a lack of intimacy and, ultimately, isolation. Thus, the obsessive creates her worst fear by trying so hard to avoid it.

Repressive Triangles

The type of triangulation discussed in the case of patients who have succeeded in becoming primarily repressive is only a subset of triangles as they are discussed in family systems theory. In family systems theory, the typical triangle consists of a third person who can be projected upon to end a conflict between two others, thus allowing a family or group to regain systemic balance. Although repressive triangulation can occur that way, so can paranoid-schizoid level triangulation. What differentiates the repressive triangle is that defense is aimed at protecting the repressive individual from feeling he is a cause of conflict, either between two significant others or between himself and another person. It is this possibility, that he might be the cause of problems, that makes the repressive tendency so necessary. If he can hide his shame, whether it is about specialness, badness, or weakness, he feels less threatened about the loss of others who might be damaged. Triangles created at a paranoid-schizoid level protect the individual from experiencing threats to his own interpersonal existence, not threats of loss (further discussion of triangles from a family systems perspective can be found below).

Some patients who primarily exhibit obsessive or hysterical features often have difficulty with the opposite end of the relatedness continuum. A person who tries to take a lot of responsibility to feel strong and who sometimes feels guilty will, in times of extreme stress, throw up her hands and uncharacteristically decide not to care about anyone or anything. A person who tries to avoid responsibility and present himself as weak so that responsibility will not be expected of him will sometimes, in times of stress, suddenly give up being indifferent and take over. It is not uncommon, for example, to find a hysterical patient taking care of her overly responsible, alcoholic husband who has fallen apart. Just as was described with the self-protection and sustenance continua, at any particular time the most threatening side of the affective role-representation will be projected and the strength of that threat can suddenly change. These shifts occur far less readily in personalities fixated at the paranoid-schizoid position than in those fixated at the depressive position due to the differing intensities of threat at those two levels. The paranoid-schizoid character typically makes this shift only developmentally, meaning that the adult personality compensates for childhood experience only after it is no longer threatened. The depressive character, although it is also compensating, does sometimes fluctuate with ambivalence that results from threats that are based more in compromise than in truly traumatic interpersonal contacts.

In the example of the codependent couple described above, when the alcoholic husband is no longer able to be in control of things, it can become quite threatening for the hysterical wife, who is used to being taken care of (which makes her feel as though she is close to someone), to find herself suddenly not taken care of and feeling completely isolated. At this point the threat of isolation becomes stronger than the threat of responsibility fragmentation, and the patient starts to obsessively take care of the husband. It is notable that it is impossible to find out where this process started. In contrast to the direction of process described above, the wife's general emotional isolation may have made the husband feel that his efforts to maintain ties by being a responsible caretaker were failing, thus leading to his excessive drinking behavior. That is, when he felt isolated despite his greatest efforts he likely redoubled his efforts until finally responsibility fragmentation became a stronger threat to him than isolation. He thus started drinking to isolate himself at an emotional level rather than continue to take responsibility.

Working Through to Balance and Authenticity

As the depressive position gets worked through, a person becomes better able to balance responsibility with loneliness. Although working through in the depressive position is limited by the extent to which the paranoid-schizoid position has been worked through, it is possible for a balance and a sense of confidence in one's identity to develop if paranoid-schizoid issues are, in fact, relatively well worked through. A person can come to know when to feel responsible for others and when she needs alone time or independence. With luck, this feeling of balance initially occurs in one's family, where others are not too devastated by independent behavior or appropriate interdependency and are also not threatened by one's special qualities or fears. Such a person learns to be with others who treat her like she is special and capable of being independent because such treatment is the only kind of treatment that feels consistent with her view of self. Likewise such a person treats others with this same kind of care when they have spent enough time with her to know that such treatment will be reciprocated consistently. At this point of development, affective role-representations are so numerous and combine the primary affective continua in so many ways that perception of reality is very accurate. Where real threat is perceived it is avoided and where real intimacy is possible it is developed.

The outer depressive-position boundary can function at this point in a far more flexible manner. The way that the person feels about others is based on reality in that intimate relations are more highly valued than relations that quickly soothe threats to existence or that aid in repressing feelings of badness. Because a person can trust the self not to overreact, the inner boundary gets increasingly flexible, to the point that inner boundary and outer boundary become one. As the true self can be revealed without excessive fear, the false self is no longer necessary. To the extent that a person is able to truly care only about what he really cares about, and to the extent that repression is no longer needed, authenticity grows. How a person feels inside is how he acts on the outside. Confidence within reveals itself in a special outer confidence that simply demonstrates that a person knows himself, knows what he is capable of, and enjoys living in a manner that is unencumbered by unnecessary concerns about things for which he is not responsible and cannot control. This level of flexibility of boundaries allows for freedom of affect and spontaneity; many emotions are available to experience at appropriate times because the experience of those emotions is no longer threatening. Both Mitchell (1988) and Greenberg (1991) have emphasized flexibility, lack of restrictiveness, and lack of rigidity in one's character as the hallmarks of mental health.

Beyond mental health, perhaps even a unique spirituality is reached as a person becomes able to remain balanced within relations and reality, attuned to what is truly most important to individual and relational vitality. Although such a level of health, spontaneity, and/or authenticity may never develop completely, it is the goal of mental health and signifies the greatest flexibility of boundaries and the most versatile mental health growth pattern. The closer a person comes to attaining this level of mental health, the more likely he or she is to succeed at attaining realistic goals in life. Flexibility of boundaries and confidence in one's reactions leads to ultimate adaptation.

Valency

With an understanding of boundaries at the paranoid-schizoid and depressive position levels, it becomes possible to explain the intrapsychic and behavioral process of valency, from projective identification, through normal interaction, and to extractive introjection. Valency occurs at various strengths as expressed behavior reflects the unified functioning of the two boundaries. To the extent that the boundaries limit communication with others, others feel themselves limited as to how they can communicate. Efforts at communication are met with resistance and bewilderment unless they fit the definitions of the paranoid-schizoid and depressive boundaries. Thus others soon behave in a way that allows for communication in this specific pattern to the extent that, because of their own characterological makeup, they feel a need to connect with the other individual. What must be perceived as outside the self and that which must be extracted from outside sources must be found somewhere, thus making people with complementary needs and weaknesses more attractive to each other. At levels of greater and greater health, there is more flexibility in boundaries, less need for extremely specific kinds of interpersonal communication, and greater variability in the understanding of interpersonal involvements.

DIFFERENTIATING MAJOR CONCEPTS AT THE PARANOID-SCHIZOID AND DEPRESSIVE POSITIONS

Because they have different meanings at different levels of mental health, many concepts in the field of psychoanalysis and object relations therapy require clarification. Many of these concepts can be clarified through an understanding of the paranoid-schizoid and depressive positions. Perhaps the most confusing of all concepts is anxiety, a term that has been used to connote both paranoid-schizoid and depressive position concerns. Likewise, guilt has been a focus of classical psychoanalysis, but Fairbairn (1941) and his followers (Guntrip 1969) have been very persuasive in their account of shame as the more fundamental, but related construct; the relational systems model is very useful in differentiating these two phenomena. The need for control and the experience of agency are also very common issues within psychoanalysis that can be differentiated by the model's two primary levels of functioning. Perhaps most important to the interactional emphasis of the relational systems model is its ability to differentiate levels of defense and the interpersonal pressures that are associated with them. This issue has been a confusing one within psychoanalytic theory, probably because there is such great overlap between repressive defenses and splitting defenses. Again, however, the relational systems model helps in differentiating these levels of defense and shows how they interact within one individual, even if that individual's defensive system is more characteristic of one level than the other. What makes all of these concepts especially confusing is the fact that the extent to which they are involved in any particular mental operation is directly proportional to the level of mental health, either the paranoid-schizoid or depressive position, at which a person is operating at any one time.

Anxiety

Anxiety, as stated above, is specifically related to the threat to the individual's attachments and relatedness created by his having what he continues to think of as bad impulses. If a person has failed to work through the paranoid-schizoid position, he will not experience anxiety. However, he will experience fear. The fear experienced by the paranoid personality, for example, is not primarily anxiety from the perspective of the relational systems model. Such a person feels extremely afraid, but that fear is not anxiety, because anxiety requires a failure of repression as part of its very definition. Rather, the paranoid personality defends against the threat that he might destroy the whole world by maintaining the affective part-self role representation more closely associated with the threat of being anni-hilated. That is, he maintains the feeling that he is fearful (perhaps terri-fied). Repression is not well enough developed within such a personality for anxiety to be experienced. Perhaps the fear that is experienced could be called mortal fear, as opposed to anxiety, to suggest that it is related to a threat to existence, not the threat of loss. There are, of course, depres-sive-level paranoid fears as well—fears that take the form of thinking one will lose someone else if some bad or shameful characteristic is discov-ered. To the extent that repression operates in holding down such fear and fails, such paranoia has anxiety as its cause.

Differentiating Guilt and Shame

A related issue is the differentiation of guilt and shame. As it is under-stood within the classical psychoanalytic model, guilt is associated with great distress. Guilt is an essential element within the relational systems model as well. In the relational systems model, guilt must be worked through in the depressive position before a person is capable of differentiating appropriate levels of responsibility for others. In contrast to the classical psychoanalytic focus on guilt, Fairbairn (1941, Guntrip 1969) and his followers have pointed out that shame is a far more uncomfortable and deeper issue. The relational systems model also views shame as deeper and more troublesome than guilt. The feeling of guilt presupposes some level of agency for which the person can feel regret. The person has had some effect upon the world for which remorse is felt. Shame, on the other hand, is related to some sense of inner weakness or lack of control, a feeling that the experiencing person is bad.

When a person is ashamed of the true self, the outer boundary and false self develop to hide the true self and protect relatedness from inner badness. Guilt only occurs after a person becomes afraid that something shameful within has been revealed and has damaged a relationship. Guilt occurs, in other words, when an individual feels some responsibility for doing something that revealed a shameful weakness of some kind. With respect to the paranoid-schizoid and depressive positions, characters caught primarily within the paranoid-schizoid position develop the outer boundary at rudimentary levels due to shame. They either care about everyone and everything or care about no one and nothing because inner weakness and need, about which there is great shame, must be hidden from the world. On the other hand, only characters who are primarily caught within the depressive position, persons who take responsibility for themselves and for their effect on others, are capable of experiencing true guilt when their inner badness seems to have shown itself.

Issues of Control and Agency

Another area of psychological functioning that is clarified by the relational systems model is that which concerns the difference between issues of control and those of agency. When a person is primarily positioned at the paranoid-schizoid level of development, control is a central issue within all relational experience. Klein (1948b) considered the use of projective identification as being a way of controlling oneself by projecting an aspect of the self into the object and then controlling the object. The need to soothe the self from threats to existence is so imminent that others are sought, and considered necessary, to play the part of controller or controlled. In this way the threatening affects are alleviated immediately.

Agency, on the other hand, is a concept related to the idea that one can control oneself. According to Winnicott (1963b), the first experience of agency is the fantasy of injuring cared-for others, which then brings on the development of concern, a sense of responsibility, and the capacity for guilt. In order to feel a sense of agency a person has to have achieved some level of relatedness. Needs are still met to some extent by others, but the fact that confidence has developed in knowing that these needs will be met means that the need to soothe the self has been internalized to that same extent. This leads to an ability to delay gratification and to see one's actions as choices.

When needs are seen as imminent, as they are in the paranoid-schizoid position, no choices are recognized. Thus the feeling of agency is not possible, and the need to control the self and/or others is exaggerated. It is interesting, however, that the need for (and fear of) control at the paranoid-schizoid level of functioning is so complete that it remains unconscious. Perceived threats to existence immediately lead to splitting defenses, and efforts to control self and other are ego syntonic.

Control becomes an issue of discomfort in the personality only when its purpose is to manage anxiety. This problem can be seen in the cases of the obsessive or hysteric discussed above, who use control to fend off fear of loss and loneliness or fear of connection and guilt, respectively. Issues of control are acted out more chaotically in the passive-aggressive personality and the histrionic personality, both of which are examples of difficulty with developing relatedness at a lower level. The passive-aggressive is desperately trying to figure out how his impulses and true self fit into a world in which it seems only particular behaviors allow him to stay related to others, an uncertainty leading to issues with authority and a tendency to become easily overwhelmed with responsibility fragmentation. The histrionic desperately avoids responsibility fragmentation by focusing all her attention on pleasing others in the world only with aspects of herself to which she attributes no real human value, and in doing so will not allow her true self to be controlled or accountable.

Splitting Defenses and Repression

Finally, all of these concepts are related to the difference between paranoid-schizoid, or splitting defenses, and depressive-position defenses based in repression. From the point of view of the relational systems model, there is no defense that is purely based in repression. Nor is there any defense that is purely based in splitting and projection. Although one can talk about the defenses in a way that artificially separates these levels (and such differentiation can be helpful), in actuality the mental and behavioral actions involved in defense are simultaneously expressed, and all defenses have components that evince both paranoid-schizoid and depressive-level purposes. To our purpose here the most important examples involve projective identification and extractive introjection, which are typically thought of as defenses based on splitting (paranoid-schizoid position), as well as projection and introjection, which are thought of as based in repression (depressive position).

Although the more advanced defenses, including projection, introjection, and identification, are primarily repressive in nature, they nevertheless involve some level of splitting and projective identification or extractive introjection. At the surface level, they are associated with these paranoid-schizoid, depressive-position splitting defenses by having some behavioral influence. The influence involved in these depressive-position defenses, however, has far less strength. Also, this behavioral influence does not directly correspond to the intent of the projective or introjective identification as it does when the defense is primarily centered around splitting.

Take for example a situation in which an individual projects fear on another person because he cannot stand to perceive the self as fearful. Furthermore, imagine that in this situation the reason the projector cannot stand to perceive the self as fearful is because fearful others are perceived as incapable of sustaining relationships due to avoidance of responsibility. In a situation of projective identification and extractive introjection, this projecting individual would have to behave in a way that pressures the other person to act fearful. That is, the inducer would be aggressive toward the targeted recipient in some way. But with projection it is more likely that the projector would behave disdainfully or avoid the other who is perceived as fearful. Neither disdain nor avoidance directly corresponds, behaviorally speaking, with fear. A person does not act fearful because someone else acts disdainful or avoids him. However, and although the effect is less direct, there does remain a behavioral effect on the other, who likely perceives the inducer's disdainful or avoiding behavior. In this case, where projection is the primary defense, the effect of the projective identification and extractive introjection might be a feeling of loss of the other or responsibility for something that has occurred. Thus the content of what is projected is fear, but the content of what is projectively identified or extractively introjected is loss or responsibility (loss of a connection with the disdainful other, or guilt for allowing something bad to happen).

When projection is primary, projective identification or extractive introjection are still operative, but with less pressure and less direct meaning. Therefore, another important component of the interaction becomes the sensitivity of the projector's target, in an interaction whose intensity depends upon the extent to which the exchange involves projection or introjection as opposed to projective identification or extractive introjection. Here the target or recipient becomes as much a part of the interaction as the inducer or projector. Both parties interact using both projection and introjection as well as projective identification and extractive introjection in a cyclical manner. For instance, in the example above, perhaps before the identified inducer projected fear the identified target projected strength. In the identified target's view of the world, perhaps strength is associated with inability to maintain relationships due to being too aggressive. Thus there is no way to identify where the process begins, or who is demonstrating the stronger need for extractive introjection or projective identification.

With respect to affective role-representations, at the level of repressive defenses, as opposed to splitting defenses, the affects and part-selves or part-objects are more multifaceted and more likely to involve issues that are less threatening to the self. In the example above, projective identification and extractive introjection can be viewed as the communicative link between the role of one part-self that can handle responsibility and a part-object that cannot. The affective continuum between these two roles represents the extent to which others are viewed as having the ability to maintain relationships. So it can be seen that affective role-representations can be infinitely complex, with varying amounts of projective identification and extractive introjection. The combinations among the three continua described earlier provide an infinite array of types of affective role-representations. Combinations of defenses at many levels reveal the underlying representations to varying extents, based on varying levels of maturation.

The relational systems model thus differentiates levels of affective discomfort and demonstrates those parts of mental functioning that are related to these different levels. Anxiety causes guilt and is far less disturbing than threats to existence, which are shameful and perceived as weakness. Control and splitting defenses are needed when threats to existence continue to be perceived, but agency and repression develop as one learns that the threat to existence is not as much at issue as the threat of loss. All mental functioning can be differentiated at these two levels but both levels are involved simultaneously in all mental functioning as well. Threats to existence at the paranoid-schizoid level are never fully worked through and the need for repression at the depressive level is directly proportional to the extent to which threats to existence are still at issue. Even when repression is primary, there remains some behavioral influence related to defenses intended to make the world fulfill the expectations of the defended person. But these influences are less powerful and less directly related to paranoid-schizoid threats, resulting in a more flexible personality that can change its expectations.

GROWTH PHENOMENA: SEXUALITY, EFFECTANCE, PAIN, AND PLEASURE

The tension between individual growth and the community is expressed within the vicissitudes of personality development discussed up to this point. That is, the various threats to the self that constitute the three affective continua represent various tensions that arise between individual growth and the place of the individual within his or her community. I have argued, however, that the growth that is possible when those tensions are balanced provides the foundation for intrapsychic structure. Emotional growth occurs to the extent that those tensions are balanced, a phenomenon that I have called confidence. Within the individual personality system a combination of factors lead to balance and growth.

Those factors can be summed up in two categories. First, growth occurs to the extent that others, and the environment as a whole, react to the individual in a balanced way. This has been discussed in detail above. The tensions of the paranoid-schizoid position continua are balanced when the hungry, voracious, fearful, and aggressive affects are reacted to with understanding, the giving of space, caregiving, and a sense of safety. The tension of the depressive position continuum is balanced when others in the environment take adequate responsibility for themselves and the circumstances of their relations with others and allow for independent action as it is warranted based on maturity. Secondly, growth occurs to the extent that the individual system is able to balance and experience itself as confident. And attempts at balancing exist from the earliest stages of life. Even before true confidence is developed, experiences in which an individual is most likely to engage are those that allow the individual to pursue balance.

Balance

In a general sense, those actions that lead to comfort involve balance on the sustenance continuum, while actions that lead to efficacy involve balance on the self-protection continuum, and actions that involve mutual caregiving or interdependence involve the balance of the relatedness continuum. But the closer any experience is to a balance of one of the affective continua, the more likely it is to tend toward balance of the other two. For example, the experience of successfully asserting oneself, which precludes the presence of too much aggression or fear, also leads to a feeling that one has been satisfied, thus obviating hungry or voracious states. Such assertion also soothes threats at the relatedness level. That is, to the extent that one has successfully asserted oneself (meaning one has not been too aggressive or fearful), one will not feel guilty or lonely because important relationships will not have been damaged and, in fact, there may be a feeling that relationships have been strengthened. Balanced experience involving any one of the continua results in positive feelings within the other continua. This hypothesis leads to a new understanding of several concepts that have been central to psychoanalytic and object relations theory.

Pleasure

The concept of pleasure has been essential to the psychoanalytic model of intrapsychic functioning. In the relational systems model, pleasure is the emotional experience that occurs when there is a likelihood of experience resulting in growth. Pleasure leads to a feeling, even if it is only momentary, that satiation, desire, and safety are at hand, and that one is also balanced within one's environment or community. Of course there are kinds of pleasure that are more visceral than others, and that have more immediate positive consequences. The more visceral a pleasurable activity is, the more likely it is to be needed by an individual who is less well-developed and who is both very needy and very threatened. Nevertheless, the experience of extreme visceral pleasure is, perhaps even most enticingly, one that promises (even if falsely) the experience of growth and balance on all three continua. In substance abuse, for example, the individual may often have the feeling that he is sated, safe, and at peace with others; however, those feelings require the presence of the substance, and thus make the feeling of confidence and balance false. In contradistinction to those more visceral pleasures, at higher levels of personality integration pleasures that require patience and hard work can be aspired to. These pleasures are considered by the healthier individual as far more rewarding than immediate gratifications. The important point to make here is simply that pleasure is a growth experience that is pursued by the personality as a system because it has a balancing tendency. Individuals are driven toward pleasurable experiences *because* of that balancing tendency.

This view has some similarity to an object relations view in which "pleasure" has been considered by many (Jacobson 1964, Kernberg 1976) to be the beginning of the "good object" and "unpleasure" has been considered the beginning of the "bad object." As has been stated, in the relational systems model there is no good object per se, but rather complementary self and object affective role-representations. There is also no bad object, but rather a tendency to project or projectively identify those affects that threaten one the most. The model does, however, have similarities to the pleasure–unpleasure view in that buildup of good experience is explained as allowing the person to perceive herself in a more balanced way (roughly equivalent to the internalized good object). Also, buildup of bad experience is seen as interfering with growth and requiring that the most threatening affects be projected (roughly equivalent to the projection or projective identification of the bad object).

Effectance

A related issue has been made central by Greenberg (1991), a relational theorist who has promulgated "effectance" as a drive. Greenberg's intention is to explain the experience of drivenness (and he uses the term "drive" only for lack of a better word), which he does by describing two primary drives. Other than effectance, Greenberg describes a "safety" drive that includes all drivenness included within the sustenance and self-protection continua as they are described in the relational systems model. He separates effectance from those aspects of drivenness because of the strong evidence that once certain kinds of accomplishments or milestones are achieved by an individual, the continuance of that behavior no longer seems connected to safety, libido, or aggression. The relational systems model explains this phenomenon by growth and balance.

To the extent that a milestone has been reached, activity involved in the effort to achieve that accomplishment no longer has a quality of growth. Where there is no longer a hunger or a need to control, a fear or a need to destroy, there is nothing to be overcome or balanced and thus the behavior is no longer, or not as strongly, pursued. It is not pleasurable. Greenberg (1991) brings as evidence the tenacity with which a child will refuse to engage in previous behaviors after having accomplished a milestone. One of his examples is the child who has learned to read and no longer wants others to read to him. In the relational systems model this is explained by the new need to pursue the growthful and balancing behavior of reading independently. The child wants desperately to become better at putting ideas into his own head instead of being fed or controlled by outside influences. He is hungry for independent action and fearful of someone destroying the level of growth that has occurred.

Until this child gains some sense of confidence with respect to the new behavior, any outside suggestion or contact will be viewed as unbalancing, unpleasurable, and as a denial of growth. But with confidence, the child might want to engage in behaviors that appear to others to be regressive. Rather than being regressive, however, such behavior indicates that the child is finding a new task balancing and rewarding. For example, after a child has been reading to herself for a time, her confidence in that ability will likely grow to the extent that being read to can again be pleasurable. Now, however, the child likes being read to because she is finding interpersonal intimacy pleasurable, an aspect of being read to to which she became blind for a time because of a perception that balance was being threatened. In the relational systems model Greenberg's "effectance" appears to be driven behavior because such behavior promises growth and balance of the intrapsychic system.

Sexuality

Sexuality is another essential element within classical psychoanalytic theory that finds a very different viewpoint in the relational systems model. Sex or "libido" was one of the two original drives within Freudian theory. The term libido is also used by object relations theorists in describing the push toward interaction with others. In the relational systems model, sexuality is, just like pleasure and effectance, related to a tendency within individual systems toward activities that are likely to lead to growth and balance. Sexuality is singularly potent with respect to all the affects involved in the three continua of the relational systems model. There can be no doubt that sexuality involves issues of hunger or desire, feasting and devouring, aggression, vulnerability, the threat of isolation, and the responsibility for the partner's pleasure. In supporting his view that sexuality is so potent because it involves so many aspects of humanity and not because it is a drive, Mitchell (1988) makes the following statement as support for his "relational-conflict" model:

> In the relational model forms of relationship are seen as fundamental, and life is understood largely as an array of metaphors for expressing and playing out relational patterns: discovery, penetration, domination, surrender, control, longing, evasion, revelation, envelopment, merger, differentiation, and so on. The body is centrally important. Sexuality and bodily experiences are viewed as particularly

apt arenas for this activity, since sexuality is enormously multiform and plastic. [p. 91]

The relational systems model is completely consistent with Mitchell's views here. But adding to his viewpoint, the model suggests that sexuality is so potent because it produces an opportunity for growth and balance, not just relational experience.

In the vicissitudes of paranoid-schizoid level functioning, sexuality can become a balance for perceived threats to the individual system, but it also involves the opportunity for intimacy and working through of higher growth at an intimate level. Sexuality involves pain and pleasure, effectance, hunger, control, fear, aggression, loneliness, and responsibility. It offers so many possibilities for growth that it is an exceptionally powerful intrapsychic phenomenon. But from the viewpoint of the relational systems model, it is not directly related to any one kind of drive. Rather, it is a diffuse expression of many kinds of drivenness that may together have more power than any one specific kind. It is certainly no biological mistake that sexuality and intercourse are necessary for propagation of the species. Sexuality is an irresistible combination of opportunities for balance and growth.

The tension between community and individual growth as the primary force forging the individual personality at an intrapsychic level cannot be explained without discussing the ways growth is expressed within the system. In this section I have suggested that growth is pursued because of the need to balance threats within the intrapsychic system. To the extent that an activity gives the opportunity for, or feels as though it is supporting a balance of threatening affects, that activity will be engaged in. I have argued that pleasure, effectance, and sexuality are all phenomena that are related to opportunities for balance. These phenomena, however, cannot exist without the vicissitudes of the affective continua. If the continua were totally balanced, that is, if total confidence were achieved, the need for interpersonal interaction would cease, and no more growth would be pursued. Such an individual could not develop. The intrapsychic system develops because of the tension between individual and community. It functions in an ongoing way because of the tension between growth and the vicissitudes of growth that are found in threats to existence at the paranoid-schizoid level and threats to relatedness at the depressive level.

DIAGNOSTICS

One of the most intriguing benefits of the relational systems model is the clarity with which diagnostic categories, and the dynamics that cause them, can be described. This is particularly true of character disorders but also has extensive application to psychotic, dissociative, depressive, bipolar, anxiety, and trauma disorders. In this brief section Figure 6–3 and Figure 6–4 will be referred to in diagramming the most common disorders in the simplest fashion. The diagrams in Figure 6–3 are specific versions of the diagram in Figure 6–1 and the diagrams in Figure 6–4 are meant to depict the functioning of boundaries as depicted in Figure 6–2.

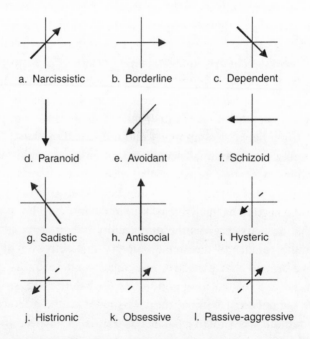

Figure 6–3.
Diagramming personality disorders. Personality disorders are depicted as having one primary affective continuum that generally maintains a unidirectional orientation so that behavior and thought can be illustrated as being at the arrowhead end of each arrow, and what is being defended against is at the other end. The axes shown represent sustenance (x axis), self-protection (y axis), and relatedness (z axis as shown by broken arrows). Only the last four disorders involve enough development at the relatedness level to require the z axis in the diagrams.

The personality or character disorders as shown in Figure 6–3 are made particularly intelligible by the relational systems model in which three primary affective continua can be oriented to each other in perpendicular orthogonal fashion to create a three-dimensional understanding of psychopathology. As discussed earlier, affective continua can be understood as being derived from two points connected by a line. One point is given the value x, y, z, and the other -x, -y, and -z. Such a line will always run through the middle of the diagram. Disorders of character that develop due to the vicissitudes in working through the paranoid-schizoid position are diagrammed as though the relatedness continuum has not developed (even though the relatedness continuum always develops at least to inchoate levels). The first eight diagrams are thus shown with only the x and y axes. The values of the points that are connected in those first eight diagrams are x, y and -x, -y. In Figures 6–3i through 6–3l, the relatedness or z continuum is drawn with a dotted arrow. In the individual diagrams, arrows are used to show the orientation of the primary affective continua of any one character disorder. This orientation is the most superficial layer of the personality. In Figure 6–3a, the narcissistic personality is depicted as an arrow that leads from a point between extremes of fear and hunger (or vulnerability) to a point between the extremes of voraciousness or dominance and aggression. The primary affective continuum of the narcissistic personality is in this way illustrated to be an orientation of dominance and aggressiveness that defends against extreme vulnerability. In Figure 6–3b, the borderline personality is shown as an arrow pointing toward voraciousness or control from a point that represents hunger or abandonment. This affective continuum demonstrates the borderline's extreme avoidance of abandonment with a general orientation of control or voraciousness.

It is important to understand that the behavior of any one personality disorder is not limited to what is represented by the arrowheads. Rather, this point merely shows the most common general orientation and likely behaviors that can be expected to range, in most cases, from the extremes of general orientation found within the quarter of the diagram that is bisected by the arrowhead. Furthermore, because the orientation is in opposition to some strong force within the personality, the threat that is opposed is typically manifest within the personality in hidden ways that are less threatening to the personality system. For example, the narcissist can be expected to be comfortable with behaviors that are aggressive (as represented by the destructive side of the self-protection continuum or y axis) or controlling (as represented by the voracious side of the sustenance continuum or x axis). There are, however, aspects to narcissistic character that express fears and hunger, such as marked paranoia and emotional isolation. The borderline personality can be shown to evince behaviors that are narcissistic (controlling and aggressive) or a mixture of controlling and fearful behaviors, which is the characteristic behavior most common in the dependent personality as shown in Figure 6–3c. The borderline also, however, experiences extreme emptiness that disguises the threat of abandonment.

Descriptions of these two pathologies are typically consistent with this view. Masterson (1981) describes the narcissistic personality as a grandiose defense against extreme vulnerability. Klein's description of envy (1957) closely parallels this view of narcissistic pathology in its description of the devaluation of others who must be perceived to be weaker and less worthwhile so that an omnipotent self image can be maintained. The cycle of the borderline in Masterson's work (1981), in which clinging and dependent behavior transforms into cold and distant behavior when there is a threat of merger (and then back to dependent again when withdrawal or disapproval is sensed), is also consistent with this model. Each of the personality disorders, with the possible exception of the schizoid whose hungry and empty orientation is maintained with little if any emotionality, can be understood this way.

The end of the continuum that is defended against, as shown by these diagrams, is understood as the least likely emotional orientation for any of the personality disorders. Even though aspects of this end of the continuum are often experienced in indirect ways, the direct feeling state is so tenaciously defended against that it is rarely, if ever, experienced (if it is experienced it becomes part of a regression to earlier times). Of course the problem with regard to such defense is that the avoided feeling state is exactly what must be experienced if the personality disorder is to be cured. Such experience can only occur within a context in which the personality-disordered individual is exposed to these feelings when they are not appropriate to reality or when they indicate a misinterpretation of reality that can be corrected.

In the case of the narcissist, for example, transference works to perceive others as voracious and aggressive, and the threat of being vulnerably hungry and fearful makes the narcissist need to be better than others. The narcissist is only comfortable surrounding himself (Kohut 1971, Wolf 1988) with others who can be thought of as equally great and similar, as in the "twinship" transference, appropriately admiring as in the "mirroring" transference, or so great that even the narcissist can learn from them as in the "idealizing" transference. Only by very slow introduction to the reality of the other person in their imperfect but not despicable form, so that severe narcissistic injury is avoided (Winnicott 1963a, Kohut 1977), can the narcissist begin to integrate some level of the vulnerability that comes with the reality that others are not always less than, or admiring of, the narcissist. That is, the narcissist must be allowed to feel vulnerable in realizing he is not so extremely special while with someone who seems to accept and appreciate his vulnerability and his overdetermined need to be special.

In the case of the borderline personality, the patient's transference has two faces. On the one hand, the patient's transference works to perceive others to be controlling and aggressive and creates a need to be better than others (similar to the case of the narcissist). On the other hand, the patient's transference works to view others as having the strength (as in the tough or strong front) and self-control (as in maintained hunger or lack of emotionality) to which the borderline must cling (which will be shown to be descriptive of the dependent personality). Through action that maintains these two orientations, jumping from one to the other, the borderline avoids states perceived as abandonment (the abandonment depression). These two alternate orientations also allow the borderline to perceive the self as independent, since merger is avoided and at times self-definition becomes strong and in control. The threat of real independence, however, leads to the threat of abandonment and the resultant clinging behavior of the dependent side of the transference. Ultimately, the riddle of the borderline's personality can only be solved within a relationship in which the other is finally understood as separate and not under the borderline's clinging or aggressive control. Within such a relationship the possibility of abandonment that comes with others being seen as truly separate can be experienced within a context in which such abandonment does not occur.

All of the personality disorders can be described in similar fashion by using the relational systems model. Although it is beyond the scope of this study to describe all the personality disorders in depth, it is useful to briefly outline the understanding that is offered by each diagram. The dependent (Figure 6–3c) can be understood as maintaining a clinging, voracious, and fearful orientation as a defense against hungry and aggressive feelings. The paranoid, as diagrammed in Figure 6–3d, can be understood as maintaining a fearful, hypervigilant orientation as a defense against rage and destructive tendencies. (Discussion of the paranoid personality disorder has led some authors, notably Millon (Millon and Davis 1996), to include many narcissistic personalities within the paranoid category. In my own classificational system, however, the paranoid personality corresponds to only those individuals who primarily evince a fearful and somewhat avoidant suspicious nature. The aggressive and grandiose versions are, in my view, subcategories of the sadistic, antisocial, and narcissistic personality disorders.) The avoidant (Figure 6–3e) maintains a combination of fear and hunger to defend against aggression and voraciousness or desire to control objects. The schizoid (Figure 6–3f) defends against merger with voracious, controlling others by maintaining a hungry, empty, emotionless state. The sadistic (Figure 6–3g, here thought of as an especially dangerous and somewhat schizoid antisocial personality) defends against fear of voraciousness or being controlled by being aggressive and relatively emotionless (and often needing to victimize others to maintain this orientation). The antisocial (Figure 6–3h) defends against fear with aggressiveness. The hysteric (Figure 6–3i) (here the relatedness or z continuum comes into play, and the shortness of the continuum depicts the presence of more balance in the hysteric than in the case of the histrionic) maintains emotional distance by denying true emotions and intimacy as a defense against the experience of guilt. The histrionic (Figure 6–3j) maintains an extreme false self and hides true emotions to defend against responsibility fragmentation. The obsessive (Figure 6–3k) (again, brevity of the axis depicts greater balance) defends against loneliness by maintaining a responsible but guilty orientation. The passive-aggressive (Figure 6–3l) varies between rudimentary, undeveloped guilt or responsibility fragmentation and voracious aggressiveness (as a narcissist with slightly built-up relatedness) in defending against isolation on the one hand and vulnerability on the other.

The last four personality constellations depicted above (Figures 6–3i through 6–3l) are also notable for difficulties with control of self and other. As discussed in the section above where agency and control were differentiated by the depressive and paranoid-schizoid positions, these disorders are marked by incomplete but partial working through of the depressive position. Thus agency is not completely developed and issues pertaining to agency or control become central to personality conflicts. In personalities fixated primarily at the paranoid-schizoid level, the need for control is part of most interactions but is not an issue that the person is aware of. In cases where the depressive position has started to develop, control is often the primary issue. For example (to take them in the same order as they were presented above), the hysteric fears guilt and maintains an emotionally lonely existence partially due to fear of being controlled by responsibility. Responsibility has become threatening because that responsibility suggests guilt for the troubles of an attachment figure, thus causing anxiety. (Often the hysteric attempts to control others so that they cannot get close, making the control issue one of agency, that is, based on maintaining self control, not on meeting sustenance or self-protection needs.) Emotional loneliness, however painful, allows for freedom. The histrionic maintains a wildness and carefree attitude to prove his freedom from responsibility. Often this wildness is in direct proportion to how responsibility fragmented the histrionic fears becoming if he were to take responsibility for damaging relations of an attachment figure. The obsessive, in contrast to the hysteric, feels a need to control everything to fight off the possibility of loss (the obsessive focuses efforts at controlling on the self, again connecting the controlling attitude to agency). The passive-aggressive fights against being controlled while at the same time allowing others to control her from a fear that asserting individuality or specialness would result in complete isolation from relatedness.

In Figure 6–4, psychotic, dissociative, depressive, bipolar, anxiety, and trauma disorders are illustrated as conditions involving boundary dysfunction or failure. The prototypical diagram follows the same configuration as depicted in Figure 6–2, in which the paranoid-schizoid and depressive position boundaries are shown as an inner and an outer boundary respectively. All of these disorders involve failures of the false self, repression, or the outer boundary (or all of these) that occur under certain conditions.

Earlier, in the section entitled Paranoid-Schizoid and Depressive Position Boundaries and the Relatedness Continuum, the working of the inner boundary in prepsychotic conditions was described as inflexibly permeable due to an individual's inability to differentiate him- or herself from the environment. Psychotic conditions are caused by the existence of this state of the inner boundary at a time when the outer-boundary, false self is no longer successful in managing to adapt to the environment.

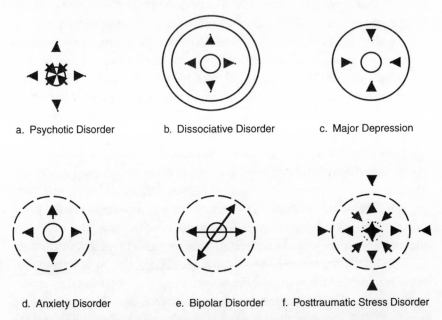

a. Psychotic Disorder   b. Dissociative Disorder   c. Major Depression

d. Anxiety Disorder   e. Bipolar Disorder   f. Posttraumatic Stress Disorder

Figure 6–4.
Disorders that involve failure of the false self or repression are depicted as they involve the inner (paranoid-schizoid position) boundary, and the outer (depressive position) boundary (compare to Figure 6–2). The disorders that involve boundary dysfunction are generally referred to in the *Diagnostic and Statistical Manual of Mental Disorders* (*DSM-IV*) as Axis I disorders. These disorders are caused by inflexibility of the outer boundary that required the environment to coincide with very specific needs of the individual based on inflexibility of the inner boundary. The outer boundary fails when life circumstances change or become overwhelming and affects controlled by the inner boundary become problematic.

Boundaries and Psychosis

Individuals who become psychotic have always maintained themselves according to a specific external structure such as a family with very specific and intrusive expectations. The false self that has been erected and the barely developed, inflexibly permeable outer boundary that allows the environment to define the individual, fail when the environment changes, such as when there is a departure from home or a new expectation of independence. As the false self and outer boundary fail following contact with the new rules of the social world, the permeable inner boundary perceives the world as threatening existence in one or more ways, and as evoking one's own destructiveness, fear of annihilation, engulfment, or starvation. The only possible defenses against these threats are various ways of retreating from reality which, if prolonged, include a shift from inflexible permeability to inflexible impermeability of the inner boundary. As stated earlier, examples of unguarded permeability include disorganized states in which a sudden psychotic break has occurred with wild projective processes that make the world conform with exactly what is needed to balance inner threats.

Examples of psychotic states that involve inflexible impermeability of the inner boundary and failure of the outer boundary include delusional states and catatonic states. Delusional states continue the projective process but become organized around particular emotional issues. The extreme withdrawal of the catatonic state occurs when inner affects become so threatening that practically no connection with reality can be tolerated and inner boundary impermeability resembles an implosive collapse. The prolonged version of psychosis is depicted in Figure 6–4a as an impermeable inner boundary thrusting projections either inward or outward and with no perceivable outer boundary.

Dissociative Disorders

Dissociative disorders are related to psychotic disorders in that the afflicted person's orientation to the world is determined almost entirely by the false self or depressive-position boundary. In the case of the dissociative, however, there has been enough development of the paranoid-schizoid position for the inner boundary to become inflexibly impermeable in daily interaction, as opposed to the prepsychotic, whose inner boundary is inflexibly permeable until there is a change in the environment. The dissociative needs the world to be a specific way that is consistent with paranoid-schizoid needs and at the same time tries to be exactly as the world wants him to be so that these inner needs are held in check. Much as in the case of the psychotic, the dissociative has episodes when environmental expectations seem to change dramatically. He becomes desperate to continue hiding extreme affects that push for expression and that were held in check by the particular compromise forged with the previously known environment. These affects are so dangerous to the dissociative that rather than experience them he shuts out awareness of them while they are being expressed. The depressive-position boundary becomes completely impermeable, allowing for no conscious experience of the effect of these affects upon the environment. Dissociative disorders are depicted in Figure 6–4b as an inner boundary pushing powerful affects toward the outer boundary that then redoubles in impermeability, causing a complete denial of the inner threat.

Major Depression

Major depression is illustrated in Figure 6–4c as the outer boundary collapsing upon the inner boundary. In cases of severe depression a feared total failure of repression that would allow extreme badness to surface and destroy relationships results in an outer boundary that inflexibly defines all others as being affected by, and affecting, the self. The outer boundary attempts to squash the affects that threaten to come into consciousness. An afflicted person thus isolates to protect others and continues to wallow in feelings of inferiority, weakness, and guilt as a way of denying feelings that could hurt relatedness. The feelings of badness further exacerbate the need to withdraw, which in turn reinforces feelings of badness, and there appears to be no defense against this cycle. Psychotic breaks occurring due to depression involve dynamics similar to the prolonged psychotic disorder of Figure 6–4a, except that depressives typically have a well-developed depressive position boundary. When that boundary fails, however, the inner boundary becomes especially impermeable requiring the world to fit into those definitions that can balance inner badness.

Anxiety Disorders

Anxiety disorders, depicted in Figure 6–4d, also involve bad affects leaking through the repressive barrier. This similarity explains why there is so much overlap between anxiety and depressive disorders. When anxiety disorders worsen they often become major depression. When major depression clears, there is often a period of anxiety. In Figure 6–4d, anxiety disorders are portrayed as involving pressure from affects originating within the paranoid-schizoid boundary and leaking into awareness. The outer depressive–position boundary is shown as a broken line, indicating that it becomes more permeable as more situations and a greater variety of others are allowed to affect the anxious individual. Anxiety disorders also involve a cyclical pattern. As situations are interpreted as connecting to inner affects which then threaten relatedness, more and more situations become applicable by association. If too many situations become associated with the threat to relatedness based on the leak of inner badness, the anxious individual will become depressed.

Bipolar Disorders

Those with bipolar disorders, Figure 6–4e, are afflicted with a failure of repression and the outer boundary, a condition that allows for concerns at once paranoid-schizoid and then depressive to alternate. Bipolars have typically developed into the relatedness continuum with rudimentary repression, guarding cared-for others from bad affects. However, the specific nature of these bad affects involves maintaining strong narcissistic or voracious, controlling needs at the paranoid-schizoid level. Bipolars are considered to have been especially vulnerable to disappointments and failures because of these paranoid-schizoid position needs. When there is some kind of failure that forces them to question their strength, greatness, mastery, or control, efforts at regaining those feelings for fear of experiencing vulnerability, emptiness, or abandonment can result in manic states. In the manic phase the outer boundary becomes extremely impermeable as the bipolar cares about no one but his own accomplishments and grandiosity. Further failure, often exacerbated by problems involved in behaving manically (such as ignoring others, lack of attention to detail, and risk taking) will lead to a depressed phase that, much like that of the major depressive, involves the collapsing of the outer boundary in an effort to protect others who could be hurt by the inner badness that sometimes surfaces. Thus, the bipolar's outer boundary fluctuates from inflexible impermeability to inflexible permeability depending on which phase he is in (illustrated here by the broken circle of the outer boundary). It should also be noted that the psychotic break in the bipolar disorder involves dynamics similar to those seen in Figure 6–4a. Just as the psychotic break of major depression involves the inner boundary becoming especially impermeable, so too does the psychotic break of the bipolar.

Posttraumatic Stress Disorder

Posttraumatic stress disorder, Figure 6–4f, involves a particular reaction to the experience of trauma. During a serious trauma the threats of the paranoid-schizoid position are stirred up as the possibility of a real threat to existence (death in some cases, but emotional existence in the case of abuse or torture) is experienced. Because the threatening situation cannot be ignored and pushes itself through defenses, both boundaries are weakened and the afflicted individual loses the ability to differentiate real threats from those that are associated with the original trauma. The bad affects that were stirred up during the trauma leak into consciousness and cause anxiety and depression to the extent that such anxiety becomes overwhelming. The ability to integrate experience becomes labored because stirred-up affects remain unacceptable at an interpersonal level. These affects typically involve a connection between the level of responsibility the traumatized individual takes for what occurred, and inner affects that this individual associates with taking or not taking responsibility. In the diagram, weakened boundaries are depicted as broken concentric circles. Arrows pointing out from the center, in from the outside, and both ways from between the circles portray the pressure from within to think and feel about the trauma, pressure from outside as daily experience is automatically associated with aspects of the trauma, and efforts at holding down feelings and thoughts that will not go away.

GROWTH AND THE VICISSITUDES OF THE AFFECTIVE CONTINUA: POSITIVE AND NEGATIVE FEEDBACK

Family systems theory has been based in general systems theory (von Bertalanffy 1968), cybernetics (most notably the work of Wiener [1954], Maturana [1978, 1980], and Maruyama [1963]), the physical sciences

(Prigogine 1976), and communications theory (Bateson 1958, 1972, 1977, Watzlawick et al. 1967), as well as various theories that involve triangulation in relationships (Bowen 1978, Haley 1977). The relational systems model is fully compatible with these theories and adds to it by describing the functioning of the intrapsychic system.

The relational systems model posits that intrapsychic functioning involves various tensions. The tension states within the intrapsychic system always involve the superordinate tension between individual growth and the community. Homeostatic patterns or balance within the intrapsychic system are, by necessity, consistent with the larger systems of which they are a part. The balancing tendency and homeostatic patterns at both the individual and community level, as ruled by the tension between individual growth and community, encompass the functioning of cybernetics within the general system of community.

Intrapsychic and interpersonal are in constant communication through projective and introjective identification that involves logical types in communication (Whitehead and Russell 1910), and that is directly related to the need for consistency between individual and community-level homeostatic patterns. The less healthy a system is, the more likely it is to dissipate tension in the quickest manner, and triangulation of a third person who can hold the conflictual tensions that occur within a dyad is a common way of quickly restoring balance in a system. What follows is a brief excursion into family systems theory for the purpose of comparing and contrasting the relational systems model at the intrapsychic level with theories of interpersonal communication. First, the natural development of mental growth within the intrapsychic system beginning in infancy will be examined. This examination will naturally lead to an analysis of logical types in communication and how these are related to the paranoid-schizoid and depressive-level boundaries and projective processes. Finally, the effect of hierarchy and the functioning of triangles will be discussed from the perspective of the relational systems model.

SYSTEMS THEORY AND THE INTRAPSYCHIC SYSTEM

The infant is part of the larger system of mother and child, which is, of course, part of the larger system of family, which is part of community, and so on. In the natural state of growth, the infant gives feedback to the environment indicating need. This feedback is deviation-amplifying or positive feedback. That is, the feedback, if properly understood, says "give me more, give me more, give me more." But at some point, when the infant has had enough, deviation-correcting or negative feedback is communicated from the infant. Such feedback indicates, "I've had enough, I've had enough, stop." These two tendencies are related to the tendency toward balance within the infant's intrapsychic system and roughly comprise the intrapsychic cybernetic model. For the sake of simplicity I will refer to the larger system, of which the infant is a subsystem, as the "community system" or the "environment" (denoting tension between individual growth and community) even when specifically referring to the infant/ primary parent dyad.

Positive and Negative Feedback

There is an essential difference between this cybernetic system and the typical model. Typically, negative and positive feedback phenomena are separated. A common example of a negative feedback system involves a thermostat. A thermostat is set at one particular temperature and when a room is too cold the heat stays on until the thermostat reads at the proper setting, at which point it shuts the heat off. Negative feedback, then, stops something. Positive feedback, on the other hand, makes something continue. It is normally thought of as making things escalate out of control (like Bateson's [1958] "runaway"), until the system changes in some significant way. For example if a man shouts at his wife who then shouts louder and in turn the husband shouts louder and so on, eventually one of them will lose their voice or leave or add in another family member, and so on, thus changing the system into a new system.

The human personality differs from the typical cybernetic system in that balance is maintained at a level of comfort between two values of discomfort. That is, both positive and negative feedback are used within the intrapsychic system. What is most unusual is the use of positive feedback (in the form of pleasure and equanimity) to maintain or increase the response that is already occurring in the environment. Positive feedback is not needed within most mechanical systems but is very common in biological systems.

From the point of view of the relational systems model, positive and negative feedback within the intrapsychic system create positive and negative feedback to the environment. Need states of the individual are constantly regulated by the threat to interpersonal existence, and balance provides the greatest opportunity for growth. Take for example the hungry infant (hunger for food, attention, and comfort all fall on the sustenance continuum; see Figure 6–1). At the intrapsychic level, hunger is negative feedback based on the threat of starvation. That is, sustenance is needed by the system and that need grows until it is perceivable as hunger by the infant, who will be uncomfortable to the extent that this hunger approaches the threat of starvation. At some point hunger is so uncomfortable that the infant must do something (like the heat turning on in response to negative feedback by the thermostat) and the infant cries. This cry serves to signal to the environment that sustenance is necessary, and can also be understood as negative feedback to an environment that is failing to provide it. In effect the cry signals "stop failing to provide sustenance." The environment then, ideally, perceives this negative feedback, that is, that lack of feeding has gone on long enough, and begins to feed the infant. The infant now feeds while giving positive feedback to the environment that feeding continues to be necessary. The pleasure the infant experiences serves as intrapsychic positive feedback, and the consequent expression of experiencing pleasure serves as positive feedback expressing a need for the environment to continue feeding.

This positive feedback cycle will continue until the infant begins to experience some sense of being full, which will be uncomfortable to the extent that such fullness approaches the threat of engulfment, experienced as crowding or being stuffed. This intrapsychically signals negative feedback that says "enough," and consequent negative feedback is relayed via behavior to the environment. There will then be positive feedback both intrapsychically and interpersonally for lack of feeding from the environment in the form of independent play, sleep, and so on. Thus a natural process of positive and negative feedback within the intrapsychic system communicates with the community system.

But the intrapsychic system is only a subsystem of the community that has its own need for homeostasis and balance. Thus, the infant's communication via positive and negative feedback to the environment will not be responded to perfectly. The infant will sometimes be more hungry or full than his system would ideally desire. He will sometimes be left hungry without sustenance and will sometimes receive sustenance when it is not needed, thus interrupting other opportunities for growth. The needs of larger systems will take precedence over the needs of the smaller system, which will require that the infant adapt to the vagaries of environmental response.

Imperfect responding, however, is also necessary for the infant's growth. With perfect responding there would be no adaptation. The infant would not have to develop the ability to balance himself. No self would develop. This concept is roughly equivalent to Kohut's (1977) and Winnicott's (1963a) ideas that growth requires an introduction to the reality of imperfect empathy in the environment. Negative and positive feedback would simply smoothly balance the infant who would cease to be human. In classical physics the perfect balancing of a system to the point that it becomes static is called entropy. What is needed is a good-enough environment. The concept of the "good-enough mother" (Winnicott 1960a) is one level at which this is true. The mother cares for the infant and tries to perceive his needs and take care of him but because she has her own needs and is herself affected by the larger system of which she is a part (which includes her child as well as everyone else who affects her), she is not able to handle his needs perfectly. The good- enough environment is that system of which the mother is a part and can be more generally understood as handling the infant's needs, to varying extents, well enough. The infant develops his personality based on the adaptation he makes within this environment. How the personality functions, then, is based on this adaptation.

Adaptations to the Environment

Returning now to the workings of negative and positive feedback as governed by the affective continua, it is important to examine what these adaptations entail. If the infant's environment responds in a good-enough way to his sustenance and self-protection needs, small adaptations will be made that change the thermostat of the individual in ways that are not seriously detrimental to overall functioning. In the example of our infant, perhaps we might imagine a mother who enjoys breast-feeding so much that she sometimes has a desire to breast-feed that is more expressive of her own needs than those of her child. So she feeds her child for too long, in too many situations, and often when he is not expressing a need for sustenance. This infant thus starts to feel too filled up, controlled, and crowded, and changes his thermostat to put him further away from this existential threat. To a small extent, equal to the extent to which the mother overfeeds her child, he makes himself a person who maintains a hungry position without perceiving a need for sustenance. This position allows him to maintain balance with more independence than he would otherwise have, but it also leaves him hungry and dissatisfied. In small amounts, this sort of tendency can be part of a healthy personality.

More extreme adaptations, however, can be expected when the environment is not good enough. If this mother not only continues to feed this child when he is clearly no longer hungry, but also takes care of all his needs before he can do things for himself, and effectively gives him no freedom, his adaptation might be to leave himself in an extremely hungry state without asking for or acting as though he needs sustenance. Such an individual (likened to a schizoid personality) cuts himself off from emotion altogether for fear of being controlled if he should express any need.

This cutting-off process can be understood as occurring to a dyadic-level deviation-amplifying feedback loop that arises because of the failure of a deviation-correcting feedback loop within the infant's intrapsychic system. At the point that the infant experiences discomfort due to the threat of engulfment, his cry or withdrawal expresses to the dyadic system that sustenance is no longer needed. If the parent's system misunderstands this signal owing to a need that is satisfied by caring for the infant, and continues to provide the same level of care for the infant, the infant's distress will be more extreme and the signal more intense. In the scenario of deviation amplification, this system could become a "runaway," until some major change creates an entirely different system.

In the case of the schizoid what is changed is the definition of equilibrium. That is, the parameters of comfort must be changed so that the infant can continue to grow given the specific tendencies of the larger system. So the schizoid cuts off emotions and maintains a state of withdrawal that makes the threat of engulfment less threatening. Although he maintains independence, however, the schizoid never allows for the maturation that can only take place with sustenance. Such an orientation is an extreme adaptation, but nevertheless, maintains individual homeostasis at the most comfortable possible (although compromised) level, given interpersonal system parameters.

Equifinality and Homeostasis

Another important systems concept comes into play here. The principle of equifinality (von Bertalanffy 1974) states that in open systems, homeostasis is based on the parameters set, independent of the original state of the system. Systems authors often interpret this concept as suggesting that the etiology of mental dysfunction is unimportant because the current homeostatic pattern of the system is the problem. That is, systems therapists believe they can readily reset the parameters of the system through intervention. In the relational systems model, however, the principle of equifinality is important in a different way. By knowing how certain parameters become set, the particular need for those parameters can be discerned. In the case of the schizoid, for example, the homeostasis has been reset so that there is little emotional contact with the environment. Although it is not a pleasurable balance, the intrapsychic system of the schizoid is sustained with little emotional sustenance because, as stated above, any expression of need brings with it a severe threat of absorption, enmeshment, or loss of personhood.

Furthermore, the personality will be crystallized and unavailable to intervention to the extent that the individual is unable to come into contact with situations that are automatically perceived as threats. If the individual is afraid, it follows logically that there is something to be afraid of. Threats to existence are projected and the fearful behavior of the individual reinforces her tendency to believe that the environment should be feared. Because contact with the environment is interpreted as threatening, changing the parameters of the intrapsychic system becomes very difficult as such an interpretation of the environment continually reinforces the perception that the parameters are correctly set.

The cost of maintaining such a homeostatic pattern, however, is that the possibility of mental growth is extremely limited. If the world is interpreted as a place where any contact with others might result in ceasing to be an individual (engulfment) then the growth that could occur through contact is impossible. Etiology is important because it suggests not only what is needed within the system but also what is being avoided. In the example of the schizoid, it could be speculated that she needs to be in a relationship where she is allowed and encouraged to be an individual. Hunger could be viewed as the primary problem. The schizoid maintains hunger while most of the people she feels comfortable with maintain voraciousness. Since voracious others are the ones who most readily accept her projections of threat, they are therefore the only ones the schizoid understands, trusts, or feels comfortable with. In essence her parameters for equilibrium have been specifically designed to withstand such a relationship and other relationships are far more awkward for her. The schizoid, as well as those with whom she associates, confirm in one another the perceptions of the world they have developed.

The Basis of Interventions

If there is to be an intervention, this hunger must be addressed, and the level of existential fear involved suggests that changes would be very difficult, given the self-fulfilling nature of the need to project affects that are most feared. In the relational systems model, the principle of equifinality suggests that a particular etiology has resulted in the parameters that are now set. Interventions must aim at demonstrating to patients in treatment that the perceptions of the environment they automatically project, and the interpersonal cycles they automatically recapitulate, are incorrect in a world where there is an infinite variety in human character. In other words, the parameters of the intrapsychic system can only be changed if they are demonstrated to be unnecessary or inaccurate. This change can only occur if two systems join and interaction between the two makes the old parameters of at least one of them impossible.

Feedback and the Narcissistic Personality

The kinds of problems described above result primarily from problems with deviation-correcting feedback or negative feedback. The intrapsychic system, prepared to respond to the environment of childhood, either reacts too soon or not soon enough to interpersonal situations. Deviation-amplifying or positive feedback loops also become very important at points in individual development where a breakdown occurs. The narcissistic personality who has failed is perhaps the best example of this phenomenon. The two threats most avoided by the narcissistic personality are annihilation and starvation, and thus these individuals typically maintain an aggressive, voracious style. Maintenance of this aggressive, voracious style is a relatively permanent adaptation to the threat of annihilation and starvation that was perceived as very much a part of the system in which the individual developed. But this general adaptation, based on negative feedback that makes the system stop aggressive consumption only when the narcissist is extremely confident that fear and hunger cannot come close to hurting him, can break down. The narcissistic personality requires acquisition, achievement, and success because these attributes earn him admiration for being the opposite of what most frightens him. In situations of failure such personalities can fluctuate wildly into needy, fearful states, at which time they attempt to again regain admiration with even more grandiose schemes and wild acquisitions (as depicted above in Figure 6–4e, although some level of relatedness was suggested there).

For the narcissistic personality, such a phenomenon involves positive feedback as bigger schemes lead to greater failure and more fearful hunger until something changes in the system. Often failures eventually lead to very deep depression, substance dependence, or, alternatively, new sustaining relational involvements. Sometimes what occurs is a recognition of the need to change and the chance to work through the most feared affects with someone who slowly proves it safe to do so, as in psychotherapy. Family systems therapists, in fact, have been known to intentionally create interpersonally driven deviation-amplifying feedback loops within families for the purpose of creating a new, hopefully healthier, system.

It is clear that positive and negative feedback loops, along with the concepts of homeostasis and equifinality, are compatible with the relational systems model. Although this discussion primarily used the sustenance continuum as an example, there are an infinite number of possible combinations between the sustenance, self-protection, and relatedness continua, just as there are an infinite variety of human experiences. The greater the health and integration of any individual, the more varied these combinations and the closer they are to a balanced and healthy homeostatic pattern of the kind ideal for growth. The less healthy the individual the less varied are the combinations and the further they are from a balanced homeostatic pattern. We have discussed the way pathology necessitates a particular view of the environment that attempts to exclude from awareness those experiences that are most threatening, and it has been suggested that deeper pathology within the intrapsychic system makes such a view more desperately held. I would now like to turn to a discussion of the behaviors that actually reinforce expected outcomes in the environment.

PROJECTIVE AND INTROJECTIVE IDENTIFICATION AND THE THEORY OF LOGICAL TYPES IN COMMUNICATION

Systems theorists, most notably Bateson and colleagues (1956), used Whitehead and Russell's (1910) theory of logical types to explain how communication tends to bind behavior. The relational systems model is able to clarify the systemic process involved in the double bind by differentiating what occurs in the intrapsychic system of the binder and what, in turn, occurs in the intrapsychic system of the bound. The theory of logical types suggests that human communications include messages at different logical levels. The relational systems model also postulates that communication occurs at different logical levels. The paranoid-schizoid and depressive position boundaries determine what kind of messages will be communicated.

Logical Levels of Communication

In the theory of logical types, sometimes these logical levels of communication are in conflict, a situation that creates very confusing communications. In their seminal book, *The Pragmatics of Human Communication*, Watzlawick and colleagues (1967) have described a common form of logical typing as the "report" and "command" levels of communication. From their point of view, what is verbally stated can be considered the report message and the underlying emphasis, suggestion, or emotional behavior associated with that verbal message can be considered the command message.

A particularly confusing, and sometimes destructive, example of conflicting report and command levels of communication is the double bind (Bateson et al. 1956). An example often used in this regard (L. Hoffman 1981) is the irritated parent who says "Go to bed; you're very tired and I want you to get your sleep." If the child interprets this to be a caring statement and draws close, rejection will ensue. If she challenges the parent by stating, for example, "I'm not tired," the result will also likely be rejection. In this message the report level appears to be a caring statement, but the command level will readily become known to be rejection or irritation. The message is thus very confusing to the child and the only possible response is confusion.

Double Binds

The double-bind hypothesis, which was developed to describe communication in the most severely pathological families, the families of schizophrenics, included a total of five necessary components that made such communication especially pernicious. These components were discussed in the last chapter. To review, not only would there be two levels of communication in conflict, (1) report, conflicting with (2) command, but (3) comment on or escape from the process would be forbidden, (4) the situation would have survival significance, and (5) after the pattern of communication was established, the entire process would result in panic, rage, or frustration with only the smallest provocation. In the example of the child above, (1 and 2) a seemingly caring comment really expresses rejection, (3) her comment in fact results in rejection, (also 3) she cannot leave her mother, (4) her mother's love, approval, or acceptance has survival significance, and (5) after it is established, even the smallest hint that her mother's niceness might betray irritation or rejection will result in self-negating rage within the child. All of these components are necessary for the full effects of a double bind. However, it is interesting that less severe forms of the double bind, forms that do not in reality include all of these components, cause very similar reactions.

The final component of the double-bind theory has significant ramifications for the concepts of transference, projection, introjection, and projective and introjective identification. When a person is used to communicating in a particular way within the family, that communication pattern occurs more readily in future experiences. A person reads new situations as if they were like original family situations, and the person then requires only very minute parts of the process to be evident in order to assume that the whole meaning of the process is the same as in the patterns already established. To the extent that double binding occurred in one's family of origin, where interactions with parents are readily viewed as necessary to survival, escape is unlikely, and where comment merely exacerbates the confusion by creating anger in the parents, the environment will tend to be readily viewed as double binding. The person who has been put in double binds is also more likely to double-bind others.

This phenomenon requires some explanation. From the perspective of the relational systems model, the result of the double bind within the personality system of the bound person is a change in parameters, as was discussed above. That is, when the environment impinges upon the individual with its needs in a way that ignores his needs but also suggests that it is his needs that are primary, a particularly confusing situation results, and there is a change of internal parameters for equilibrium. To continue with the example of the schizoid, the mother needs, for her own reasons, to continue "caring" for the infant when the infant no longer needs such caring. Thus, this "caring" is not really caring at all, but is, rather, sustenance for the mother. The schizoid tendency is thus to maintain self-integrity through withdrawal so that the environment's response will not be as damaging.

Double Binds and the Schizoid

This manner of maintaining equilibrium will, by necessity, require a particular kind of communication with the environment. The schizoid who, contrary to his own self-knowledge, continues to need relationships (relationships that appear not to be relationships), double binds others in his environment to sustain those relationships. His deepest fear is that others will control him, so he never even allows himself to experience the feeling that he cares. Others do, however, come into contact with him. Because he is not consciously afraid, if another person shows interest in him, he will associate with that person. He will do whatever that other person wants because doing it does not noticeably bother him. Within this situation, he actually double-binds the other person into being voracious and controlling. At one level of communication, the report level, he is willing to associate and, in fact, is willing to do whatever the other person wants. But at the command level of communication, the other has absolutely no emotional impact on him. To the extent that the other person brings her own personality to the situation needing to get close to others out of some kind of desperation, she will read this confusing message as if neither leaving nor commenting is an option, and the situation has survival significance. Ever-increasing efforts at getting to an emotional connection will be attempted, and these will appear to be controlling, voracious behavior. Thus, the schizoid double-binds those who choose to associate closely with him into behaving in a voracious manner.

Double Binds and the Dependent

Perhaps an example of another diagnostic category would help in the generalization of this process. Imagine the double-binding behavior of the dependent personality. The dependent's behavior can be understood as a combination of voraciousness and fear that fends off experiences of starvation and destruction (see Figure 6–4c). The dependent comes into contact with many people and is always willing to do what those others want due to his tendency to consume what others have to offer (staving off hunger) and his fearfulness of the possibility of conflict or aggression. There is a report-level message given to others that says "You are sustaining and so strong." But the command level message says, "If you don't give me all your love I am worthless and will fall apart." To the extent that another comes into contact with the dependent, and feels such clinginess is difficult to brush off (and also feels some responsibility to take care of this fearful other), there would be some sense that leaving is difficult, commenting is hurtful, and there is survival significance for this dependent. Within the relationship the dependent can never be satisfied. Efforts to soothe and make the dependent feel better only lead to more dependence and clinginess. The engulfment and inadequacy feelings of the involved person that result from failure to bolster the dependent are likely to create a reaction of withdrawal and aggression as these are the responses that are least likely to allow one to be engulfed or fearful. Thus the dependent double-binds others into aggressive and withdrawn responses.

It is interesting to note that the most likely person to be a target for such interaction is someone who already has characteristics that are associated with what will tend to be double-bound. In the case of the schizoid, for example, only people who want to draw others out will attempt contact, and these others will generally fit the schizoid's understanding of others as voracious since they will try so hard to get an emotional connection. In the case of the dependent, others who appear confident, stoic, and tough tend to be attractive, but their confidence is actually overconfidence and their toughness is an aggressive overcompensation for feelings of weakness. Thus the vagaries of the double bind involve all aspects of valency, not only transference, projection, and projective identification, but also introjection and introjective identification, as attractions of persons to each other tend to be defined by attributes that are connected to what must be projected or introjected.

Report and Command Messages in the Intrapsychic System

Finally, it becomes possible to discuss how these report- and command-level messages are engendered within the intrapsychic system. The relational systems model suggests that two boundaries develop, one at the paranoid-schizoid level, the other at the depressive level. The paranoid-schizoid boundary determines, through varying levels of flexibility between permeability and impermeability, the extent to which an individual will experience need states. As discussed earlier, permeability and impermeability are understood as the level of specificity in the definition of what will be experienced by the individual. In the case of personality-disordered individuals, as has been explained, the paranoid-schizoid position boundary becomes very impermeable. Only perceptions from the environment that seem to immediately soothe a threat are experienced. Likewise, only affects from within the personality that seem to immediately soothe a threat are acknowledged within the personality. The depressive-level or outer boundary of the personality-disordered individual is either extremely permeable or extremely impermeable, meaning that the individual is either emotionally affected by almost everyone and everything, or is emotionally affected by almost no one and nothing. In understanding projective identification, or the double bind, we can now examine *why* report and command messages are communicated. Report messages are created by the functioning of the depressive-level boundary. Command messages are created by the functioning of the paranoid-schizoid boundary.

We can now return to the examples of the schizoid and dependent personalities discussed above. In the case of the schizoid the report message, "I will do anything you want," is the result of an impermeable depressive-position boundary that does not allow anyone or anything to affect the intrapsychic system. This could be confusing at first, but in the context of being the pursued person, the schizoid actually is not aware of caring about a connection to the other person and does whatever the other wants only because it does not affect him and it seems so important to the other. The paranoid-schizoid level boundary is also impermeable and only allows perceptions of others as having no emotional impact due to the fear associated with allowing anyone near. The command-level message is therefore, "You have no effect on me." As stated above, this leads to a deviation-amplifying process in which ever-increasing efforts to connect at an emotional level lead to voraciousness. Thus the projective identification of the schizoid uses a double bind created from messages of differing logical types that result from the report of the depressive-position boundary and the command of the paranoid-schizoid boundary.

In the case of the dependent personality, the report level message, "You are sustaining and so strong," results from an extremely permeable depressive position boundary. The dependent cares about the opinions of everyone, any and all of whom are considered stronger and more substantial than the self, and all of whom directly affect the affective system within the personality. But the dependent's paranoid-schizoid level boundary, which creates the command level message "I must have you and will fall apart without you," is just as impermeable as the paranoid-schizoid boundary in the schizoid personality. The dependent only allows perceptions of others who are seen as able to protect and sustain him. And they only allow themselves to be conscious of affects from within that are weak and needy because they are so threatened by inner aggression and hunger. The primary projective identification or double bind of the dependent is caused by the functioning of the depressive and paranoid-schizoid level boundaries.

Healthier Systems

It has likely become apparent that neurotic systems have not often been covered in explicating the relational systems model. This is because the healthier the personality system, the more complicated it is. Two factors contribute to this difficulty in explaining healthier systems. As explained above, as paranoid-schizoid threats to existence reach increasing levels of integration (become less threatening and thus more balanced through more empathic than unempathic experiences), depressive threats become more dominant and issues of relatedness become more central. This added dimension makes the functioning of the personality far more varied in terms of the number of affective role-representations. The development of the depressive level also changes the character of boundaries, which become more flexible between permeability and impermeability as more possibilities for caring about others, and more acceptability of inner affects become possible. Secondly, the desperation with which the intrapsychic system needs to double-bind others or use projective identification is lessened due to the felt decrease in threat to existence. Others can be seen more as individuals and the intrapsychic system allows for more variability in interaction.

Although I will not attempt to explain the interactional process involved between healthier systems, the relational systems model applies equally to them. I have argued above that the projection and introjection of the healthier personality maintain a component of projective and introjective identification that is different only in that the decreased level of desperation within the personality decreases the strength of projective and introjective identification or of the double bind. Report and command levels of communication will still be inconsistent, but to a smaller degree. The experience is less likely to take place in a context of survival significance, and both the ability to comment and to escape are likely to be possible. Others who experience the pressure are far less likely to respond in the manner expected by the projector and are far less likely to have been chosen for attributes that make such influence powerful. The projector is also far more likely to experience the response as it really is and allow the difference to influence the impression that was already constructed. Finally, an important corollary must be added to the discussion above: the more intimate involvements are, the more likely that situations will be interpreted as having survival significance and that options for escape and comment are limited. Thus, even between relatively healthy personality systems, when intimacy is involved (as in a marriage), communication at different logical levels can lead to strong projective and introjective identifications or double binds.

TRIANGLES AND HIERARCHY

Theories of triangles and hierarchy are crucial in understanding how human systems reach states of equilibrium beyond the dyadic level. Each of these concepts helps to dissipate the destructiveness of deviation-amplifying processes by offering paths of least resistance for dealing with conflict. When the interpersonal aspect of one person's intrapsychic negative feedback is ignored by another person who then proceeds without stopping some behavior, an escalation of behaviors that were initially intended to be negative feedback can occur in a process of positive feedback loops, each behavior leading to more of the opposed behavior in the other person. Although I have so far only discussed this process leading to a parameter change within one of the individuals, which in a dyad, occurs due to the inferior hierarchical position of one member, it is also possible for the dyadic system to add another individual to balance the first two.

Triangles are the path of least resistance when a third person is available. Consider, for example, twin brothers who compete to be the smartest. Each tries to say the smartest things and simultaneously disparages what the other says. When their younger sister walks into the room and asks a question about something one of the others has said, both twins turn to her, call her an idiot, and start to laugh together. She now feels that she is less smart than her brothers. Obviously, what has occurred is a kind of narcissistic struggle between the two brothers in which both of them needed to feel strong in their intelligence to fend off feelings of weakness and dullness. Their behaviors were escalating in the fashion of deviation-amplification until finally their sister unknowingly offered a compromise solution. They could both be smart and she could be dull.

Notice how hierarchy worked in this solution. It is unlikely that the same outcome would have occurred if the boys' father walked into the room (although it could occur if his place in the family was below theirs, a not terribly uncommon situation). The boys clearly felt they had more power, and more control over needed sustenance and self-protection attributes, than did their sister. The sister, perhaps needing the affection or sustenance and self-protection attributes of the brothers, was an easy target.

It is instructive to discuss what would occur if the father (one who has a higher place in the family hierarchy) came into the room rather than the sister. If we imagine this father to be a person who values intelligence to such a degree that his sons make great efforts to please him with their own intelligence, and we also imagine that he has a strong need to be the most intelligent person in the family, what might we expect to occur? This father might start questioning the boys about their argument, and might become boastfully instructive, with the consequent feeling in the boys being that they are not respected and are not intelligent. This is another good example of the influence of hierarchy on the likely flow of projections and introjections after a deviation-amplification takes place. In this case the amplification occurred between the boys and was escalating to a point that the father's attention was drawn to it, thus bringing a family member in so that family homeostasis would assuredly be restored. The father's particular way of restoring homeostasis was consistent with a hierarchy in which he held a place of authority.

But the particular type of homeostasis in the family developed in a way that was consistent with particulars of the father's personality, and without the intervention of his authority (or someone else's), deviation-amplification processes would likely result in either the triangulation of a weaker member, like the younger sister, or some change that creates a new kind of system. If the family remains intact, the most likely change due to runaway amplification is a change in the emotional parameters within one or both of the boys so that an equilibrium state could be reached between them. That is, one of the boys is likely to concede at some point to the other's dominance in the intellectual arena.

It is also important to note in the example above that the boys' affective role-representation of respect and intelligence has as its opposite disrespect and dullness. At a point in the future, perhaps when they have left the family, if this split has not been integrated, it will likely become most comfortable to maintain the respected, intelligent side (as the father does) while projecting into others the disrespect and dullness, just as happened with the younger sister. Authority and control over resources within a hierarchy make projections go one way, because the most threatening affects are generally related to losing the love and support of the authoritative figures. In other words, because the strength and control of authority figures is so definite, lower members of the hierarchy will maintain within themselves the uncomfortable affects involving annihilation (fear) and starvation (hunger) whenever they are in interaction with those authorities. Because it is more comfortable to feel strong (assertive) and in control (sated), however, when in interactions with others who do not hold perceived authority, like the sister, a person who has held the lower position with authorities often fights to maintain the higher position elsewhere.

Hierarchies Outside the Family

It also often becomes important to seek higher authority and higher positions in hierarchies outside the family. The pain of the lower position is considered so threatening that a person seeks situations in which they never have to be in that position again (the classic situation of identification with the aggressor is one example). This switch occurs along the lines of the affective role-representations. But it only occurs if there is a way to make oneself more comfortable. Personalities that ultimately fear aggression and/ or control to extreme degrees often never make such a switch and take low positions in hierarchies even outside the family and even when they become parents. Examples include dependents and avoidants, who often have children who hold higher hierarchical positions in their families than they do.

As members lower in the hierarchy move up in that hierarchy, that is, as they gain authority and control, threats related to annihilation and starvation become more threatening than threats of destruction and control. As these members see themselves as stronger and having mastered more of life, the affects they have maintained throughout the years become increasingly uncomfortable and they are likely to challenge authority. This development can be seen in the common struggle that occurs within families as children become teenagers. Healthy resolution of this struggle requires parents to balance their authority with healthy respect for their teens who are, in fact, becoming more and more capable. The common struggles of this period, however, have led theorists to many discussions of the way amplification processes lead to changes in homeostatic patterns that may either involve someone leaving (without a change within the system when they are present), or a re-establishment of hierarchical dominance when the escalation leads to the negative feedback of drastic measures such as physical violence.

Healthier Resolutions of Conflict

It is necessary at this point to discuss healthier resolutions of conflict. Families of all levels of health and integration make use of triangles at times. But there are different ways that triangles come into play, with healthier ways occurring more frequently in healthier families. For the sake of simplicity, personality disorders have been used to explain how systems function, but at the point that depressive-level phenomena begin to develop, that is, when the capacity for concern becomes possible, an individual has become less desperate about threats, perceives her own ability to control herself, sees her impact on others, and is less afraid to see that the feelings engendered in her can just as easily be created by her. Thus, the development of shame about the residual bad impulses that continue to exist within her occurs. Although these bad impulses are less threatening now than before the depressive position began to develop, because of the development of concern, a person is more likely to perceive herself as responsible for the relationships between others. In other words, at this level of development, a person becomes more likely to view herself as the part of a triangle that either causes conflict or resolves conflict between others.

Of course the prototype for the other two members in this triangle is the parents (even though many triangles occur and the prototype is more related to positions of hierarchy than whoever is actually parenting). Although there are many ways that this process occurs, if we look again at the examples of the hysterical and obsessive personalities (discussed in the section above on depressive-level development), the process becomes clear. In the case of the hysteric, patterns within the family take place in such a way that the child's feelings of specialness seem to him to cause conflict between the parents. When the parents are in conflict, the hysteric thinks that in some way one of the parents' preference for him, and perhaps his preference for one of the parents, is the cause of the conflict.

Such an interpretation by the child might have some validity although this description is overly simplistic. In families of neurotics, it is not uncommon to find that parents seek closeness to a child when they are in conflict with each other. It is also common in families of neurotics that parents like their children more than they like each other. So, the triangle within the neurotic family is sometimes created by parents who insinuate their children into their conflicts. But an interesting phenomenon occurs when the child starts to see these triangles as troublesome due to new feelings of responsibility related to understanding his control over himself, and he starts to hide his feelings of specialness as though they were bad.

For the hysteric, a great conflict exists between the desire for recognition of specialness and the likelihood that such recognition would disturb the balance between others. The way this conflict is typically dealt with is for those feelings of specialness to be denied, but in their place comes behavior that gains attention in some way even though it is not considered special to the hysteric. Hysterics often gain attention by their dress or by neediness, but hide true feelings of specialness from others and themselves. They get involved in romantic triangles by enjoying special attention from others, but not truly connecting emotionally (since the true self is denied). Because they are not emotionally connected to these others they are not conscious of the problem created by enjoying the attention of someone who is involved with another. They think, "I'm not doing anything wrong, I'm just being a friend." However, this friendship is often characterized by the other thinking the hysteric is special in some way.

Thus the triangle that existed with the parents is recapitulated through a process of projective identification. At the paranoid-schizoid level the hysteric accepts and communicates only messages consistent with neediness and desire because specialness and strength are thought of as damaging to relationships. At the depressive level the hysteric finds others to care about who are strong and helpful so that he does not have to feel responsible himself. Others are attracted to the hysteric but denied real contact with the assertive special self so that the hysteric believes he is not responsible for the feelings of the other or the relationship in general. However, recognition for competence and strength, the recognition that is needed by the true self, cannot occur because the threat of responsibility fragmentation prevents all expression of those qualities.

The case of the obsessive also involves triangles. Like the hysteric, the obsessive also removes her true self from relationships to compensate for the possibility that it could damage others' relationships. However, in the case of the obsessive, what is denied and shameful is weakness and badness. The conflict of the parents is believed to be related to this weakness or badness. Often the obsessive has paid most attention to the area of conflict between family members that is related to the way each parent handles her. That is, when parents have a difference of opinion about discipline or handling homework or, less directly, whether or not kids should be allowed to stay up, go out, or clean their rooms, the obsessive begins to believe that those parental conflicts can be corrected by her "perfect" behavior. If it is perfect she will not need the parents to be concerned about any of these matters. Again, the true self is pushed down, but instead of specialness, it is weakness and badness that are most threatening because they appear to cause the most conflict between the parents.

The obsessive, like the hysteric, also gets involved in triangles throughout her life (although in the case of the obsessive this is far less obvious). The obsessive insinuates herself in the lives of others in conflict out of a sense of responsibility. She drives others apart from each other by being so good and perfect that others' relationships seem to pale in comparison to what would be possible if the obsessive were not in the relationship. Just as in the case of the hysteric, the obsessive is unaware of her tendency to triangulate others in this fashion. But projective identification, born of contradictory messages communicated at the paranoid-schizoid and depressive levels, results in repeated entanglement in triangular interactions. At the paranoid-schizoid level the obsessive accepts only communications that say she is strong for fear that if she were weak it would hurt others or others' relationships. At the depressive level the obsessive cares about people who need help so that her strong and perfect action can solve problems and she can maintain her feelings of goodness and strength. The weak and hungry self of the obsessive is hidden from others so that the possibility of loneliness and isolation, which could occur if her badness were exposed, is avoided.

Family Homeostasis

Patterns of relationship triangles do not recur because of "repetition compulsion" (Freud 1920), a concept that suggests there is a need to work through the problem, but rather because personality styles have become adaptive patterns in situations where there has been conflict. The responsible behavior of the obsessive truly does help her parents have less conflict. The emotionally distant behavior of the hysteric really does dissipate conflict in his family. The intrapsychic system fits naturally with interpersonal systems within which a child must fit as he or she develops. Homeostasis must be achieved or, alternately, positive feedback will result in change to a new kind of system. If no equilibrium is possible within the family, other changes will occur such as one family member leaving.

Different kinds of triangles are used to handle conflict, and healthier triangles involve some connection to or responsibility for the relationships of others. Family homeostasis involves the trading and exchange of affective role-representations, within the limits of the structural hierarchy in the family and the environmental pressure on the family from larger systems. All systems reach some kind of homeostasis, sometimes requiring intervention or interaction with larger systems to reach that homeostasis. When family homeostasis is reached, every member of the family has a role that makes it possible for the others to maintain their roles. A family's homeostasis involves both adaptation to the environment and previous adaptations made by each of its members. The intrapsychic system is the adaptive optimal growth pattern effected within the individual, given the homeostatic patterns of which he has been a part.

Crystallization of the Intrapsychic System

The relational systems model describes a pattern of adaptation within a world of relationships. The world of relationships for which the intrapsychic system develops, however, is only a small subgroup of all possible relationships. Nevertheless, the specific adaptation is generalized. This generalization occurs because the individual personality solidifies at a time when sustenance, self-protection, and relatedness are all dependent on the significant others with whom the individual attaches and grows. This dependency is so complete that the individual is extremely malleable with respect to the needs of others within the family. Since family members have made their own adaptations, they have their own ideas of how relationships work and they defend themselves by pushing their most feared affective role-representations on others in the family. The individual takes on these roles (as well as their opposites) as they are seen in other family members, for the sake of survival. The intrapsychic system maintains affective role-representations as reality, adapts to them, and becomes especially suited to maintaining an inner equilibrium based on the idea that these representations truly fit reality. Giving up these ideas, which are transferred to others in every interaction, means giving up one's identity. If the intrapsychic system is somewhat crystallized, what kinds of interventions are efficacious in helping people change? This is the topic of Chapter 7, in which the use of self or the use of countertransference will be discussed with a special emphasis on using countertransference in family therapy.

CONCLUSION

One additional comment seems necessary in concluding. Many psychoanalytic theorists have postulated stages of development that are beyond the scope of this study. Of special interest here is the work of Mahler and her colleagues (1975) on the separation-individuation process, Kernberg's four stages of normal development (1976), and Stern on the developmental progression of the sense of self (Stern 1985). The work of these theorists is more detailed and specific than what has been presented here. However, the developmental understanding given here does not contradict the observable aspects of those theories (most notably, it is likely obvious that the emphasis here has been on the relative working through of developmental positions, leaving room for continued experience within those realms throughout life, very much like Stern's views on developmental stages as epochs). Rather, the most essential aspects of psychological development are highlighted within the relational systems model due to their interpersonal significance. The stages of development that have been emphasized are those that are most central to the creation of defenses that affect the interpersonal context. They are thus the stages that facilitate an integration between the intrapsychic domain of psychoanalytic theory, and the more interpersonal world of systems theory.

The relational systems model has wide applicability and generalizability for many models of therapeutic intervention. It is a system that works from so many points of view because it accurately describes processes of human communication and development. Like systems theories and many analytic interpersonal theories, it postulates that there is no such thing as growth in the individual without corresponding meaning attributed to relationships at every level of functioning. Unlike other theories, however, it describes the process of growth within the individual as a systematic pattern that includes drivenness. The model is consistent with analytic theories in describing processes of splitting at less mature levels of development and processes of repression occurring at more integrated levels of development. Systems theory benefits from psychoanalytic theory with its more specific understanding of the intrapsychic mechanisms that produce interpersonal pressures like projective identification. Psychoanalytic theory benefits from the understanding of behavioral observation in systems theory, which has produced ideas like the theory of logical types and the double bind. Beyond systems and psychoanalytic theory, the relational systems model has broad applicability in the treatment of human suffering, which can now be understood to be patterned interpersonal communications that have developed as adaptations that are no longer adaptive. The goal of therapy then, of no matter what kind, is to bring about greater adaptation, integration, and flexibility, in a world with multitudinous possibilities for relatedness. In that vein, therapy must be a microcosm for infinite possibilities.

7

Relational Systems and the Therapist's Use of Self

By describing the relationship intrapsychic tensions and affects have to the common experience of emotions and their interpersonal expression the relational systems perspective brings great emotional understanding to family therapy. Through it, the interplay of intrapsychic and interpersonal phenomena becomes integral to the systems approach. Powerful interventions are discovered in a way that is consistent with the emotional experience of system members. Those interventions are found by using countertransference to dip into the emotional melting pot that is created within the therapist–family system. In formulating specific authentic, empathic interventions that aim to correct and complete organismic functioning, the therapist is part and parcel of everything that occurs, so that every aspect of the therapist's contact with the family is in actuality part of a larger relational intervention.

GENERAL CLINICAL IMPLICATIONS OF THE RELATIONAL SYSTEMS MODEL

The relational systems model detailed in the last chapter has implications for behavioral, psychodynamic, and experiential therapies, as well as family systems therapy. Exposure, the most common technique of behavioral approaches, is related to the relational systems model in that treatment occurs through a process of exposing the patient to a relationship in which the threats to interpersonal existence, exaggerated within childhood, are no longer present. Assimilation and accommodation (Piaget 1954), concepts that have been used in the integration of behavioral and psychoanalytic theory to explain the treatment of transference (Wachtel and Wachtel 1986, Wachtel 1987, 1997), can be used to understand how exposure works within the therapeutic situation. With exposure, changes occur in the personality as it accommodates to a new person and to emotions that have long been disavowed. But assimilation in the form of transference limits that change by attempting to fit new experience into old patterns. Insight, considered important by psychodynamic therapists, is helpful in the treatment process in that it helps a person begin to consciously recognize patterns of interaction which, when aided by will power to the extent that a person has developed a sense of autonomy, assists the process of accommodation.

All of these phenomena, however, require a particular pattern within the therapeutic relationship if personality change is to be effected. In order for the patient to be exposed to a different kind of relationship, the therapist must not only be different, but must also be able to enter into the patient's world of affective role-representations. At the same time the therapist must resist succumbing to the pressure from the patient to enact the projected role-representations to a degree that reinforces the threats for which they were developed. This kind of therapy can only occur through a style of concerned authenticity that requires a high degree of personality integration and self-reflection within the therapist. I will now expand on the interplay of these clinical processes.

The Experience of Exposure

Simply put, exposure is the only possible cure for the personality. Because personality systems are maintained with orientations to relationships that are just the opposite of the affects that are most threatening, there is no opportunity for the individual personality to experience those affects without being threatened and thus taking the opposing position. Working through the abandonment depression, for example (as in the case of the borderline patient), is the same as exposure to the object of a phobia as in systematic desensitization. But instead of being exposed to a thing or a situation, in working through the abandonment depression the patient must be exposed to a relationship in which caring is involved but the other person in the relationship is not always present. The borderline activates herself in any way possible to avoid abandonment feelings, from behaviors similar to narcissistic withdrawal and control to behaviors similar to dependent clinginess. But she never allows the experience of abandonment to occur because in all her clinging or narcissistic activity she never truly connects to others nor is she ever independent. In the therapeutic relationship, however, her activity can be confronted in a caring manner. She can connect to the therapist as a person who respects her ability to care for herself but will be there when needed. Through an exposure to a person who cares empathically and balances responses without overreacting, over time the borderline can grieve for what she has missed because she is able to experience abandonment feelings. That is, she must deal with her independence but experience the grief of being alone. The experience of abandonment feelings within a context in which there is really no emotional starvation is similar to that of the phobic individual who is being exposed to the object of a phobia while in a relaxed state. A new association must take place because now caring about someone no longer always means being controlled or abandoned by them or, on the other hand, controlling or clinging to them.

As discussed in Chapter 4, Wachtel (1987) describes transference in Piaget's (1954) terms: "assimilation," "accommodation," and "schema." The worse a person's pathology, the more likely that he will assimilate almost all relationships into the maladaptive patterns with which he grew up and to which he adapted. The threats perceived as possible if he were to be in a position that had always been painful to him are so great that he will only interpret events as though they fit into a schema with which he is more comfortable. Accommodation, or changing the schema to fit new information, must occur for an individual to adapt to new levels, but requires that a person react in unfamiliar ways. In psychotherapy, the relationship itself can be different than what has been experienced by the patient and thus cause accommodation within the patient's schema or transference. There must be exposure to relationships that prove old schemas to be incorrect, and emotions must be experienced in a context where they (ultimately) turn out to be not so threatening as to require immediate defense.

Insight and force of will are helpful in this regard. Wachtel has discussed how insight is conducive to change, but is insufficient by itself (1987, 1997). Insight can show a person where change is needed but it can't force him to change. Will is also conducive to change in some cases, but tends to fail in accomplishing permanent change of issues that involve strong urges related to sustenance, self-protection, or general relatedness. Only exposure to the threatening affects within a relational context where the threatening affects apply by way of transference to the person to whom the patient is relating will dissipate the urgency of that threat. When that urgency is lightened, freedom to respond in new ways becomes possible. Insight helps in showing where these threats are, and force of will helps the patient maintain the relationship even though it is painful at times; however, only maintenance of that relationship with a person who responds in new ways can lead to curative exposure.

Experiential Aspects of Therapy

Experiential aspects of therapy are thus central to clinical applications according to the relational systems model. Two areas of special importance are the character of the therapist and the activity level of her therapeutic approach. If the therapist is to react in a different way, she must have certain attributes. Although the relationship cannot be completely mutual (Burke 1992) because it is a treatment relationship in which the object of change is by definition the patient, the therapist must be as authentic as possible (Hoffman 1992a,b). The therapist must be able to feel the role that is being pushed upon her, but react in a healthy manner (Sandler 1976). The therapist must empathize with the need that is hidden even when the patient's behavior evokes threatening feelings in her by way of projective identification. The therapist cannot be afraid of her own hungers, voracity, rage, fears, guilt, or loneliness because those feelings will be evoked within the therapy and must be properly understood as threatening to the patient. The therapist must teach by example that emotions are natural and need not lead to shame or guilt. The effective therapist must be a relatively healthy person or the patient's exposure to the therapist will not lead to cure.

The activity of the therapist is also essential. However, because the relationship is, by design, a therapeutic relationship, activity must be used in amounts that are most helpful. Greenberg (1991), in discussing the analytic concepts of "neutrality" and "abstinence," as well as activity level, has discussed the tension that exists for the therapist in being both a new object for a new relationship and an old object for transference. The choice of the right amount of activity is based on the extent to which a new object or an old object is needed. The therapist must sense this tension. With more severe pathologies more activity is expected, as the person desperately needs a new object and the transference patterns must be changed. With less severe pathologies it is necessary to be less active as it takes longer for transference to develop and for some level of intimacy to exist between patient and therapist. But whatever kind of personality therapy, in the end the cure will involve exposure to the new object that is the reality of the therapist as he truly is. Regardless of the type of personality therapy practiced, if a therapist attempts to act as if he were something other than what he *truly is,* such action can only produce greater confusion in the transference. The therapist's authentic and real caring toward his patient will lead toward the right balance since it will allow the therapist to feel whether a less or more active approach is necessary at any particular time.

SYSTEMS THEORY, PROJECTIVE IDENTIFICATION, AND COUNTERTRANSFERENCE

Family systems theory gives an excellent description of whole systems and their subsystems. But systems theorists have not often extended their paradigm to the intrapsychic level of individual functioning. That the individual might have relatively fixed aspects to his personality has been considered contradictory to systems therapy because systems approaches emphasize that family problems are strictly failures of the system as a whole. Systems theory thus predicts that the individual subsystem is relatively plastic in the way it will respond to changes in the greater system.

To ignore the extent to which a lifetime of personality patterns becomes fundamental to an individual's functioning, however, is to ignore the individual. Although individual personalities are not fixed, they are also not plastic. Personalities function in the larger system of the world, and every smaller system of which they are a part, in patterned ways. The relational systems perspective uses the concept of projective identification to describe how the internal, intrapsychic subsystem functions in interaction with dyadic and larger systems. And although the intrapsychic system may have rigidified somewhat over the years, the fact that it communicates through projective identification means that when the projective identification is not allowed to occur some shifting must take place. Either the internal system must maintain equilibrium without projection or a new target for the projection must be found. Family systems theory has largely ignored this second and most likely possibility.

Concepts parallel to that of projective identification have, however, been described in family systems theory. "Logical types in communication" and "the double bind" are examples of ideas that are helpful in clarifying the way in which projective identification takes place from a behavioral point of view. But the interpretation of these phenomena given by systems therapists demonstrates how their approach, since it views the individual within the system as having a relatively plastic internal structure, fails to grasp the somewhat rigidified constitution of the individual's patterns. Theories such as logical types in communication and the double-bind demonstrate the extent to which intrapsychic patterns, once manifested interpersonally in behavior, become very important to systems functioning. Any intervention meant to bring on relatively permanent change in the dynamics described by these concepts must address the ongoing needs they express if it is to have an ongoing effect. If the need remains the same, the dynamic will continue in some context that was not addressed by the intervention used. Systems approaches have presented the shifting of projective patterns as though the shift indicated a permanent holistic change. They have not addressed the intrapsychic issues that are systemically central to those patterns.

Nevertheless, just as systems theory predicts, if the larger system changes, then so too must the internal, intrapsychic system. The rigidified nature of the internal, intrapsychic subsystem itself indicates that changes in larger systems must be relatively permanent to bring about change at the intrapsychic level. Because of the crystallized nature of the intrapsychic system, it can be quite difficult to change its functioning and quite difficult to change the larger system of which it is a part. Whatever kind of intervention is used to change a family system must aim at bringing about permanent change in its process by addressing the overall needs of the greater system as well as the subsystems within. Permanent change can occur in the system when both intrapsychic and interpersonal needs are addressed.

Because families do function in a coherent, systematic manner, and because the greater system finds a balance (often referred to as homeostasis, and not necessarily a healthy balance) to meet the particular needs of its members, its subsystems, and itself as a whole, there *are* interventions that address those needs for the whole system and all its members at the same time. The therapist's countertransference, since it reflects the particular way in which the therapist's personality becomes part of the therapist–family system, can be used to uncover the interlocking dynamics of the family and its members at interpersonal and intrapsychic levels.

The Therapist's Use of Countertransference

The use of countertransference always exists, at least prereflectively, and is always affected by the therapist's system of affects and boundaries, as well as by the systems of affects and boundaries that surround her. The therapist's intentional use of countertransference can be refined with an understanding of the intrapsychic system as described by the relational systems model presented in the last chapter. The therapist can use this model in self-reflection to uncover the intrapsychic phenomena that necessitate and regulate projective and introjective identification. Interventions formulated will always involve both prereflective and intentional aspects of countertransference as the therapist aims to understand her part in the system with the family, how much the family can tolerate from her, and whether or not the family will benefit from the uncovering of powerful family processes.

With respect to expectations of responsibility, ability, and of understanding limitations at whatever level the client or client-family is functioning, the therapist's role and use of countertransference are analogous to the activities of the parent who must care for a child. The generative process in the healthy family naturally leads to teaching increasing independence with a basic empathy toward the infant's relative capabilities (which can be viewed as empathy toward specialness as well as functional ability). The infant must grow toward independence as an individual system for survival, and also for better functioning of the larger family system whose members desire their own independent functioning within the system. Caretakers of the infant, by the very fact of doing a good job, create a system in which the definition and integrity of the infant largely depend on their relationship with him. Such responsibility for another taxes the individual caretaker and thus provides added impetus for increasing levels of independence to be encouraged.

When a family comes to therapy, projective and introjective identification are used in the relationship with the therapist, who is open to helping and who has her own unresolved conflicts, and thus is deeply affected by such communication. In spite of the inflexible nature of the client-family's boundaries, with the consequent difficulty in modifying what will be introjected by the family members due to their need to perceive the environment in only specific ways, the therapist is tasked with understanding and changing family perceptions. The therapist's position with respect to the family, as analogous to the healthy parent to the young infant, necessitates a high degree of personality integration and flexibility for a salutary change in the therapist–family, and then in the family system's functioning.

THE THERAPIST IN THE FAMILY SYSTEM

Consider the following example. A family comes to therapy with difficulties that reflect a level of projective identification and extractive introjection that have set into a homeostatic pattern that causes pain. In whatever way the primary problems are presented, they reflect a certain emotional economy in the family. Tradeoffs are determined according to where real power lies and how it is exercised. A narcissistic father requires some family members to be inferior in keeping with his projective identification of vulnerability and his need to maintain grandiosity. He not only possesses, in reality, the physical size, and the monetary resources, but he also controls the emotional economy because, as part of his projective identification, his approval or disapproval is held as the benchmark of quality. An adolescent son, developing through a period in which his body and mind are changing rapidly, and who is struggling with his independent identity, has a valency for complying with his father's wishes based on years of experience, and at this point becomes especially vulnerable.

This adolescent has always been affected by family pressures that suggest that the father's accomplishments are great, no matter how great they may be in reality. The family unconscious holds the possibility that recognizing the reality of the father's accomplishments, or lack thereof, may lead to disaster. Although the father is extremely agitated by the son's recent failures in school, his own worthlessness resides in the son, which allows his own grandiosity to remain intact. Empathy fails in the family as everyone struggles to understand why such an intelligent child should *wish* to fail. The whole family holds extremely high standards, in keeping with father's views, and the boy has worked hard to emulate his father, but has never been considered good enough. Other family members are approximately as successful as the boy, but they are seemingly not held to the same standard even though they all believe they are. Mother idolizes father, does whatever he wants without much concern for herself, and often loses control when she gets angry at her younger children. Everyone in the family believes the problem resides within this one son. They are extremely resistant to hearing anything else. No family member realizes that, in accordance with family pressures, any real success the son might attain would make the father reintroject his own feelings of worthlessness and/ or reproject them toward another family member, and the whole family would perceive itself to be in jeopardy.

How does the therapist get involved in the family system? The therapist is not a family member with years of shared experience in the family. Nor does the family's current functioning affect the therapist daily and hourly as it does family members. But the family functions as a unit when with the therapist, and therapy is a challenging situation for any family. Thus under stress, the family will use modes of communication with the therapist similar to those used within the family. When the therapist is sensitive to these communication patterns, thus creating within herself a kind of valency for family emotions, she can then feel the pressure of projective identification and the suction behind extractive introjection. In the above example, the therapist feels condescended to by the father, feels she must instill hope in the adolescent boy, and feels feared by the mother and other family members. The family as a whole feels like change might destroy them, and so there is a rigidity to the family's responses. Subgroupings within the family will also put pressure on others and the therapist with projective identification. If the therapist is able to be sensitive to these forces, the emotional existence of the family is laid bare in the consulting room.

The process by which the therapist becomes involved happens at an unconscious, prereflective level, even if the therapist eventually attempts to gain access to the meaning of that involvement with self-reflection. The therapist is as affected by boundaries and his own psychological makeup as family members are, even though the family's boundary and personality characteristics are interconnected and the therapist is the newcomer to the system. The primary difference lies in the therapist's effort toward understanding and openness, which creates additional valency within the therapist. This valency cannot be underestimated in importance because the therapist opens up to those threats to self-protection, sustenance, and loss that continue to live in her personality no matter how worked-through the paranoid-schizoid and depressive positions might be. In fact, it is the level to which these positions have been worked through that allows the therapist to open boundaries and empathize temporarily with such terrifying possibilities, without acting out. Once the therapist has experienced the raw projected emotion, or the emptiness created by extractive introjection, she self-reflects upon that experience and formulates an idea of what that experience might mean within the context of the therapist–family system. When formulating an intervention, it is absolutely necessary that the therapist's experience be claimed as her own. These feelings cannot be considered pure derivatives of projective identification because they exist only as a result of the therapist's unique personality coming into contact with the personality systems of the family within a context of therapy. The therapist can become involved at such a level with either individual family members, subgroupings, or the entire group.

Bion's "basic assumptions" (1970) have been used by several authors as a way to understand group-level projective identification and are one way of understanding the therapist's countertransference reaction. These theorists view a group's need for hope in someone as a leader as an indication that the group is expressing (1) the need to be creating together as a "pairing basic-assumptions group," (2) their need for a strong leader as an indication that the group is fighting for mastery or definition and is functioning as a "fight-or-flight basic-assumptions group," or (3) their need for a nurturing leader as an indication that the group is in need of sustenance and is functioning as a "dependency basic-assumptions group." Scharff and Scharff (1987) added to this list the "fission/fusion basic-assumptions group," which represents the developmental stage of fusion with paranoid-schizoid anxiety, and they postulated that the other basic-assumptions groups, as well as the work group, represent oral (dependency), anal (fight-or-flight), genital (pairing), and oedipal (work group) stages of development. They did not speculate on the kind of leader necessitated by the fission/fusion basic assumptions group but it seems consistent with their view that the wished-for leader would encompass characteristics of all the other leaders. The fission/fusion basic assumptions group would be expected to make the therapist an integral part of the family until disappointment occurred, at which time extreme protest would be expected much like what occurs in what could be called the fused relationship between the newborn and its primary parent. Although these needed leaders are not always the therapist, such pressure can occur in family therapy and can lead to an understanding of what the family's experienced deficit at that particular time might be. These pressures on the therapist can also indicate the developmental level of the family.

Basic assumptions that create leaders for particular purposes within the family can also be sensed via countertransference. For example, a mother might be permanently installed as the nurturer and therefore the leader of the dependency basic-assumptions group within the family. The eldest daughter might be the rebellious member and thus represent the leadership role in the fight-or-flight basic-assumptions group. Often the therapist's observation of countertransference will come as the result of projective or introjective identification from the active basic-assumptions group leader and thus the therapist will be able to have some insight about the entire family. The eldest daughter may indicate to the hard-working therapist that therapy is "bull," and the therapist notices the feeling that her efforts are shackled despite great effort, thus allowing her to understand that the whole family is perhaps feeling shackled by her interventions. Through this interchange the therapist may formulate an intervention aimed at demonstrating how control has affected her in the family and how it affects family members—or she might simply change her behavior and thus change the therapist–family system.

In family therapy, whatever the group (or any subgroup) may project has correlates in all other family members. Thus, the therapist is able to formulate interventions based on what has been perceived as originating in one family member by discussing its relation to the whole group, including himself, or he might simply base an intervention on what happened between himself and that family member. However, in my view the therapist cannot be taken out of the system as though the countertransference he is experiencing has nothing to do with his own personality functioning. And as part of the system with the family, the therapist's mental health or high level of personality integration is essential, because he must, as accurately as possible, perceive the process of projective and introjective identification between himself and the remainder of the therapist–family system. The therapist aims to be as genuine and authentic in his responding as possible so that he can be confident that he understands his own behavior and attitudes within the process. Behaving in any way that is not natural, such as aiming for abstinence, can only cloud such clear understanding. Being a self-reflective person can be a developed asset, however, and taking on the relational systems perspective cannot be accomplished without developing such self-reflectiveness.

Finally, the relational systems model points to particular meanings of specific affects. The combination of feeling afraid and observing a family or family member as aggressive likely indicates warded-off vulnerability in a family member or sector of the family. Likewise a feeling of being ineffectual and useless combined with the observation of a capricious, demanding nature on the part of a family or family member can suggest warded-off depression or abandonment in family members. The relational systems model presented in Chapter 6 demonstrates that primary affective role-representations exist within certain family members who project the most threatening aspect of their personality into others. It is often the case, as the therapist gets closer and closer to core family issues, that the therapist becomes the target of these types of projective identification. This can occur as the result of triangulation, as two family members or parts of the family use the therapist to make each other okay and the therapist "bad," or it can occur in a dyadic mode between the therapist and one specific family member. When it occurs it has meaning for the whole family and the therapist must realize that he is being used in a way that occurs to other family members when he is not part of their system. Most importantly, his formulation of what is occurring can begin with the knowledge that his experience is likely similar to something that is too hard to tolerate within the family. If he can determine its likely origin and its purpose within the family, he can use it to provide deep understanding of family pathology that also allows family members to feel understood.

Consider the family presented at the beginning of this section. As I stated, the therapist simultaneously feels condescended to by the father, knows that she must instill hope in the adolescent boy, and feels feared by the mother and other family members. An almost infinite number of possible interventions based on countertransference are possible depending on the most pronounced emotion experienced by the therapist. An example of such an intervention that I used with a family similar to the one presented above took place in the sixth session when I was relatively confident about the family's commitment.

I've been noticing today in the way you've been talking to me, Mr. H, that you've made subtle references to me making mistakes, as though you think I just don't know what I'm talking about, and to tell you the truth I've often thought, in my treatment with you, that maybe I'm stuck or not doing the right things. But before I noticed this feeling, I was feeling kind of, ... well, almost afraid, but also needing to demonstrate my knowledge. And it made me wonder if you somehow don't like to, but come close to, feeling this way yourself sometimes, but then because it's so uncomfortable you try to be the opposite, which makes the feeling occur in others, like Johnny, or like what seems to have happened with me. I think you learned somehow that to let others know you feel vulnerable would mean you'd end up being especially hurt, like with your father who always wanted you to be great but didn't really recognize anything you did. So now you make sure you're not vulnerable but in the process you make someone else feel those vulnerable and worthless feelings. I was wondering if maybe you sometimes exaggerate the side of you that knows you're good, so you won't have to think about that other side that doesn't feel so good? And I think you even share some of that goodness with others when you tell them they're good. But the problem is, *you* control your own feeling good, and theirs, by being the one and only one who is able to judge whether something is good or not.

An intervention like this typically requires much processing afterwards and runs the risk of being completely denied, especially if it is perceived as accurate. But in family therapy, even if the one person with whom you are speaking denies an accurate statement, someone else in the family will invariably pick up on some aspect of it, which can lead to more processing. The most essential ingredient in the above intervention is that the therapist must remain empathically attuned to the primary subject (if there is one) as well as other family members, and demonstrate that attunement by making it clear that the processes of projective identification and extractive introjection do not indicate that any of the participants are in any way bad. People have many words for badness, such as weak, vulnerable, pleasing, and so on, to all of which the therapist needs to be attuned. Often, in making such an intervention, the most important ingredient is that the therapist expresses understanding for what is so painful about the projected aspect of self or the need that creates an introjective vacuum. If the therapist is successful in understanding this aspect of family life, the original projector is able to draw that part back into the self and the whole family is able to begin the process of healing.

THE INTENTIONAL USE OF COUNTERTRANSFERENCE AND THE RELATIONAL SYSTEMS PERSPECTIVE

The intentional use of countertransference, which requires self-reflection, is the only way to achieve some of the interventions discussed thus far. Although the therapist's prereflective tendencies might lead to calm assurance or naturally derived interventions, as suggested earlier, his intentional self-reflection, understood through a particular theoretical model, leads to more precision. The use of empathy, whether its countertransference aspects are consciously used or not, always requires self-reflection to the extent that separation from the patient is necessary for accuracy. But beyond the accurate empathy that results from maintaining relative objectivity, the application of theory allows the therapist to understand the relationship between emotions evoked in him and the warded-off emotions in the client or client-family that have been transmitted through behavior. In this model self-reflection means more than understanding one's relationship to another because it includes the understanding of why emotions are warded off and created in others, and why the therapist is likely to experience these warded-off emotions.

With such an understanding, self-reflection on countertransference re-actions can lead to interventions that fit any family therapy approach and ensure that both interpersonal and intrapsychic dimensions are being ad-dressed. A strategic therapist might interpret the intervention in the above section as indicating to the father that if he continues to ridicule his son, he will be guilty of being unable to manage his own emotions, an insult that would be intolerable to a person who demands control. A narrative therapist might see such an intervention as remapping the effect of a prob-lem and suggesting that family members do have influence over it. A struc-tural therapist might believe this intervention works because he has ob-served that a rigid boundary had formed between the mother and son, and now, with the realization that her husband may be hurting her son, sees her tighten the boundary between herself and her husband and open up to the son, allowing him to feel worthwhile in spite of the father's attitudes. From the relational systems perspective, such an intervention, based on self-reflection, simply describes a picture of family reality that has here-tofore been unnoticed, but that must now be noticed for the sake of all family members. Such an intervention works because the family feels deeply understood while at the same time they learn how their suffering transfers from one family member to the next. The assumption is that family members care about one another, and that if they can be shown this trans-fer process, then they can begin to change it. To the extent that such an intervention works for the reasons postulated by other systems therapies, it is important to notice that an intervention of this kind, nevertheless, presents none of the awkwardness characteristic of inauthentic behavior of the sort that often occurs in systems therapies due to subterfuge or trick-ery.

The therapist who views himself as part of a system with the client or client-family can recognize how his own tendencies have combined with the tendencies of the client or client-family, and then formulate an inter-vention. That intervention will include the ways in which the therapist was responsible for the dynamic that played itself out, as well as the client or client-family's responsibility for it. The therapist with a high level of personality integration, however, can be confident that his perception of the dynamic that has played itself out in the therapy is characteristic of other situations in which the client or client-family regularly find them-selves, even though it occurred in a particular way with him as a unique person. It should also not be an embarrassment that the therapist learns about himself in the process of doing therapeutic work. Any new system with which a therapist comes into contact will undoubtedly be both similar and different from others. Within every new therapist–family system that is formed via the therapeutic situation, the therapist should be able to expect that his prior experience will be of value and that new experiences will arise. New experiences can be expected to help the therapist learn about new aspects of his character, and growth in directions previously unimagined will undoubtedly occur.

The integration of interpersonally oriented analytic theory and systems theory, which I call the relational systems perspective, allows for complete use of countertransference in a way that has not been adequately portrayed in any other model for family therapy. The following listing of propositions encompasses the relational systems perspective and summarizes its utility. From this perspective, the therapist is viewed as inside the therapist–family system. The inner workings of that system are viewed as being comprised of subsystems that use projective identification and extractive introjection as their dynamic interactional mechanisms. Projective identification and extractive introjection are also viewed as expressions of intrapsychic dynamics that aim at relieving intrapsychic and interpersonal difficulties but that paradoxically also maintain current levels of functioning that interfere with personal and interpersonal growth. Interventions in the system are aimed at intrapsychic as well as interpersonal functioning and are informed at least partially by the therapist's countertransference. The relational systems perspective includes the therapist as a full member of a system with the family. The therapist is seen as a unique person who adds uniquely to that system. The therapist's countertransference within that system can be used self-reflectively but is understood to be in operation prereflectively at all times. The prereflective use of countertransference demands a high level of personality integration because self-reflection alone cannot completely prevent the potentially deleterious impact of the therapist's personality on the therapist–family system. Personality integration is also important in the self-reflective use of countertransference because the therapist must have a relatively accurate understanding of his or her part within the system with the family. The accuracy and empathic attunement of that understanding also require the application of a theoretical system that explains how and why emotions are transferred from individual to individual and from group to group.

The relational systems model, in its entirety, offers a relatively complete understanding of the processes involved in the use of countertransference in family therapy. Knowledge of a theoretical model such as this one can become integrated within a therapist's personality. The therapist's capacity to self-reflect upon his part in the therapist–family system, combined with the extent to which the theoretical model is integrated within the therapist's personality, allows for a spontaneous and genuine use of countertransference.

THE THEORETICAL MODEL APPLIED

In Chapter 2, the examination of countertransference in family therapy through the lens of the totalistic perspective revealed that its use is ubiquitous. Countertransference has not been thought of as a tool by many authors in family therapy, and its self-reflective use has only been emphasized by a few. But the prereflective use of countertransference is important within several schools of family therapy. In most psychoanalytic family therapy approaches it seems countertransference is used somewhat indirectly as a consequence of avoiding countertransference problems. Object relations family therapists have attempted a relatively complete integration of the use of countertransference but have not examined the impact of the therapist's unique personality within the therapist–family system. In contrast, systems and narrative and solution-oriented therapists do not describe any use of countertransference. Of course the prereflective use of countertransference cannot be eliminated from any kind of therapy, and, if systems epistemology is fully applied, the recognition of the therapist's part in the therapist–family system would bring recognition of the prereflective use of countertransference in systems approaches. Experiential therapists have not applied any theory to therapeutic process, but have asserted that the therapist's personality is central to a therapeutic effect. Thus experiential therapists emphasize the prereflective use of countertransference. Integrationist approaches have shown the greatest potential for a comprehensive use of countertransference. Among the integrationist approaches, the most promising recognize both the prereflective and self-reflective uses of countertransference by emphasizing both an experiential aspect to therapy, and an application of interpersonal theory to the therapeutic process.

In this section, I will present vignettes from each of these four views for the purpose of demonstrating how the relational systems perspective, and the use of countertransference with that perspective, can enhance family therapy work of any kind. Thus, the examination of analytic models will show how the therapist's active part within the therapist–family dynamic could be better integrated within countertransference interventions that take account of the therapist's unique personality. In examining systems and solution-oriented approaches I will emphasize the maintenance of those basic philosophies, with the addition of therapist self-reflection in making interventions more cohesive. The focus on integrationist and experiential models will show how theory and spontaneity can be better integrated.

From the relational systems perspective, interventions can be formulated that closely parallel the analytic, systems, and experiential interventions, but, unlike interventions in some systems approaches, indirect or tricky communication is not necessary. Simply put, many interventions that focus on the true pain of human experience often have the result of changing motivation and changing behavior. This change can occur in a "strategic" sense because family members resist understanding their pain or how it is caused. This change can also occur because family members care about each other, want to understand, and want to be understood.

THE PSYCHOANALYTIC/OBJECT RELATIONS VIEW

The following vignettes from the work of object relations family therapists demonstrate both self-reflection and a broad understanding of countertransference. However, the assumption of perfect mental health in the analyst precludes a holistic use of countertransference that takes into account the therapist's part in the therapist–family system.

David Scharff

What follows is a clinical vignette used by David Scharff (1991, pp. 433–441) to demonstrate the way in which the interface between the family and the therapist can be understood through the therapist's countertransference.

The Simpsons had been in treatment for approximately a year. They had initially come for therapy because of sexual difficulty: Mrs. Simpson said that she hated sex, while Mr. Simpson suffered from premature ejaculation. In addition, Mrs. Simpson was recurrently depressed, while Mr. Simpson had so much trouble with his memory that it interfered with his work as a computer programmer. They readily agreed to a family evaluation as well because of difficulty with their middle child, 5-year-old Alex, who soiled and wet his pants and was generally immature. The evaluation revealed that 3½ year old Jeanette was also immature, seductive, and overexcited, perhaps oversexualized. The oldest boy, Eric, initially appeared to have solid latency development, but later revealed some unsublimated aggression.

I recommended a combination of family therapy, sex therapy for the parents, and individual therapy for the mother and Alex. The parents at that time elected to make individual therapy for Mrs. Simpson their priority. A year later, when I saw them again, the parents were in better shape: The year's intensive psychotherapy with a colleague had allowed Mrs. Simpson to flourish so that she was less frequently depressed, although she still had severe regressions and had been hospitalized for a few days several months ago. She had taken and maintained a part-time job, and she was now interested in sex. The couple agreed that they still needed sex therapy for their dysfunction, but the first priority for them now was family treatment, which we began while Mrs. Simpson continued in individual therapy.

The family therapy session I will describe came after approximately eight months of weekly family treatment. We had not been able to meet the previous week, but in the session two weeks earlier, we had investigated the centrality in the family of the mother's depression and had been able to understand the role of each of the other family members in relation to it. Today, two weeks after the previous session, they came in, the children leading eagerly as usual. Eric began by showing me pictures he had drawn of transformer robots called demolishicons, the most powerful of which was Demolishicor. He then began to build with the collection of colored blocks that all three of the children liked to use. Alex began to draw. The father suggested he draw Donald Duck. When he said he could not, the father said "He can *be* Donald Duck, but he can't draw it." Alex drew a Mickey Mouse face while Jeanette ate candy from a packet. They were all whispering.

I asked about the candy and the whispering. "Is there a secret that leads to the whispering?"

They denied that there was a secret. They had arrived a half-hour early, and Mrs. Simpson had bought the candy because her mouth was dry from her antidepressant medication. Further discussion of Mrs. Simpson's medication brought forth memories of her recent hospitalization and the panic that had led to it. As she talked, Alex handed her a second picture he had been drawing of "Monstro the Whale," who, he said, had swallowed Geppetto, Pinocchio's puppet-maker father. Jeanette handed her mother a picture of the primary colors, which she then listed.

Thus far I felt that the activity in the room was avoidant, although not unusu-

ally so for the opening part of a session that followed an emotionally charged session and then a missed one. I was absorbing the experience of avoidance without comment.

Eric was now building a small building, which he said was a museum. It was the same sort of structure he had built the last time, and he told me that the same sort of thing was going on there—namely, "Nothing!" Eric wanted more cars and blocks to complete his design, which meant that Alex should surrender some of his. Mr. Simpson and Alex tried to help him think of how he might finish his project with what was available and without taking something from Alex.

Mrs. Simpson said, "Eric, if you can't have it the way you want it, it would be nice to try to have it another way."

Eric rejected her advice and began to pout.

Noting with some amusement that the museum was loaded with toy soldiers holding rifles aimed at me, I said half jokingly, "I see that all those guns are pointed right at me!"

The family laughed.

"Why am I the enemy? What bad thing am I about to do?" I asked.

Eric then took the Incredible Hulk, a great, green, unfriendly looking figure, and had it menace me playfully. It was coming to fight. I thought about the way in which the Hulk had often represented anger in the family. In a session some weeks previously, we had talked about Mrs. Simpson's feeling that she was an uncomfortable Hulk who wreaked damage on the family when she meant to work for its good. I felt I had now penetrated a quietly menacing anger which had first been expressed in Eric's trying to confiscate Alex's supply of toys, but which belonged in the transference to me.

I said, "Wait a minute while I find a toy to talk to the Hulk."

Mrs. Simpson handed me a baby doll, saying "Babies have been known to be vicious."

Her offer seemed to indicate her identification with me as the object of Eric's anger, so I handed the doll back to her and said, "Maybe the baby can find out what I've done wrong."

In retrospect, I could see that handing the doll back to her was also a wish to avoid Eric's anger, to aim it at the mother instead. In this wish I had joined the family pattern of directing angry accusation at the mother.

She obligingly took the doll and, through it, said to the Hulk, "Okay Hulk, what have I done?"

Eric said for the Hulk, "I'm mad because you won't let me rule."

Mrs. Simpson replied, "You can't always have your way, and pinching won't help." The doll and the Hulk wrestled.

Alex interjected, "The baby lost her diaper and she's going to poop all over the floor." He stepped in to fight playfully with the Hulk himself. The parents and I were all aware that Alex's encopresis had now entered the discussion about anger.

I said, "Alex said that when the Hulk attacked the baby, she would lose control of her poops. Can people control their poops when they fight?"

Alex did not answer, but a minute later he stopped the fight and, taking a car, knocked over the museum Eric had built.

Eric got angry, "Alex! Why did you have to do that?" He dropped the Hulk and began to rebuild the museum.

I felt a wash of sadness that the anger had gotten out of hand and that I could not help them stop it. My feelings were complicated. On the one hand, I felt a kind of glee that Alex had been able to be directly angry instead of soiling his pants. On the other, I felt identified with Eric and the beating he was taking. In this confusion of my own feelings, I could sense the family's confusion. I turned to the family to work on it with them.

I said, "When Alex got between the Hulk and the baby, he talked about people losing control of their poops. But instead of losing control of his own poops like a baby this time, he destroyed the museum and Eric got mad. How does this relate to family events?"

Mrs. Simpson said, "Eric acts aggressive, but if you return it in kind, he doesn't like it. He thinks his own actions are okay, but in others, they're wrong."

Lightly touching Eric's shoulder to get his attention because I felt this discussion would be hard for him, I said, "So you're saying Mom, that Eric expects that he can play like the Hulk without objection. Then he's surprised if someone else gets mad."

Eric said, "Dr. Scharff, please don't touch me on the shoulder. I'm sunburned."

I realized that Eric was hurt, that he was not experiencing what I was saying as sympathetic, and that he'd like me to "lay off."

Eric was now rebuilding the museum. Alex put a family of small dolls in a car and drove over to visit the museum. I realized that Alex was continuing to act maturely, not like a soiling baby, but was playing out the aggressive problem in an age-appropriate way. Eric had Demolishicor attack Alex's family.

Mr. Simpson said, "Jeanette and Alex can't stop Eric. He ignores it when they try to defend themselves, and he overwhelms them."

Mrs. Simpson had now turned red, and she spat out, "I'm livid. When he does this, I get so mad. Right now, I just want to leave the room!"

I said, "Tell me about it instead."

She said, "I can't discuss my anger yet. I feel he's so stubborn, even after you point it out to him. It causes everyone else to be unhappy. He monopolizes things like the blocks. I just want to knock over that museum."

I turned to Eric, with whom I was again suddenly feeling thrown into sympathy as the victim of his mother's anger, and said, "Eric, does this happen at home?"

Nodding slowly with tears in his eyes, he acknowledged that it did.

Mr. Simpson said, "Usually things break down at this point. Eric, give some of the blocks to Alex and Jeanette."

Mrs. Simpson added, "Eventually we intervene. Then he's upset that we have forced his hand."

Mr. Simpson said, "Then Eric feels we favor Alex and Jeanette."

"Is that right?" I asked Eric.

He nodded sorrowfully, putting his head down on a table and becoming inert.

"What is this like from your growing up, Mrs. Simpson?" I asked.

"It's like my father," she said. "We would dread the time he came home. He'd line us up and yell at us, looking for someone who did something wrong. Then if one of us admitted something, he'd yell at that one. It was awful. He had to be in charge. He made the rules, and no one else mattered. And my mother didn't protect us from him. Just like I can't protect Jeanette and Alex."

"So you feel that Eric is like your father—so destructive?" I asked.

She nodded, beginning to sob. "And when I feel that and I get so mad at him, then I feel that I'm like my father, too. I hate that worse than anything in the world. I hated that man. And now I'm just like him. And then I hate Eric worse for making me feel that way."

I now felt sympathy for Mrs. Simpson, too, no longer identified with Eric against her "tyranny" but able to see the internal tyrant that victimized them all and that they dealt with by projecting it into one another. I felt sympathy for all of them, for the suffering they shared.

Seeing Eric now slumping over the table, his father said to him, "Come here, Son."

Eric got up slowly and was comforted by a loving hug from his father, draping himself across his chest while his father stroked his arm and back. I felt comforted watching them. At the same time, it did not get in the way of the work that was going on. I felt grateful to the father for taking care of Eric in a way that let the mother continue to speak. He was managing to hold the family in holding Eric. It let me keep my attention on Mrs. Simpson. Jeanette now went to her and climbed in her lap, comforting her, while Alex continued to play with the remains of the museum.

I said to Mrs. Simpson, "When you feel you're bad like your own father, you hate Eric, but you also hate yourself."

"Yes," she sobbed. "And I feel I've damaged him just the way I felt my father hurt me. And I can't undo it. There isn't any way out."

It was excruciating for me to remain in the room. I wondered what despair I had wrought. And at the same time, I felt almost exhilarated that the family was managing to hold a steady course through these straits of despair. I felt we were beginning to get a whole-family view of the trouble, and I felt less torn between competing sympathies and thus less angry at one family member for seeming to victimize another. I was drawn now to enlarge my understanding of the father's role, a feeling spurred by gratitude to him for comforting Eric so effectively a moment earlier.

Wanting to enlarge the field at this moment to include the father, I thought of how he tended to remain outside emotional moments, so I turned to him and asked directly, "Does this have any echoes for you, too, Mr. Simpson?"

He said, "My childhood wasn't so dramatic. At least I don't remember any event like that. Sometimes we'd be spanked with a belt for doing something wrong. I can't remember anything more."

Thinking of Mr. Simpson's inability to remember so many things, I said, "Of course, you not being able to remember is one of the things you struggle with. What kinds of things did you get spanked for?"

"I only remember one time," he said. "I was spanked for going over to a little girlfriend's house when I was about Eric's age. My dad womped me with his belt. It hurt. I can relate to Eric's sulking now when I think about it."

I turned to Eric. "Did you know about your dad's being spanked with a belt?" I asked. Eric shook his head, but he looked partially revived. I felt he was in touch with his parents' moving histories. Over the next couple of minutes, we established that in a sexual connotation: He had been strapped at least partly because he had disappeared with a girl.

I had been working to locate each individual in the family struggle. Now I felt I could draw the events of the hour together, to offer the elements of a "because clause." I said, "Mrs. Simpson, you get so mad at Eric because he reminds you of your father. Then you feel like the bad parent yourself when you get so mad. He feels destructive and hopeless about getting your love. Mr. Simpson feels that insisting on any sexual overture will make you hate him like your angry father. Therefore, he tries to deny those interests to be "the good father," but he ends up feeling he's been strapped by his own angry father that he sees in you. So the two of you have a similar struggle, Mr. and Mrs. Simpson, when sexual matters are at issue. But in the setting with the children, it is often Eric who is in the role of bringing up the bad father. When he wants something for himself, he feels bad about it, and he becomes a Demolishicor. But he also does it in a way to protect you, Mrs. Simpson, from feeling that you are the Hulk or the Demolishicor yourself. Strangely, his way of behaving seems at first to protect you from those feeling of hating yourself by taking it on himself."

Mrs. Simpson said, "Yes, you're right. But when I want to bust up his museum because I don't want him to be so high and mighty, then I get to feel awful." At this moment, Alex took the car and broke down the last remains of the museum.

I said, "And it's at those times that Alex takes on Eric for you, Mrs. Simpson. It is part of the reason Alex is so hard to stop in his impulsive destructiveness. He used to do it by becoming an angry, pooping baby. These days he is getting more directly angry."

Jeanette climbed down from her mother's lap and began to play sweetly among the ruins. *In looking back on the session, I realize that Mrs. Simpson had said that it was the baby who could best take on the Hulk, and that I might have added that Jeanette was often put in the role of becoming the sweet baby who could save them from these issues. But one never thinks of all the things that might be said during a session.*

Mr. Simpson was rubbing Eric's head. I asked Mr. Simpson, "What do you think is happening now?"

He said, "Eric's hurt. He has a hard time when his mom's so unhappy with him. There are things he wants to do better and doesn't know how to change."

I asked Eric, "Is that right?"

He nodded.

Mrs. Simpson said, "He probably hates me back."

I said, "So you're afraid he'll hate you like you hate your father? But is there anything else you feel for Eric?"

"Oh, yes! I love him. Really I do. He's a wonderful kid. I don't know what else. I feel hopeless, like all the damage is done. He's already been hurt. I've done it. I hate myself." And she began to sob again.

Alex began to build a simpler house from the blocks, one to house the family car.

I said to Eric, "Do you still feel like crying?"

"Yes," he said. "I feel sad."

"I know you do," I said. "And I think this has been painful for everyone, your mom included. But it's important we talk about all this because it's underneath so much of what goes wrong at home. It gets in the way of the loving. In your family, Mrs. Simpson, you felt your dad hated you and you hated him, but you also wanted his love. What's so painful about being so mad at Eric is how much you care about him too, and feel for him being in a situation like yours. And you also envy him being so competent, getting so much from you and his father, and then wanting more. It makes you remember how you've felt that you had so little. This image of the bad father comes out at these moments of breakdown. It often keeps you, Mr. and Mrs. Simpson, from feeling that you can be good parents. Each of you has felt that you couldn't get enough to go around. It gets played out in the way we've seen. If someone wants too much, it's as though he is taking it from the rest of the family. And finally, I have a lead from Mr. Simpson's memory that this might also be operating in the sexual relationship. But that we'll have to explore with the two of you alone. What's important today is the way each member of the family plays out the anger over what's missing, and the pain when it goes wrong."

This vignette is an excellent example of the combined use of prereflective and self-reflective countertransference. The therapist appears to be genuine with the family and reflects on his own experience in understanding family dynamics. Perhaps best exemplified in the vignette are empathy and the ability to delay action or interpretation until family dynamics fully play themselves out. Nevertheless, the full benefit of a use of countertransference never seems to take place. In spite of the fact that it is the sole presentation of the use of countertransference given within this paper about using countertransference, David Scharff never discusses with the family his own experience and therefore does not appear to share the impact of family dynamics in a way that would clearly demonstrate to the family what behaviors must change. That is, the kind of intervention that describes one's part in a complementary identification, and therefore highlights how the therapist came to feel a certain way, which could be used to demonstrate how family members come to feel how they feel, is never brought forth despite the fact that such an identification clearly occurs. Perhaps one reason such an intervention is not formulated is that accepting one's own responsibility for negative countertransference reactions is not possible within analytic models that assume perfect mental health in the therapist. In my own view, one reason that mental health is so necessary within the relational systems perspective is that the therapist must assume that she does *not* have perfect mental health.

Two opportunities for an intervention that would more deeply address family vulnerabilities within the vignette are most obvious. At one point, early in the session, Scharff describes the feeling of avoidance within the family. At another point Scharff reports feeling that it is "excruciating" to be in the room due to the "despair" he has caused, but "exhilarating" due to the family's apparent ability to hold themselves during such a difficult moment. Although Scharff's final interpretation is delivered with empathy, and appears to encompass a more holistic view of family experience replete with genetic meaning, it seems distancing in its lack of a cohesive description of what has just occurred in the room with the family.

An alternate interpretation, indicated by the relational systems model, would attempt to incorporate the same degrees of history and empathy within an intervention and to also include the therapist's experience. Such an intervention would use the strongest currents of emotion experienced by the therapist as its focal points. The following example relies on some fantasized empathic experience with the family and the assumption that the therapist's clinical skills would be sharp enough to elicit a similar enactment:

This has been a tough session for me as it seems to have been for all of you. Right at the beginning it almost seemed like there was some vacuum of emotion when everyone was playfully destructive, and I noticed myself feeling like some of you were even a little angry with me as if I'm forcing you to look at things that you'd rather not see. Sometimes that's most obvious when the kids are playing, like when Eric seemed to be pointing all those guns at me. Usually that typifies more of a whole-family feeling, but it's interesting how it seems to come most powerfully from Eric. It's sort of like the anger some of you are feeling is felt to be so destructive to the family that it's simply not expressed—or if expressed it only comes out indirectly. I got caught up in it, too, when I passed that baby doll to you, Mrs. Simpson. Right then I sure didn't want to be the one fighting or bringing up angry feelings. I'm also aware of how automatic it was when I handed the doll to you (Mrs. Simpson). I knew somehow that you were the one who takes the heat— you carry that burden and you become the one who supposedly has the biggest problem. But it seems like it's your ambivalence about anger that causes it. When you're crying we all feel bad that you're upset. It was especially hard for me when both you and Eric were feeling so bad. I felt like *I* was the cause of the family's pain then. My guess is that Eric feels like he's what causes the pain sometimes and yet it's the whole family's anger he's expressing. Everyone avoids anger because they know how upsetting it is to you, and yet, in a way, you express your anger all the time. Like when you said you think the damage has already been done with Eric. Even though you say it while you're crying, it's an expression of unreconcilable disappointment with Eric, and it's a way of passing on anger to him that probably feels even more excruciating to him than what I felt in meeting up with your despair. Yet he has no way of appropriately expressing this anger because you're already so upset. So you have this burden that you partially create for yourself, but which is also given to you by the rest of the family. Mr. Simpson, you seemed kind of absent in this session. I liked the way you held Eric when he was feeling bad, but somehow you seem to stay out of the fray. Your inability to remember makes me feel frustrated, and I wonder if you often feel frustrated, and then pass it on to others, as if you don't have a problem at all. By not remembering, you take yourself out of the picture as though you are just here to help the other family members who are suffering. But you're suffering, too.

But I think the most important thing for all of you to know is that even though damage has been done, all of you can feel better. Both of you, Mr. and Mrs. Simpson, have suffered in your childhoods. You experienced how destructive anger can be when it's mishandled. Mrs. Simpson, you seem to think of anger as a monster and I felt that monster lurking in this room today. But you're not your father, Mrs. Simpson, and neither is Eric. I think the need to see your father in yourself and others, and to even create him sometimes, is related to a continuing need you have to recover from your father's behavior. Mr. Simpson, always being there to soothe anger still won't make it go away, and until you recognize your own feelings rather than just taking care of others' feelings, your family will have to *have* those feelings for you to take care of. And you're right, Mrs. Simpson, Eric is a great kid. You all can see that something is already changing in the family by the way that Alex can now be destructive without pooping in his pants, which was the only way he could be angry when the family treated it as so awful. What is necessary now is that both of you, Mr. and Mrs. Simpson, learn to express anger appropriately. Along with that will come the ability to express other emotions in more evenly tempered ways. If you knew that you could express anger right when you felt it, Mrs. Simpson, you wouldn't start to feel the need to either blow up or get depressed. Mr. Simpson, if you started saying that certain things bother you, you might find that your family can handle it even if they do get a little hurt. I can tell you it's clear to me how much love there is in this family— just because you are all able to handle coming here and going through so much.

This intervention would likely occur over many sessions and would require explanation along the way. However, what is important to notice in it is the difference in point of view. The therapist is part of a system with the family and reports his experience in a way that is congruent with his part. In the relational systems model the therapist openly recognizes the part he has taken in the interaction and uses his own personality and theoretical understanding to formulate the intervention. The therapist's desire for a healthier family system is partially generated by his own desire to feel better when with the family. His maintenance of boundaries when with the family requires honesty and openness from within the system of which he has become a part.

Samuel Slipp

Slipp's (1980, 1984, 1988) approach bears many similarities to that of the Scharffs (D. Scharff 1991, J. Scharff 1991, Scharff and Scharff 1987). An important difference lies in Slipp's belief that countertransference reactions require intimacy and that when the therapist recognizes a countertransference reaction it is only the result of especially powerful forces within the treatment relationship made possible through the creation by the therapist of a trusting relationship. Slipp attempts to be objective in delivering both systemic and genetic interpretations. But he does not think of himself as part of a system with the client or family, nor does he believe that the therapist's personality is an important component within therapeutic enactments. The following vignette, (from Slipp [1988], pp. 204–206) like the Scharff (1991) example, deals with the destructive nature of aggression, and exemplifies Slipp's approach.

In object relations family therapy, a safe holding environment needs to be developed in order to lower defensiveness and to increase the level of trust. Here, the most important factors are the therapist's genuine concern for all the members of the family, refusal to take sides or to be judgmental, and willingness to consider each member's perspective and feelings. The family members also need to develop confidence in the strength of the therapist to contain the expression of aggression. The therapist acts like a referee to prevent low blows and the occurrence of a free-for-all. This is particularly important for families in which there is the fear that aggression will get out of control and will be destructive to the cohesion of the family.

At one point in treatment, Harry came close to openly expressing his aggression by making a cryptic remark that thinly masked his hostility toward me and the treatment. He made a joke about the lack of effectiveness of the treatment process. I saw this as a derivative of the transference, in that I represented his ineffectual mother from whom he could not expect help, and instead whom he had to help. I acknowledged Harry's efforts to be open and honest about his distrust and anger toward me, and his concerns about how effective I might be in helping the family. (I felt it was too early at this point to make a transference interpretation.) I further stated that I realized how difficult it was for him to express his anger, and I acknowledged his effort to do so.

In this way I attempted to establish a corrective emotional experience. I could show him that I was able to accept and contain his anger without retaliation (like Rose) [the patient's wife] or falling apart (like his mother). I would not abandon him emotionally or physically. This had been exactly his fear concerning his weak and depressed mother; she would become sick and abandon him again if he expressed rage. Thus he did not need to deny responsibility for his anger now but was entitled, and indeed encouraged, to express it openly and honestly, *himself.* This undermined his false self and the need to use projective identification as a defense.

The systemic level of interaction was dealt with by describing how Rose and Harry's conflict became escalated by the very way they dealt with each other. The more Rose demanded, the more Harry withheld; and the more Harry held back, the more Rose demanded. This created a vicious cycle—a circular process in which each one of them reacted to the other, a process that ran away with itself. An objective description was made of their interaction, which prevented the focus of blame from falling on either one of them: "Both of you are victims of this process; it is a no-win situation. It may be that this is how each of you have felt since childhood, as if you've been a victim of others." This sensitizing of them to the fact of their bouncing off each other defensively alerted them to the systemic process, to its transferential significance, and contributed to their working on controlling it.

One way of resolving Harry's use of projective identification was through the use of the objective countertransference he evoked in me. I experienced a sense of frustration and annoyance with him which I contained. When I felt that Harry was sufficiently engaged in treatment, I revealed my own countertransference feelings. I did this in a way that was calm and not accusatory. I reframed my countertransference feelings in a positive way and tied them in with a genetic interpretation that described the source as well as the purpose they served. In this way, I tried to diminish Harry's defensiveness, guilt, and loss of self-esteem.

I said, "I sincerely have been trying to help, but at times I've experienced myself feeling helpless and frustrated in my efforts. Then as I was mulling over these feelings in my head, I realized that you must have felt this same way when your father died. Perhaps you wanted me to feel the same way, so that I could empathically understand how helpless and frustrated you felt then. Your mother became sick, and there was no one there to help you mourn the loss of your father. You were alone and unable to express your feelings openly. This continued even when your mother returned, for fear that she would become sick again and leave. This must have left you feeling trapped, impotent, and angry."

The conflict was thus placed back into Harry. He could now own it and did not need to project it into others and act it out through them. He then began working through his fearfulness about being openly expressive and taking responsibility for his anger. He acknowledged that he had feared that if he expressed his anger at his mother, she was so narcissistically vulnerable that she would only become sick and leave again. Thus he could not get his own need addressed, and felt he had to function as a protector of his mother. This same conflict, this fear of being open and honest in expressing his feelings, was reflected in his distant and angry relationship with his wife.

In the past he had dealt with his helplessness and anger by projecting this aspect of himself into another, thereby rendering the other person helpless and enraged. This solution gave him some sense of mastery over his own helplessness and rage by externalizing these feelings and controlling the other person. But he did not really address the underlying issues of his rage, insecurity, and lack of self-esteem, which continued to be acted out in the interpersonal sphere. The obsessive defenses Harry erected were constricting his freedom of expression and his vitality, and were punitive and self-defeating. Insight into the genesis of his obsessive behavior enabled him to recognize the source of it, ventilate his rage, and stop taking it out on his wife. In turn, Rose had grown sufficiently in her self-esteem to feel entitled to receive better treatment. The marriage would not have lasted much longer had Harry not changed and become more considerate of Rose's feelings and needs. Harry and Rose continued on in individual therapy with separate therapists, to work through the conflicts that each of them had become aware of in marital therapy.

Slipp's (1988) use of the system when working with husband and wife is unique among object relations therapists. His connection of the therapeutic enactment with genetic causes clearly helped the patient gain a better understanding of his behavior. But a more complete understanding of this patient's acting out via projective identification can be derived if the therapist is willing to take responsibility for the emotions that have become engendered within himself. The following intervention is again my own, and takes liberties in assuming clinical skills that make the enactment possible, and time enough to create an adequate holding environment within the therapy:

"Harry, I've found myself becoming increasingly frustrated by your need to control the therapeutic process and what seems like your hesitance to reveal your anger and distrust with me openly. I know that my frustration is partly caused by my desire to help you—perhaps it's sort of a need to help you. But my feelings of frustration have been so strong that I'm realizing how it must be for you to feel like you can never be helped. When you constantly helped your mother, who should have been there to help you, you became less and less trusting that anyone would help you or even care about you. And now, when you get into an intimate relationship, unless you're helping the other person, you feel like you'll be abandoned. So you're constantly frustrated. The important catch is that someone, like me, might really want to help you and won't abandon you. That's when the possible pain you anticipate stops you from ever giving someone a chance, and you keep yourself at a frustrated level. The tough thing is that even if you do decide to be open and trust, you will be hurt sometimes. Although I'll always be willing to see you and give you my best, you'll probably sometimes experience my self-absorption, or inability to meet at a certain time, as pain. And with your wife, of course, she needs to have her own independent activities—and everyone is selfish sometimes. What you'll eventually have to come to realize is that others really do care. I really care about you. Rose cares about you so deeply that she's extremely hurt by the frustration you pass on to her. But neither of you will ever be happy unless you allow yourselves to feel the pain that goes with being truly intimate."

Such an intervention cannot be reached without the therapist recognizing and revealing her part in the interactional dynamic. The primary patterns that affect the patient's life will occur in the therapy no matter how intimate the relationship as long as the therapist is trying to treat the patient. But the therapist's frustration does not occur without the therapist desiring to be somewhat intimate with the patient, and the intervention cannot work without the therapist admitting that desire.

THE UNIMPORTANT VIEW

Structural, strategic, solution-oriented, and narrative models of therapy do not recognize any importance in countertransference. Because the therapists who work with models in the area I have called the unimportant view do not value or recognize countertransference, and in fact, even suggest that there is no place for reflectiveness in the process of family therapy (Haley 1976), it is likely that prereflective uses of countertransference are especially prominent in their work. And, among the purists in these approaches, it is especially unlikely that there would be any interest in integrating analytic thinking in their work.

But such an integration offers some of the very strengths that these therapists prize. Rather than pathologize people, as many systems and narrative therapists suggest is problematic in analytic models, the relational systems perspective suggests that the key to change is in recognizing that the current family system functions as it does because painful or uncomfortable emotions are avoided unnecessarily. The goal of the relational systems perspective is to have people recognize that they need not have so much pain or put that pain into others within the family. The goal is to have family members interact with one another in a more comfortable and loving pattern that can take the place of old, hurtful patterns that continue because they are not understood and because they provide a temporary fix for the pain that is felt. The key to change, in other words, is to perceive the world and one's interactions differently. Transference is not a permanent, unchanging view of the world, but constitutes a habitual emotional economy that, although providing immediate gratification or avoidance of pain, is inefficient in the long term.

The relational systems model aims to replace old patterns with more efficient new patterns, and to do this relies on demonstrating the inefficiency of old patterns to the family. Interventions that simply attempt to describe accurately the process of emotional transfer between family members and what those transfers mean about the intrapsychic patterns of family members, often have structural, strategic, and even solution-oriented or narrative effects. The relational systems model allows the therapist to challenge dysfunctional structures and boundaries, harness emotional family dynamics strategically toward positive effect, and co-create new narratives of family emotional life. These interventions are best formulated by recognizing emotional dynamics within the family as a part of the therapist–family system.

Salvador Minuchin

In Minuchin's structural therapy the goal is to encourage appropriately flexible boundaries, a process that returns the family to a more functional hierarchy through interventions that make flexible boundaries more likely. Minuchin concentrates on joining with the family so that his interventions, aimed at restructuring the family toward systems understanding rather than individual pathology, will be accepted and acceptable. In the following vignette, Minuchin (1974, pp. 158–171) comments on the therapist's maneuvers with the family and categorizes interventions as either accommodation "Ac."—(joining and/or accepting family dynamics so that resistance will not become too strong) or restructuring "Re."—(presenting a systems view or changing current family behavior to enact a more appropriate family hierarchy and appropriately flexible boundaries).

The Smiths were referred to a family therapist for consultation by a psychiatrist participating in an introductory seminar on family therapy. Mr. Smith has been a psychiatric patient for ten years, having been hospitalized twice for agitated depression. Recently, his symptoms reappeared. He is restless, unable to concentrate, anxious, and has again requested hospitalization. The family interview is an attempt on his psychiatrist's part to find an alternative to hospitalization.

Present at the interview are Mr. Smith, aged forty-nine, his wife, forty-two, their only son Matthew, twelve, and Mrs. Smith's father, Mr. Brown, who has lived with the couple since their marriage. The referring psychiatrist, Dr. Farrell, is also present.

The transcript of the interview itself appears in the left column. In the right column are comments and analysis. The therapeutic strategy and techniques appear in roman type; the thoughts and feelings of the interviewer and the family about both themselves and each other during the session appear in italics. The accommodation and restructuring maneuvers are designated *Ac.* and *Re.*

(Minuchin is wandering around, rearranging chairs. He knocks over an ashtray and replaces it.)

Minuchin: Do you have relatives in Israel?

Mr. Smith: Relatives in Israel? No.

Ac. Starts the session with a statement that defines him as part of the family's kinship network. ("I am like you.")

Minuchin: I know a Smith family in Israel. Okay. Let's try to—Dr. Farrell has met only you, and none of the other members of the family.

Ac. Separates himself from the previous therapist. He is a family consultant and may do things differently.

Mrs. Smith: Excuse me, but Dr. Farrell and I had a conversation several years

ago. I don't know if you remember.
Over at the hospital.

Dr. Farrell: That's right. Only once.

Mrs. Smith: Right.

Dr. Farrell: Mr. Smith was my patient
for at least a year or two—

Mr. Smith: I was your patient.

Dr. Farrell: —When I was at the psychiatric clinic. And I left there, oh, I
think four or five years ago. Since then,
he's been under the care of Dr. Post,
who would have liked to be here today
but was unable to keep—to make it on
such short notice.

Minuchin: You saw Dr. Post weekly?

Mr. Smith: Monthly.

Minuchin: Monthly. What is the problem? You know, I don't know too much
about you. And one of the ways in
which I work is, I prefer not to know
too much, so I didn't ask Dr. Farrell.
Probably you will give me your own
version of what are the problems, and
so we can go out from there. So who
wants to start?

Ac. Again, separates himself from the
previous therapist, indicating that he
will rely on his own hearing of the information the family is now to supply.

Re. Directs his first question about the
problem to the whole family, not to the
identified patient, which challenges the
notion that there is one patient.

Mr. Smith: I think it's my problem. I'm
the one that has the problem. And—

Minuchin: Don't be so sure. Never be
so sure. (*Mr. Smith is leaning forward,
very intent. Minuchin is lounging. Matthew looks at Mr. Smith, and both laugh
at Minuchin's reply.*)

Re. Counters Mr. Smith's move to maintain the structure by presenting himself
as the problem. The therapist questions
the identification of Mr. Smith as the patient and responds to his seriousness

with bantering. He also challenges the patient's and family members' reality experience.

Mr. Smith: Well, it seems to be.

Minuchin: Okay.

Mr. Smith: I'm the one that was in the hospital and everything.

Minuchin: Yeah, that doesn't, still, tell me it is your problem. Okay, go ahead. What is your problem?

Re. Challenges the patient's reality again.

Ac. Encourages the identified patient to talk, which keeps him central.

Mr. Smith: Just nervous, upset all the time.

Minuchin: You are upset?

Mr. Smith: Yeah, seem to be never relaxed. Oh, sometimes, sometimes I'm relaxed. But most of the time not. Then I got up tight and I asked them to put me in the hospital. And I have been talking to Dr. Farrell at the hospital.

Minuchin: Do you think that you are the problem?

Ac. and Re. Following the sequence of challenging the husband's claim to his role as a patient, the therapist makes a tracking statement in the form of a question, which carries a restructuring doubt.

Mr. Smith: Oh, I kind of think so. I don't know if it's caused by anybody, but I'm the one that has the problem.

Mr. Smith accommodates to the previous attack on the family structure, conceding that someone might be causing his problem.

Minuchin: Mm. If—let's follow your line of thinking. If it would be caused by somebody or something outside of

Ac. Accommodates to Mr. Smith's accommodation. As a result, a concern for issues of interpersonal causality is now

yourself, what would you say your problem is?

Mr. Smith: You know, I'd be very surprised.

Minuchin: Let's think in the family. Who makes you upset?

Mr. Smith: I don't think anybody in the family makes me upset.

Minuchin: Let me ask your wife, okay?

Mr. Smith: Fine. Okay.

Minuchin: Who do you think is—

Mrs. Smith: Well, I've tried to think about it myself, and I really feel he makes his own problems.

Minuchin: Mm.

Mrs. Smith: Because he worries about things like paying the electric bill. That's a normal procedure for every individual. And he has a steady job. He doesn't have to worry about that. He worries about the house. When he

attributed to Mr. Smith. The narrow diagnosis is replaced by the broader question: what is the problem?

Mr. Smith counters.

Re: Insists on an interpersonal framework and continues to challenge the identification of Mr. Smith as the problem. At the same time, this approach confirms Mr. Smith's position of centrality in the family. It accommodates to his position as gatekeeper while simultaneously challenging the structure.

Ac. Acknowledges Mr. Smith's position as gatekeeper. The therapist is experiencing the power of a rigid system, for his challenges have been consistently countered by the identified patient, who insists on remaining the problem. Consequently, the therapist moves to contact another member.

This long monologue emphasizes the husband's control over his wife and the extent to which she defers to him. But her elaborate description of the ways in which her husband must control her serve to define him as a sick man. As comes home—as if the house was going to go away. Well, no one's going to come in and take anything. That's why I say I feel he just makes his own problems. And I really don't feel that I irritate him, unless I don't know about it. Because I always try to go out of my way to do—I try to think like he thinks and will try to do things that—will try to make it easier for him. *(Mr. Smith begins to fidget in rather bizarre ways. He reaches over as if to touch his wife, but lets his hand drop to move along the edge of her chair instead. He "blows off steam" with a long sigh. He examines the corners of his armrest. Suddenly he leans over to extinguish his cigarette, then carefully brushes off every inch of his chair arm. He looks at his watch and examines his fingernails.)*

Like for instance, I'll ask him "Well, do you want me to go to the store?" which he says no. He wants to go to the store all the time. "Shall I go down to pay the bills?" No. He wants to. If we get a call to go somewhere, I always say, "Well, I have to ask Bob first." I just don't do it on my own. I always—because I feel he's the head of the family, and this he's entitled to. That I would always ask him before I myself would do anything. So I don't think—

Minuchin: There is nothing that you do that irritates him?

Mrs. Smith: Yeah, Well, that's why I say, unless—I don't know. I really don't know. Now, when I first went back to

she talks, Mr. Smith displays behavior that underlines the meaning of her communications.

Re. Again questions the validity of labeling the man sick without taking into account the transactional context of the family, and again questions the family member's experience of reality.

work, about fourteen years ago, is it?
Yes, About—approximately fourteen
years—

Mr. Smith: Seven—

Mrs. Smith: He didn't like the idea of
me going back to work, but when I went
back to work, it was because we had a
hard time financially, getting along. And
he was working two jobs. And at that
time he wasn't feeling good, and I said
to him, I said, maybe if I go back to
work it would help you. You won't have
to work two jobs. And so of course he
agreed, but he didn't like me working.
But he agreed to it because it was a fi-
nance thing at that time. So—

*The therapist's restructuring probes
have been deflected by the relentless
monologue and by Mr. Smith's symptomatic behavior. The therapist feels
curtailed and frustrated; he experiences
the need to regain control of the session.
However, he cannot interrupt this
woman too sharply. That would be construed as another attack on a person
already victimized.*

Minuchin: What is your work?

Ac. Confirms Mrs. Smith by entering a
dialog with her.

Re. As she has been talking about herself only in relation to her husband, the
therapist moves her from describing
herself as the victim of a sick man to
describing her life outside the family.

Mrs. Smith: I work at a bank.

Minuchin: What do you do there?

Mrs. Smith: I am a file clerk, and I type.
Everything in the office, actually. And
he—well, he never liked the idea of his
wife working. But yet it made things
easier, on the whole. It's not that we're
loaded with money, but we don't have
to worry about payments.

*Again the therapist is blocked. Each
spouse has obediently entertained the
idea that the husband might not be the
sole problem, so they cannot be accused
of not cooperating. Mrs. Smith has responded to his attempt to redirect her
attention. But after two statements, she
returns to describing her husband as a
sick man. Within this very rigid system,
the therapist's interventions are
dropped. The experience of being*

blocked leads him to develop a new strategy. He realizes that he must join more closely before any restructuring operations can be accepted. He decides to join the spouses by confirming each individually, hoping that he will then be in a position to challenge their interactions. In effect, he will be saying, "You are both nice people, but something in the way you interact is questionable."

Minuchin: Mr. Smith, why don't you like your wife working?

Ac. Makes contact by using the content of Mrs. Smith's monologue.

Re. The terminology "you don't like" is associated with normal behavior, not with being sick.

Mr. Smith: Well, I'm more or less used to it now. But at the time she's talking about, I didn't think a woman should work. And—

Minuchin: Is your family a traditional kind of family?

Mrs. Smith: Oh, yes.

Mr. Smith: Maybe it's because mother never worked. I mean outside of the house, she never worked. And I always wanted to do the supporting, and—

Minuchin: That your wife worked meant something? That you could not support her?

Mr. Smith: At the time that she said I was working two jobs. And I was complaining a little bit. And that's why she said she would do—

Minuchin: What's your work?

Re: Interrupts a train of thought headed

toward again making the point that Mr. Smith is sick, turning it into a dialog about other areas.

Mr. Smith: Where do I work? I work for a manufacturer.

Minuchin: What is your job? What do you do?

Mr. Smith: I work in the lab as a technician and an inspector.

Minuchin: That means the production aspect of it?

Ac. Although the therapist does not understand and is not interested in Mr. Smith's work, his question opens up a common area; they can talk about business together.

Mr. Smith: Well, on overtime I work in production. During the week I work right in the lab, working on samples and different tests to be made. We use the microscope a lot, reading samples under a microscope.

Re. The content is about normal aspects of the identified patient's life.

Minuchin: How long have you been working there?

Ac. Exploring the man's life confirms him.

Re. Continues to emphasize the normal aspects of life.

Mr. Smith: Thirty years.

Minuchin: Thirty years! My goodness!

Mr. Smith: Yeah. With the company. But not in this job thirty years. Just about seven years on this job.

Minuchin: I don't know. I never worked any place for more than seven years. This is the longest time I have worked. I am much more restless than you, clearly. I am a very restless kind of person. *(He scratches his head, checks his watch, and fiddles with his coat.)*

Ac. Becomes less assertive, mimicking Mr. Smith, and introduces his own personal life, talking as worker to worker.

Re. By joining Mr. Smith, the therapist suggests that the patient may not be sick. Furthermore, by becoming "restless," the therapist creates a paradoxical situation in which the weaker man, Mr. Smith, is seen as the stronger. If such confusion is possible, the identified patient's sickness may also be open to question. The rigidity of the family's schema is questioned. *The therapist is aware of pursuing a strategy that will enable him to get closer to Mr. Smith. He is not aware that his behavior is fumbling and that his stance has lost power. He uses talking about himself as a means both of getting closer and of challenging the definition of the man as sick. He feels more accepted, more relaxed, and more confident that his interventions will now be accepted by the system.*

Mr. Smith: Mm.

Minuchin: You are not, evidently.

Re. Insists on making his message explicit.

Mr. Smith: No, I wouldn't say I'm restless. I mean, I sleep. but I don't—

Minuchin: But you are steady in one—

Ac. Confirms Mr. Smith as competent.

Mr. Smith: As far as the job's concerned, yeah. Well, I went there at nineteen, and I've stayed down there.

Minuchin: You are now forty-nine?

Mr. Smith: Forty-nine.

Minuchin (hesitates, as if thinking): We are the same age.

Ac. The therapist and Mr. Smith are similar in age as well as in restlessness and in being workers.

Mr. Smith: Are we?

Mr. Smith acknowledges, accommodating to the therapist.

Minuchin: And when did you begin to kind of worry about things?

Re. Now disengages, becoming the expert addressing a person in need of help.

Mr. Smith: Ten years ago.

Minuchin: Ten years. Tell me, maybe your son—your only son?

Ac. Establishes that he has Mr. Smith's permission to contact Matthew.

Mr. Smith: Yeah.

Minuchin (to Matthew): Your father said he is the problem, and your mother agrees that he is the problem in the family. But what are the things that make your father—that irritate him, that make him upset, so he gets pissed off?

Ac. Keeps the father in the position of identified patient as he contacts his son.

Re. To explore the interpersonal transactions that may irritate Mr. Smith questions the presenting problem of intrapsychic pathology.

Having successfully established contact with two family members, the therapist moves to include a third. He uses language geared to an adolescent, approaching him as a person who observes things in the family. When Minuchin contacted Matthew, he hoped to find an ally—a pathway for restructuring interventions. Instead, the boy parrots his mother. The therapist is irritated, and his frustration becomes part of his next communication to the family.

Matthew: I don't know. I don't think it's like—anybody that puts it on him. It's just—I don't know.

Minuchin: I just can't believe that, you know. People are always part of—when people live together, then they irritate each other, you know. I am sure your father irritates you sometimes. (*Mrs. Smith nods emphatically.*) And I am sure that your grandfather irritates you sometimes. And you in turn irritate your grandfather and your mother and father. I am sure of that. Am I right?

Re. Insists that the family explore interpersonal transactions. The therapist challenged the system only indirectly while talking with the father and mother, but while talking with the son, he attacks strongly. Again he questions a family member's perception of reality.

Matthew: Yeah. But I don't irritate him that much, like really nervous. I might, you know, be bad sometimes. But I don't think I really irritate him that much.

Ac. Finishes his attack with a request for affiliation and acknowledgment.

Minuchin: What about your grandpa? Does he irritate your father?

Ac. Addresses boy as a competent observer of the family scene.

Matthew: No. He don't say much.

Minuchin: Grandpa doesn't say much. How old are you, Mr. Brown?

Ac. Makes contact with the fourth member, affiliating with him jovially.

Mr. Brown: How much do you think?

Minuchin: Oh, like fifty-three.

Mr. Brown: Seventy-eight.

Minuchin: Seventy-eight. You look fine.

Mr. Brown: No, I'll tell you now what I think. What brings it on is Bob himself. He's always worried about me. He wants everything done just certain ways, see? He's particular, in other words, see? And he sees something done, and right away, he's got to go and do it. And someone says, "I'll do it." "No, I'll do it. I'll do it," he says. That's one thing, now. Now, another—

The therapist feels a sense of respect for the elderly. He also feels protective toward the grandfather, sensing his displacement in the family. The grandfather also maintains the family structure.

Minuchin: You are saying he likes to do things instead—for other people?

Re. Relabels Mr. Brown's description of Mr. Smith's actions. Mr. Brown calls them controlling; the therapist suggests they are helpful.

Mr. Smith: I think he missed the point—

Mr. Smith insists on his position as a patient. He interrupts the dialog between Mr. Brown and Minuchin, eliciting a structure—maintaining communication from the grandfather.

Mr. Brown: No, no, no. For himself. Now, suppose there's dirt on the carpet or something like that. He'd say, "Well, there's dirt on the carpet." She'd say, "I'll clean it up." "Never mind, I'll do it." And he'd go right away and clean it up. Now I don't think he should do that.

Minuchin: He's helpful that way.

Re. Again relabels.

Mr. Brown: I don't think it's good. I don't think he should do that. There's lots of things that he does that he shouldn't do. He should let someone else do something too.

Mr. Brown seems genuinely concerned for Mr. Smith, not just in alliance with his daughter. But the grandfather is not powerful in the system. The therapist treats him with respect but decides that restructuring interventions utilizing the grandfather cannot succeed.

Minuchin: Like who?

Ac.

Mr. Brown: Any one of the three of us.

Minuchin: He takes everything on his shoulders?

Mr. Brown: Almost everything. I— pretty near everything.

Minuchin: You—What's your name, you said?

Ac. Having established affiliation with Mr. Brown, turns back to another member and seeks contact with Matthew in a more familiar mode.

Matthew: Matthew.

Minuchin: Matthew. You disagreed with that—with your grandfather's statement.

Matthew: I think he's partly right. I don't think he takes that—you know. He does try to do a lot of things. Like, somebody will offer. He'll say, "No, I can do it myself." I don't feel like he takes everything on. He'll do a lot of that. Not really too much. But he tells me to take out the trash and all, still. Stuff like that, I still got to do most of.

Mrs. Smith: But when you don't do it, he ends up doing it.

Matthew's complaint sounds quite typical of problems between adolescent sons and their fathers. Mrs. Smith joins in an alliance with Mr. Smith, defining the boundaries of the parental subsystem.

Mr. Smith: I don't think that's what's wrong. Because I don't—I could help my wife more as far as cleaning is concerned.

Mr. Smith re-establishes his position as sick and reactivates his son's treatment of him as sick.

Matthew: Yeah, like he'll come home and, like, run the carpet sweeper.

Mr. Smith: Just fast stuff.

Matthew: Yeah.

Mrs. Smith: But it's a big help.

Mr. Smith: Heavy cleaning, I don't do for her, and dishes, I don't do for her. Yeah, I do help her with the dishes ever since I've been married, but not all the time. Most of the time.

Matthew: I think he means like if something's, like, broken in the house, or—

Minuchin (*indignantly*): Wait a moment, wait a moment. Who means?

Re. Models for Mr. Smith a way of defining the intergenerational boundary, for indignation is a powerful force for separation.

Matthew: My grandfather.

Minuchin: Your grandfather. You are explaining your grandfather.

The therapist feels that Matthew criticizes his father too freely, so he decides to attack the son, showing his indignation.

Matthew: Yeah. Like if something's broken in the house or something, he'll want to do it himself, or something.

Mr. Smith: No, I'm not too handy a person that way. I want it done right away, probably, and characteristic—

Matthew: Yeah, like you want it done right away.

Mrs. Smith: He hasn't enough patience to wait.

All three statements maintain Mr. Smith as sick. There is agreement on this dysfunctional transactional pattern, which keeps the family close. Mr. Smith had again started to portray himself as sick, which activates Mrs. Smith's protectiveness, preventing further amplification.

Mrs. Smith: But I don't think that's bad. A lot of people are that way.

Minuchin: Mom was saying, "Don't be critical of Dad."

Ac. Maintains and defines the spouse subsystem boundary so that supportive, positive transactions can grow. *The therapist feels he has been too negative toward Mrs. Smith and corrects himself.*

Matthew: She what?

Ac.

Minuchin: She just said, "Don't be critical of Daddy." Because you were saying, "He's impatient," and Mom says, "Well, you know, a lot of people are like that." Is she protective of Father?

Matthew: I don't think so.

Minuchin: There is nothing wrong with that. I think it is rather nice.

Ac. Again supports spouse subsystem, dwelling on positive husband–wife transactions, which reassures Matthew that he does not have to be involved.

Matthew: She is a little bit, I guess. I don't think she's really overprotective.

Minuchin: I just mean protective, in a nice way. In the same way in which Daddy apparently is protective of everybody else, according to Grandpa. Is that true? Is your husband trying to do things, trying to do your job?

Ac. Confirms Mr. and Mrs. Smith as positive and good.

Re. Emphasizing positives in the husband–wife relationship challenges the family schema.

Mrs. Smith: Well, he worries about me excessively.

(Mr. Smith sighs loudly, then suddenly springs up, strips off his jacket, and strides away to hang it up. Then he lights a cigarette.)

The therapist feels that he is losing Mr. Smith, who has a glassy, distant look in his eyes. He feels a need to be in contact with Mr. Smith, but Mrs. Smith continues talking and he does not want to interrupt her rudely.

Minuchin: He worries about you. That you don't like?

Mrs. Smith: Yes. I don't think he should, because I feel I'm an individual, and he shouldn't worry so much. Because he has a lot of his own problems he should take care of.

Mrs. Smith's remark about Mr. Smith's problems is a distancing communication, made in response to the therapist's previous operation, which was designed to increase husband–wife contact.

Minuchin: You mean he worries about you, sometimes it bothers you. Can I have a cigarette, Mr. Smith?

Re. Counters Mrs. Smith's attempt to maintain the prevailing structure with an interpersonal confirmation supporting the husband–wife subsystem.

Mr. Smith: Sure (*offers a cigarette to the therapist*).

Minuchin: I smoke only when I don't know what to do, but by this time I don't know what to do, so I am worried. I am smoking. (*The therapist takes off his coat, hangs it up, and walks back to get a light from Mr. Smith.*)

Ac.

These are spontaneous mimetic operations, resulting from the therapist's concern. Mr. Smith's symptomatic behavior and Mrs. Smith's distancing operation have again left the therapist feeling excluded and powerless. The therapist and Mr. Smith are now both smoking and both in their shirtsleeves.

Minuchin: What's your wife's name?

Ac. Tries to decrease distance by using first names.

Mr. Smith: Rosemary.

Minuchin: Rosemary. And yours?

Mr. Smith: Bob. Robert—

Minuchin: Bob. Rosemary says that sometimes you worry too much about her. What does she mean?

The therapist has retraced his steps, having observed that direct contact with Mrs. Smith activates Mr. Smith's restlessness. He now contacts the wife through the husband. Having accommodated by honoring Mr. Smith's centrality, and mimicked by taking off his coat and lighting a cigarette, Minuchin once more feels in contact with Mr. Smith.

Mr. Smith: Well, I'm—I don't really know what she means by that. I'm concerned over her, and I'm very much in love with her, and I don't think I worry too much—

Minuchin: Let's find out. Let's find out. (*He gestures, indicating that Mr. Smith and Mrs. Smith should talk.*)

Re. Assigns task of talking to each other. *The therapist senses that the family members will now follow his instructions, so he starts a different phase of the interview, instructing the partici-*

> *pants to talk to each other so as to activate their enactment of accustomed transactional patterns. He now wants to keep himself out of the discussion as much as possible.*

This vignette does an especially good job of demonstrating the use of self. Minuchin is adept at being himself with good effect. Examples include the moment when he becomes "restless" to make himself the weaker man, and his reaction to Mr. Smith's boredom with refocusing on him, taking off his jacket, and lighting a cigarette. These prereflective therapeutic maneuvers cannot be taught and are essential to Minuchin's technique. But Minuchin's technique is indirect without reason. In a situation such as the one depicted here, a therapist could use his irritation in formulating an intervention that accommodates and restructures, while it also addresses boundary issues. The following is an example of what a relational systems therapist might say:

It seems this group has had some difficulty in understanding or accepting a different view of the family problem. You all insist on thinking Father has a big problem when, in fact, all of you have a problem. I can understand why you might do that—I mean, no one wants to think they have a problem—well some people are better at having problems than others, like Mr. Smith. I guess what's so interesting about your family is that I'm asking you all what you do to irritate each other and you're so polite about saying you're not irritating or irritated that *I'm* getting irritated. Could it be that when you're all this irritated I have to get irritated so you won't have to deal with it? I think your family works like that. Several of you know you're irritated but there's some unwritten rule that being irritated is wrong. So you all think Dad is irritating you, when actually you are all irritating Dad just as much—no, more. I think Dad is the most irritated person here. Dad actually seems to want to handle the family's irritation—I mean, that's what a good man would do, I suppose—but really you are all pretty irritating and it's not fair that Dad ends up being hospitalized because of it. Examples of this might be how, no matter what I say, somehow it seems to be ignored unless it agrees with the way you already see things. You don't say, 'Hey, that's not the way I see it, can you tell me what you mean?' Instead you just state a different opinion like what I said doesn't make any difference. Do you guys do that to Mr. Smith? Ignoring other people is one of the most irritating things to do. Lots of times it expresses the idea that listening to the other would irritate you. So, I think one way you guys deal with irritation is to irritate someone else rather than feel irritated yourself. And Mr. Smith, I think you are allowing this because you like to think the world is doing you wrong—that you're all that's good and everyone else is bad. But that means you really think your family is so weak that they can't take responsibility for their own irritability or anything else. You let them feel strong, and think you're weak, but really you think it's the other way around."

This intervention focuses on the emotional process within the family while at the same time it demonstrates to the family that the father has a role higher up in the hierarchy. Other family members are defined as too weak to handle their own irritability so that their authority within the family is decreased. Although it is not clear in the writing of this example intervention, empathy would be used as the method of accommodation. Family members' viewpoints and feelings would be attached to the intervention so that it would seem congruent to each of them even if difficult to tolerate. Perhaps one of Minuchin's greatest skills is the ability to understand a system while remaining empathic to it. The relational systems perspective aims to meet these same standards while also directly addressing the family patterns that have developed.

Jay Haley

The strategic approach focuses on using the family's dynamics in formulating interventions that require the system to realign in healthier ways. The methods used have been referred to as a sort of therapeutic judo with which the power of the family can be directed to defeat dysfunctional patterns. Often the therapeutic approach taken with a family is determined by an understanding of how the family's problem-solving has gone awry. In this next example, one of the premiere techniques utilized by strategic therapists, the paradoxical intervention, is demonstrated. This excerpt is drawn from Haley (1976, pp. 250–257). The therapist here, Mariano Barragan, M.D., is working under live supervision from a group of therapists behind a one-way mirror.

Within this session, and prior to the excerpt, the therapist has been working toward helping a boy recover from his fear of dogs. The therapist has noticed the overemphasis of the parents on the boy's problem, and has guessed that the problem is actually maintained by this focus and the parents' own need to avoid conflict within their marriage. The mother has been identified as "overinvolved," and the primary intervention used up to this point is activation of the father by appealing to his expertise in the management of dogs, which he has developed in his work as a mailman. The therapist's suggestion that the family obtain a dog has been met with some hesitation.

"Yes, I know what you mean," said the therapist. "But I want you to get together and—today is Friday, I want you to get together and talk about the dog." Turning to the boy, he added, "Then I want you to decide exactly what you have to do, and then I want you to go and do it. But first I want you to talk about it with your parents."

That ended the second interview. The following week the family had not obtained a dog, and the session was a general one on family life. At the fourth family interview, the family arrived with a puppy. The boy let it out of the box, avoiding touching it.

"I hope he doesn't go to the bathroom," said the mother. The dog did so, and the therapist and family laughed. The therapist said to the boy, "What I want to see you do is—you know that he is afraid, right?"

"Right," said the boy.

"Now, how are you going to do something about that?"

"You want me to do something? But how am I gonna do it?"

"You know that you have to get this little puppy over his fears, right?

"Right,"

"I want to see some action."

"What?"

"I don't know, you've got a problem."

"Pick the dog up," said the father.

"I can't pick him up."

"You held him."

"There are a lot of people here helping you," said the therapist. "You can ask your parents, you can ask your sister, Sharon."

"I held him," said the boy, and he added as his sister went to pick up the puppy, "No, Sharon, no, no."

The mother mentioned the boy had come a long way, "but he just won't pick up the puppy and carry him."

"I've seen him hold him," said the father.

When mother said she didn't remember that, the boy pointed out that he had held him at his aunt's house. The mother recalled it then.

The therapist asked the father what he thought of the boy's progress, and the father said, "I think he's doing all right. Maybe it may not seem like that, but I think he's doing a whole lot better."

"I feel as though he's doing good too," said the mother and she mentioned how he used to scream if *she* touched a puppy. The therapist, who did not want to review the past fears, said quickly, "So you agree with your husband."

"Yes," said the mother.

At this point the boy has improved sufficiently so the therapist can begin to shift to the next stage of therapy. There seemed to be a marital issue, and to deal with that before there is a change in the boy would be a mistake. There must be a step-by-step process. If there are marital issues, which is not always so, the therapist needs to shift to them. The way the therapist began the shift was by giving credit to the parents for improvement in the child. They deserved the credit for their cooperation, and giving it prepared for the ultimate disengagement of the therapist when he would have to leave the family system. It is easier to leave if the responsibility for the change has been placed within the family.

The therapist said, "What I want to say is whatever progress Stu has made has been basically because of you. I think it is not the time to be modest.

"I'm not trying to be modest," said the father.

"You see," said the therapist, "what I am trying to point out to you both, but especially to you," he added to the father, "[is] that there are lots of things that you have done about Stuart's fears."

"Well," said the father, "answer this, why couldn't I or my wife do it by ourselves?"

"Well, first of all, you didn't think about the business of your being an expert on dogs. Which you are. I mean, let's face it, whether you admit it or not, it seems very easy for you nowadays, and as a matter of fact it was such a part of everyday life that you never knew about it."

"Uh-huh," said the father.

"But your being a letter carrier has helped Stuart."

The mother said, "I agree, I agree. But you put it in words, that mailmen are experts on dogs."

"What I'm trying to say is that you have done a lot in here to produce whatever change has happened."

"That makes you feel good, anyway," said the father.

The therapist moved the family to the next stage by asking the parents, as a reward for having done so well with their child, to go away for the weekend. This forced a focus on the marriage. The task also shifted the mother from engaging with the child to engaging with the father. This shift often takes the form of complaints about his neglect of her and requests for more from him, and at that point the child is left out of their struggle.

"I don't know how you feel about it," said the therapist, "but I think what is important is that you get a reward for what you have done. I can think of several. For instance, how about a weekend away by yourselves?"

"Yes, that would be really nice," said the mother. "I don't know if Stuart heard that."

It is typical in this type of situation for the mother to bring the child into an issue between the parents. The therapist quickly moved him out, and father noticed that.

"Never mind Stuart," said the therapist. "This is a trip for you two." He then added, "It will be good for Stuart, anyway."

Talking of a weekend together, the father said, "Can you remember that far back?"

"That would be ideal in terms of his realizing that you are not so concerned about him. Which is what I am trying to do," said the therapist.

In the sixth interview, the parents had not gone out alone together and were not talking about any marital issue. The boy was still somewhat afraid of dogs. Because of a danger of a relapse at this point, the therapist avoided having the family shift back to the boy's fears by doing so himself. He encouraged the boy to have a relapse and asked the parents to cooperate. Such a move stabilizes the improvement and prevents the family from going back to old patterns. In a playful way, the therapist asked the boy to help the puppy by pretending to be afraid of him. The boy's response was a classical one to a paradoxical therapeutic maneuver.

"Stuart," said the therapist, "do you think that we can play a trick on that dog so that he will be all right?"

"Like what?"

"But you have to be pretty smart. And I'll show you the way in which you can measure how smart you are being. All right?"

"How are you gonna do it?" asked the boy.

"I will ask you to do something, and I'll ask your parents to participate in that. All right?"

"Like what?"

"See, actually we have to trick this little puppy into thinking that *you* are afraid of *him*. Like, you know, you have to kind of—"

When the therapist hesitated, the boy said, "Run from him? I think that would be mean to him."

"Show him that you are afraid of him."

"Like doing what? Chasing him away and everything?"

"You don't have to chase him away. You know, do you think that if you are afraid of me you are going to chase me away? No, you're just going to run from me. Right?" He added to the parents, "Do you think that you can help Stuart to get afraid of the puppy?"

"I'll try," said the mother.

"No, no, no, that's not very enthusiastic."

"Help him to be afraid of the puppy?" The mother and father looked at each other, puzzled. They were responding to the paradoxical idea that the therapist who was attempting to get their child over a fear of dogs was now asking them to encourage the boy to be afraid of dogs.

"I'm very serious about this," said the therapist, "and I'm sure you get the idea. The idea is to get the puppy to think that Stuart is afraid of him. So that the little puppy will understand that it is his job to convince Stuart not to be afraid of him. Now we all know that he is not afraid of the puppy, but it is just tricking the puppy for the puppy's benefit."

"Well," said the boy, "I think he knows that I'm not afraid of him."

"I know that, that's why it is a trick. And you only have to do it for a couple of days. I'll tell you what. I want you to ask your parents what they think about it, how they think you can do it." As the boy looks solemn, he added, "Look, you don't seem too happy about the idea."

"No," said the boy.

"Why not? Look, you are an expert on that. Weren't you afraid of dogs for a long time?"

"Yeah."

"Well?"

"I think I acted crazy," said the boy.

"You think you acted crazy, when you were afraid of dogs?"

"Uh-huh."

"All you have to do is the same things that you were doing before."

"It's gonna be hard."

"Oh, I know it's gonna be hard."

"After all this time, seven or eight years, almost eight years, I've been afraid of them, but now it's slipping off of me."

The paradoxical intervention was successful, and the boy began to touch the dog. The parents had not succeeded in getting away for a weekend, but they had a pleasant evening at home, which was unusual for them. The therapist continued to insist that they get away together without the children. A marital difficulty appeared. After congratulating them on their parenting, the therapist said, "But you haven't taken care of each other."

"We don't see much of each other," said the mother.

"You don't like that, do you?"

"No."

"When was the last time you even talked about it?"

"We don't."

"You mean you don't talk about things that you dislike?"

"No we don't."

"How come?" asked the therapist.

"Because, well, I guess that we can't talk about those kind of things really."

At this point the therapist could continue to focus on the child problem or he could explicitly make a contract to deal with the marriage, which was decided as the next step.

The mother continued, "That would lead to arguments, and rather than argue, we don't talk about some things. Right?" she said to her husband.

He replied, "I guess. I don't see why."

When the therapist saw that the father was reluctant to talk about this issue, the therapist said, "This is not my business, right?"

"Evidently it is part of the therapy," the father said.

"Let me speak very frankly with you. I feel very optimistic about Stuart's fear of dogs. That will be gone." He continued, "If you want to stop at the level of Stuart getting rid of the fear of dogs, we can do it, but what I really had intentions of asking you today is—do you want the whole thing? Or just to get rid of this?"

After a long pause, the father said, "Do the whole thing."

"Do I have your permission?" asked the therapist.

"Yes," said the father.

The therapist had them talk about their life together. The mother said, "I do need to get out of the house, but you just get tired of saying it. I know that in order to make a happy home, it's not just the children, it's time together, going places together so that when you come back you can appreciate being with them. If I went away myself, the whole weekend, I'd be happy."

When the therapist asked the father what he thought about his wife's sadness, he said that he had seen the "tiredness, the look on her face, the droop, I know."

"I am tired, and it's against my nature to prolong things."

"I think you're lonely," said the therapist.

"I know that, I admit that." She turned to her husband. "I've admitted that to you haven't I?"

"Yes," said the husband.

The mother talked about her situation and said, "After awhile you get the craving for the conversation of grown-ups, and being a woman, not only just grown-ups but the male."

The therapist decided to deal with this impasse between the spouses by paradoxically encouraging a relapse. He said, "There is a very good way to settle this situation."

"What's that?" asked the mother.

"Why don't you both try—and I'll ask Stuart to help you—try making him afraid of dogs."

"Make Stuart afraid of dogs?"

"Yes, just as afraid as he was when he walked in here, and then we can get busy working on that and we won't have to talk about this anymore."

"That's a nice waste of time," said the father. "Is that what you're saying?"

The mother replied, "He's saying that maybe that will be a mutual meeting ground. . . . "

The father said, " We don't need to talk about the dog. Stuart doesn't need the fear of the dog. And we don't need to keep on talking about it. I mean, the way you say it, that's the only time that my wife and I get to talk is about Stu, and if we don't talk about the dog, we won't have anything to talk about?"

The therapist agreed, saying, "You know, you are making me feel like a villain. I come into the picture and make you work on the problem and you get the problem solved, and all of a sudden Stuart is not afraid of dogs. I get the feeling that you worked against yourselves because there you are left kind of empty." He added, " By being so worried about losing the love of these kids, you've lost sight of each other."

The therapist talked with them about taking each other for granted, and the wife agreed that she felt that way. She added that she did not take her husband for granted, and then she said, "I *have* taken him for granted, but I don't think I do now. I know I don't."

What made you change?"

"That's a different story," she said, and she hesitated. "Just something that happened between us, which made me not take him for granted, but then I think that now he takes *me* for granted."

"Something that happened between both of you?"

"Right."

The therapist asked whether they wanted to talk about it, and they were unresponsive. In this situation there was obviously a problem in the past between these spouses. Exploring painful aspects of the past is not essential in this therapy. The problem is how to get past them and move on. The therapist handled this one in an unusual way. He said to them, "Why don't you *pretend* that you told me, and then go on."

Pretend what?" asked the mother.

"That you told me about it."

"All right," said the mother. "I'll say that we had Stuart and I was on cloud nine because this was what I really wanted. Then something happened, and I think that I started realizing that I was too wrapped up in Stuart. I wasn't giving enough attention to Tom. Which caused what happened to happen. And I wanted to, you know, maybe give him more attention, but I don't know if he wanted it. So that's the way it happened."

"All right," said the therapist. "Well, you said it."

"I think we changed, Tom changed."

"How much resentment was left?"

"A lot."

"Is it still there? Is that 95 percent of this situation?"

In this excerpt the therapist works toward change in a family that seemingly does not want to get personal. They see themselves as having a particular problem that they want solved. Their efforts to help their son before therapy was initiated consisted of being extremely concerned (a tactic that could be thought of as extractive introjection, which extracts the boy's competence and gives it to the mother instead), and the therapist recognizes that this effort is itself the problem. The reader is left in the dark about how the therapist knows that bringing father in to help the son will improve matters, except that the therapist can see that mother is overly involved. Minuchin (1974) would suggest that a diffuse boundary between mother and son, and a rigid boundary between husband and wife, violates the healthy generational hierarchy. The parental and the marital subsystem are not functioning properly, and the father is in a distant position within the family system. The first intervention skillfully addresses this problem by bringing the father closer to the son and thus putting the system in better balance. The intervention requires a prereflective use of countertransference in detecting the mother's overinvolvement and some ingenuity in formulating a plan to get father more involved.

All of the interventions after this point also involve prereflective countertransference in detecting what can be identified as resistance. Strategic therapists recognize when familial power maintains the problem focus. But the strategic model also informs interventions through a sophisticated psychological paradigm. This family provides a good example of this paradigm. When the family refuses to focus on marital issues, which in this family are considered to be the likely cause of the problem, the strategic model postulates that relapse is likely since homeostatic patterns will activate problems with the son for the parents to concentrate on. That is, the boy has fears so that the parents can focus on the boy instead of themselves. The strategic model also postulates that family problems are actually caused by the family's attempt to solve the problem in a way that maintains the status quo. In this instance, for example, the parents' concentration on their son is reinforcing because family tension is reduced. Because families want to maintain the status quo, and when faced with problems react with problem-maintaining solutions, strategic therapists often circumvent the family system's standard operating procedures by tasking families with behaviors that are likely to make those old procedures impossible.

Instead of fighting this family by drawing attention to their refusal to concentrate on the problem, which appears already solved, the therapist refocuses on the problem but in a way that redirects family energy. For example, this family always focused on helping Stuart get over his problems, but the strategic therapist focuses the family on creating the problem, a tactic which changes the basic dynamic of the family and sabotages the homeostatic pattern. The therapist prefers that the family fail, but if the family were to succeed in creating the problem the therapist would still not have failed with the family because they will have proved that they in fact do have control over the problem and can create or eradicate the problem whenever they want.

Although the strategic intervention here is quite ingenious, it is unnecessarily cryptic from the relational systems perspective. Even within this excerpt Haley (1976) comments that the therapist must ask the parents to take credit for improvement or they might have trouble disengaging from the therapist who helped them change and who might be perceived as needed for maintenance of the change. Such a comment is indicative of a problem that arises when the therapist is working so indirectly: the family may not feel responsible for the change. They do not know how or why it occurred, only that it did occur in a context of dependence upon the therapist's seemingly magical knowledge. The relational systems model can work more directly with family difficulties and does not contribute to dependence upon the therapist, although it does count on the therapist's ability to understand the family in ways it has not previously been understood. The family is informed about why their problems are occurring, and the therapist allows herself to be seen as vulnerable to the same kinds of problems when, while using countertransference, she reveals uncomfortable feelings. Rather than foster dependence, the therapist models healthy behavior in showing that vulnerability does not necessarily result in pain, and gives her knowledge to the family so they can own it for themselves.

Analyzing this family from a relational systems perspective requires a great deal of speculation owing to the lack of emotional information given in the vignette. From a relational systems perspective, this family can be seen as avoiding the emptiness, loneliness, and pain of rejection within the marital relationship by extracting the son's chance at growing maturity and confidence. Rather than accepting her own fear (exactly what she is fearful of it is impossible to know from the vignette, but is likely to be related to rejection and/or sexual intimacy), the mother soothes that fear by usurping her son's developmental growth or natural boyhood invulnerability and treating him in such a way that he feels fearful. The father's peripheral position affords him relief and complements the mother–son overinvolvement. His wife feels better and he does not need to feel guilty about the lack of appreciation he gives her nor must he think about his own emptiness. The boy, because he has the least amount of power in the system, and because he has a valency for anything that might please his mother or activate his mother out of depressed feelings, becomes the bearer of family problems. He feels fearful but desires a more complete relationship with his father, and, although he wants his mother to maintain a euthymic mood, he also desires more distance from her emotional state, and less responsibility for her emotional stability.

An intervention informed by the relational systems perspective could work in a strategic manner. A closer look at the interventions used within the vignette reveals an avenue to parallel but more direct interventions. The first intervention used by the therapist in this vignette involves activating the father as an expert. From the relational systems view, a countertransference intervention might involve a similar tactic. The therapist might experience the father's distance and need for answers as a projection of competence. In an alternative intervention, the therapist might say,

"I notice myself feeling very confident when I'm with your family and I think it has something to do with you acting like I have all the answers. But I was thinking that, in fact, you have all the ability you need to help your son, you just don't feel comfortable doing what you need to do. I think you might do this with your wife, too. You sort of let her make the rules for the boy, and you let her have so much concern, but really you are the one who is most likely to be of help. For example, you are an expert with dogs because you're a mailman. Couldn't you teach your son some of what you know about dogs?"

Such an intervention (with, of course, a bit more explanation), speaks to the boundaries between the father and mother and the father and therapist, activating the father in a helping role, without anything being hidden.

With respect to the paradoxical interventions, the connection of these to double binds and projective identification is clear. Paradox creates a kind of double bind by giving two incompatible messages at two different logical levels with only one likely behavior (of course the true double bind makes escape from the situation impossible). The parents are told that if they want to avoid their own relationship they must create problems in their child. On the surface the message is "create a problem in your child and work together to do it or you are failures." And success would mean they have the power to manipulate something that they would rather not realize they have control over. It would also indicate they had worked together. Underneath the surface is the reality that if they succeed in creating the problem in their child then they are failures at having a happy child. The parents are put in an impossible situation in which doing nothing is the only possible solution. The preferable alternative is to fail at creating the problem and be better parents.

In a relational systems model, an explanation of the family dynamics can have the same effect without the strategic manipulation. A typical intervention might occur at the point that the parents are making the therapist feel like a "villain." Here another therapist might say,

"I find I'm struggling to get you two to work on difficulties you have with each other, and I've noticed myself feeling like a villain because of it. You came to therapy wanting help with your son, which I've been giving you, but you two didn't realize how much you needed him to have those problems. Now you're looking at each other realizing that you're going to have to talk or your son will develop either the same problem or some other problem so you guys won't have to deal with each other. Stuart doesn't want to see his mother depressed, and if helping him makes her feel better, you better believe he's going to make himself be someone who needs help. He might also feel that getting into some kind of difficulty is the only way to get his dad interested at all. So, he's going to have problems. But I'm thinking, in a way, it's a good thing for you two that he does have these problems, because there's a very real possibility that your problems can't be worked out and so you need him to have these problems so that you guys can feel okay. In fact, I think we should have him continue to be afraid of dogs for your sake—so, Mom, you won't have to be afraid of discussing problems in your marriage, and you, Dad, won't have to feel guilty about hurting your wife with neglect."

This intervention does not rely on manipulation. Even the last part, although it sounds like encouraging the problem in a disingenuous way, is merely a statement of fact based on the information so far given. The relational systems model counts on the therapist to report how he feels about or perceives the system. Interventions that have a strategic effect are not uncommon. Parents are not likely to be comfortable with the idea that they are creating problems in their children. But, if presented in an empathic way that makes sense to family members, a strategic effect will occur simply because family members will want the therapist to be wrong and may try to prove the therapist wrong by solving their problems differently.

The Narrative Approach: Victoria C. Dickerson and Jeffrey L. Zimmerman

Narrative and solution-oriented therapies are similar in that they focus on solutions as opposed to problems. The approaches are different theoretically, however, so that they cannot be compared directly. Most solution-oriented therapists work within a systems paradigm. Narrative therapists, on the other hand, do not see problems as necessitated by the systems' functioning, but instead, posit that problems occur because family members or individuals perceive problems and talk about problems while ignoring the times that problems have not occurred. The basic philosophy is that calling something a problem makes it a problem. When persons see themselves as the problem, they continue to emphasize their own problematic nature. They are a problem by their own definition. However, when a person and family see a problem as something that occurs only sometimes within a wider context of problem-free functioning, the person and family do not look at themselves as people who are problems. Rather, the person and family look for ways to emphasize how the problem has been avoided and they look at problems that do occur as anomalies to otherwise healthy functioning.

In this next excerpt, the therapists talk with the family about ways that a problem, stealing and argumentativeness by a 12-year-old boy named David, has been avoided. In previous sessions, therapy had focused on the family defining the problem without making the boy himself the problem. Things that others like about the boy had been included in those discussions. In this excerpt the therapists focus on "landscape-of-consciousness" questions and "landscape-of action" questions (asking the family members to focus on times when they were aware of things not fitting the viewpoint of the child being argumentative and a thief). Awareness of a different story one or one's family could tell is the central point. If the story is positive, so too will be the future.

The family consists of David and his two families. He lives with his father, stepmother, and stepbrother, and spends weekends with his mother, Patty, and his stepfather, Larry. The first session included all involved, the second session was with his father, stepmother and stepbrother, and this session occurs with his mother and stepfather. The excerpt is from Dickerson and Zimmerman (1993, pp. 231–235).

Session III
The third session, which was 2 weeks after the initial session and was videotaped, was with David, his mom, and stepdad. David's time spent with them was mostly limited to every other weekend and some holidays. A similar direction was taken in this session in that unique outcomes were searched for and some time was spent with David in helping him identify that he might have ideas and plans for himself. This seems important in families of adolescents, although with younger (12- and 13-year-old) teenagers, the work is slower. The session followed a back-and-forth process between complaints by parents (mostly stepdad), attempts by the therapist to bring forth unique outcomes, and a beginning process of restorying. A transcript of portions of the session follows.

The session began with a review of the last session with David's other family. After checking with David that it was okay to review the last session, the therapist began:

T: We talked some about the *stealing habits*, but that those habits hadn't occurred since the time before. And it hasn't occurred since then either?

D: Yeah.

T: Well, you must be pretty pleased about that.

D: Yeah, well another week.

T: Well, another week, another day, even—it's good. And then we talked a bit about the *argumentativeness* as a problem. But what Mark pointed out, which I thought was really interesting, is that he saw some changes in David over the last couple of years ago, in ways that he was sensitive, he seems to be able to make friends and keep them, and he knows how to be in the world. You remember your dad saying that? *(David nods.)* He's sharing things. So what he said about that is that gave him confidence that he could beat these habits, too.

You talked, David, about how *not thinking* got you to do compulsive things *(nods)*, and about how you were going to try to think about that, to catch it, to think more about what was lying ahead, to think about consequences. So, did I summarize it okay? *(David nods again.)*

T: So . . . since David spends his time between two families, why don't one of you catch me up on how things are in this family?

[Larry began by spending some time talking about his relationship with David, some of his worries, and his attempts over the years to share things with him and learn about him. He also discussed how he and David clashed around chores and how he was tenacious in requesting that David do things.]

L: But a situation where all of a sudden chores need to be done, it can start; he can go from the wonderful kid that everybody sees, that everybody in my office sees, when he's helping us, to the Mr. Hyde, just like that.

T: And it tends to come up around your requesting something from him?

L: Yes, but since a lot of life is requesting things of people, you can see how often that can happen, you know.

D: I've gotten better about that, though.

T: You think you're getting better about that, huh?

L: He is; he's getting better about that.

T: Oh, all right! Do you have some examples of that, recent ones?

D: Yeah.

P: Yeah, now when we ask him to do his regular chores around the house—can't ask him anything extra, but the regular stuff—making sure his bed is made, doing the vacuuming, the yard work he is supposed to do, he will do that without a fuss because he knows he has to do it. I mean, there's no question.

T: So, it's just sort of an expectation that he does.

P: Right.

D: *(to Mom)* You hardly have any expectations. Everything's just "go."

T: So, David, when your mom says regular things like making the bed, doing the vacuuming, mowing the lawn—those aren't expectations?

D: Those are.

T: So you do them.

D: Yeah, it also goes along with cleaning the bathrooms.

P: Yes, that's right, you have to keep your bathroom clean.

D: There's nothing else, I don't think.

L: Whatever else we may ask you to do.

T: So, David, I have a question for you. How did it happen that you got so that you just did those things without having to be bugged to do them?

D: Because they started getting more regular.

T: Oh . . . so what do you like about that?

D: They're regular.

T: So regular things just become a part of your plan of life? Tell me how old you are again?

D: *(puzzled look on face)* Twelve.

T: Because I keep thinking you're older.

L: Coming up rapidly on thirteen.

T: Okay, maybe that's what it is. Because you know the reason I asked you that, the reason I got confused there for a minute is, I don't know very many regular twelve- . . . even almost-thirteen-year-old boys who do their regular stuff sort of as a part of their plan. They always see it, not as their plan, but as their parents' plan for them.

D: More of it is their plan for me.

T: Well, you just told me, yeah, maybe so, but you've incorporated it into your life.

D: Yeah, I've done it—it's part of my life—but it's their plan for me. It's not my plan. If it was my plan for myself, I would be doing something different.

T: I understand that, but let me ask you this. No, that's probably too hard a question to ask.

D: Ask it.

T: Well . . . Well, okay, I'll ask it. If you were living on your own . . . the reason I don't think I should ask this is that living on your own is a long way away.

D: Well, they've asked me this question before. *(Mom laughs: so does David.) (to Mom)* Haven't you?

T: What am I going to ask? Tell me what I'm going to ask.

D: You're going to ask me, if I were living on my own, what would I do with myself?

T: No, that's not what I'm going to ask. What I was going to ask is "If you were living on your own, would part of your plan for yourself include doing some chores?"

D: A little bit.

T: A little bit.

D: Not much.

T: Well, why would it?

D: Not as much as them.

T: Probably not. But why would it include doing some chores?

D: To keep my house clean if I was living on my own.

T: So that is somewhat important to you?

D: Yeah, I mean, I would keep it not like their kind of clean.

T: You might have somewhat different standards for yourself, but you'd have standards.

D: Yeah, I'd keep my house clean, I'd vacuum it, but I wouldn't do everything as much as they do.

T: All right. That's what I mean. That's why I said to you that I could see you've incorporated these plans into your life. Even though you might not have the same ones, you would see they were important to you in terms of living in this family.

[The therapist's intent, in this example was to work with David in an attempt to develop an outline of a story he might like to have for himself, separate from his parents' story for him. The therapist's questions can be seen as a landscape-of-consciousness questions, since they attempt to bring forth preferences, goals, intentions, and values. White (1991) points out that these questions help develop commitments in life and, with adolescents, the beginning of their own story. From a narrative perspective, David's noticing his own intentions will affect his interpretation of his parents' demands and lead to different actions.

What followed was a discussion initiated by Larry about how both he and Patty became independent early in their lives and how they expected something similar from David. These personal experiences were accounted for in the stories that influenced their response to David and led to the kinds of demands they were making. The therapist then returned to some questions around the problem.]

T: What are you thinking about? When you folks first came in here you were concerned about the *stealing habits*, and now we've had a period of time that they haven't occurred. Are you encouraged, are you a bit wary? What's your state of mind here?

P: I'm very encouraged. I felt that there was a lot of hope that came out of our first session together, just laying everything on the table. It was almost as if no one had anything to be afraid of anymore because it was all there; we all knew about it. Everyone had told David the way they felt about it. So, the worst had happened. So when David went back to school, it was like a sense of relief, like I lived through that one, it couldn't be any worse than that.

[The therapist commented on the hope and caring they showed and on the fact that they were "all on the same side, trying to fight the problem."]

T: What have you seen David do to get some charge of his life and keep that problem at bay? What have you seen him do in this period of time?

P: We've been together but in different ways than we're normally together. We went skiing and we had a lovely day. We just had a very nice day. We skied together the whole day, and David . . . it was a different David. It was not the David that was so frustrated and then would frustrate me because he'd get so angry and just not want to try anymore. He fell down a lot, but he got up every single time and never said a word about it. And, in fact, it was just the opposite . . . as I came by and said, "Are you okay?" he said, "I'm fine, go ahead."

T: What did you see . . . what do you think it was, Patty, that maybe David doesn't even see? What was it about him that he didn't even let the frustration get in there?

P: He was feeling good about himself; he was happy and confident and feeling good about himself.

T: And how did that happen? What did he do, or what happened in his family, that he was so confident?

P: I don't know specifically, but he was. It was a different attitude. [This example shows work in which the therapist is prompting the parents (mostly mom) to notice those times when David conquered the problems and to begin to pay attention to how the victories may have occurred. In addition to these landscape-of-action questions, landscape-of-consciousness questions brought forth a new description of David, with "new" characteristics to fit into the emerging new story.

The remainder of the session was spent continuing to help the parents and David notice more of how David does for himself and thinks for himself and takes charge of his own life. No subsequent appointment was made at that time. The next appointment was scheduled with David, his dad, and stepmom.]

In essence, the narrative approach is about transference and the power of projection. Family members perceive each other according to past experiences that have developed into stories about each other. Family members have a very difficult time undoing the perceptions or stories of others. No matter what they do, they continue to be perceived in old storied ways. The relational systems model allows for new stories to be told but does not focus exclusively on the positive. The therapist who does focus exclusively on how problems have been avoided runs the risk of ignoring the family's way of viewing things; family members are likely to feel that avoiding conflict and difficult feelings is the best way to interact. Despite the therapist's statement at the beginning of the above vignette that there was a back-and-forth process between the parents' complaints and the therapist's interventions, the parents' complaints did not make it into their excerpt. In such a paradigm emotions have little importance (notice that no emotional content is involved in the above vignette) and yet emotions are central to human existence. In the relational systems model the therapist could evoke a new story by using a countertransference intervention, which would doubly serve as a landscape-of-consciousness and landscape-of-action intervention.

The following is an example of a relational systems intervention as it might occur with a family like the one above. Total speculation about the feelings a therapist might experience with such a family is necessary due to the lack of emotion in the vignette, but the authors did state earlier in the paper that in the first session family members reported feeling suspiciousness and a lack of trust because of David's stealing, and his stepmother had experienced a "dungeoning" feeling from having to lock things up. The basis for this intervention is the author's imagining that the parent's complaints in this session might evoke a similar feeling in him.

 I've noticed as we've been speaking that I'm feeling sort of shut out of the family. It's almost like you're all locked up tight, and I can't seem to tell how anyone is feeling about things. You know this family has had a few difficulties in the past that maybe you don't want to share your feelings about. But we must all be aware of the amazing way you've all come through it. I wonder if this same locked-out feeling I'm getting is experienced sometimes by David, too. I know that there's a lack of trust, some suspiciousness, and stepmom even said that it feels like she's imprisoning herself in a dungeon. I wonder if when David feels that way he starts to want to steal so he can get back something that somehow he feels like he's lost. I know the more you all try to lock me out, the more I feel like I have to steal some real information from you. I also know that when David has managed to avoid the stealing and the argumentativeness, other people in the family were being less suspicious and not so locked up. I feel that too—the more you tell me freely, the more I feel like I can just relax and not try so hard to get from you what you don't want to give. So, it's obvious that everyone here is capable of not locking up, and not stealing or even arguing excessively—but we still need to look at what it is about those times that makes you able to do that.

This intervention could lead to landscape-of-action questions aiming at an understanding of how different actions lead to unique outcomes. It can also lead to landscape-of-consciousness questions about how one's intentions and preferences might lead to different unique outcomes. Focusing on David as someone who makes sense because of the feelings he has serves to take away the problem focus. His strength in avoiding the target behaviors can also help him untie himself from that focus. Where the primary focus is news of a difference, the relational systems model focuses on the news of a difference in the strength of family members to manage emotions interpersonally, even with conflict, without avoidance. Without that balance, narrative and solution-oriented models are likely to contribute to the avoidance of conflict as well as to the idea that problems should not be discussed in the future.

THE EXPERIENTIAL VIEW

Experiential therapists work in the most genuine and authentic way they can. They attempt to be themselves, and to use the fact of who they are to therapeutic effect. Two superb examples of this approach can be found in the work of Satir and Whitaker. In these examples of their work, the prereflective use of countertransference is prominent, but the self-reflective, intentional use of countertransference could be enhanced with the integration of intrapsychic and interpersonal theory.

Virginia Satir

A comprehensive application of Satir's work can be found in the book Satir co-authored with Michelle Baldwin (Satir and Baldwin 1983), where an entire session is printed for the purpose of examining the Satir method. The vignette below is found at pages 84–93 of that book. The authors' comments (found in the right column and numbered to correspond to interventions in the left column) help to distinguish those aspects of the method they consider to be most curative. Empathy and the natural use of self are the most obviously effective characteristics of Satir's work. But a subtle intentional use of countertransference is also present. This particular segment of the Satir interview was chosen to highlight that use of countertransference.

63. Virginia (*coming down to Lisa's level*)**:** OK. I noticed that you came over here when mother was crying, and I wonder what you thought was happening when your mother was crying.

63. Virginia makes it a point to move down to eye level with a child when engaged in meaningful interaction.

Lisa: Everything was so sad and everything.

Virginia: Everything was sad. Is that what you felt? (*She puts her hand on Lisa's cheek.*) Have you ever felt that before, in this family, that sometimes people were feeling sad? (*Lisa nods.*) OK.

Lisa: And unwanted.

Virginia: And you didn't want it?

Lisa: And unwanted.

64. Virginia: And unwanted? Could you tell me about what the unwanted feeling is?

Lisa: It's really when nobody cares for them, or anything.

Virginia: Is that talking 'bout Daddy?

65. Lisa: Talking 'bout everybody.

Virginia: Everybody. Sometimes you can feel that there's a feeling that people feel unwanted. Is that it? (*She holds Lisa's forearm.*) That Daddy might sometimes feel that "nobody cares about me," and Mama might feel that way, and Susie and Betty and Lisa and Lucy and Coby, too?

Lisa: Uh huh.

Virginia: When you feel that's going on, what happens with you, honey?

Lisa: I just go up in my room and lay down and sometimes I take a nap—a long nap. Or sometimes I just run out the door.

Virginia: I'd like to make a suggestion to you, because maybe this could be

64. *Virginia:* What is happening here, when Lisa states that she feels sad and unwanted, is that she is pointing to the present but unmanifested pains between the parents. In this family, as in many others, there are rules against speaking about one's pain.

65. *Virginia:* I regard this part as a microcosm of the whole family relationship. People in this family are trying to hide their feelings of being unwanted and what they do as a result of feeling those. Casey has already made hints about his wish to be wanted in the family by his earlier statement, "I don't want to be the bad guy in the family."

Comment: Virginia, when confronted by the feeling(s) of one individual, will often check with other family members to see if they know something about this feeling. By becoming aware that they share similar feelings, family members who often keep their feeling of hurt and vulnerability from one another can begin to develop a bond leading to intimacy.

helpful. I am going to find out if everybody in the family does know what it feels like to feel unwanted, but I wonder what would happen if you felt that way and you said, "You know, right now I'm feeling nobody loves me." What do you think would happen if you put words to that?

Lisa: Then my mom would probably say to me that she does love me.

Virginia: Then maybe your mother would come to you and say she does love you? Would that help some things?

66. Lisa (*nodding*)**:** It would just make me happy again.

66. There is an implicit message for the whole family that verbalizing bad feelings may help to cope with them. Note that Lisa has the answer inside her and that Virginia is only helping to bring it out.

Virginia: It would make you happy again. OK. You're sitting down here, but I wonder if you could [say], just for practice, just so everybody could hear and you could hear: "Right now I am feeling nobody loves me." Would you say those words?

67. Lisa: Right now I feel like nobody loves me.

67. Having Lisa state "Right now I feel like nobody loves me" reinforces the learning and also enables Lisa to rehearse a statement that she might feel awkward in making without some prompting. There is value in reinforcing a newly acquired skill by practicing it during the sessions.

68. Virginia: OK. Now, I want to check out something. Since there's a . . . (*looking at Lucy and pointing at her missing*

68. Even in the middle of the most intensive interaction, Virginia will not hesitate to add a light touch. Nonver-

name tag). Does Lucy hear you, too? Do you sometimes feel that nobody loves you? Sometimes, in the family, you feel that?

Lucy: I don't know.

Virginia: Have you ever felt that? *(After a long silence, Lucy smiles self-consciously and nods affirmatively.)* I don't know, I just wonder. You do sometimes? What about you, Coby, do you know what that feeling is, have you felt that sometimes? That "nobody loves me?" Not all the time, but just sometimes?

Coby: Yes, ma'am, I have.

Virginia: Have you felt it, Betty? And have you felt it, Susie? And how about you, Casey?

Casey: Sure.

Virginia: And how about you, Margie? *(She nods. Virginia asks the family:)* What would happen if, when you were feeling it, you were to put words to it like Lisa just did? What do you suppose would happen with you, Casey, if you put words to that? "Right now I'm feeling nobody loves me."

Casey: I have. I've put words to it before.

Virginia: Those words?

Casey: Well, nobody gives a shit about me.

69. Virginia: Oh, that's a whole different thing. *(Getting up and pointing a finger at Casey:)* Because you know

bally, she is joking with Lucy for having removed her name tag.

69. This is a good example of the difference between an "I" statement, which lets the other person know about my what that means—"You should give a shit about me," and that doesn't say, "I'm feeling, at this point, unloved." *(Sitting down, she still maintains eye contact with Casey.)*

feelings and makes it very clear that "I own the feeling" and "I am responsible for it," and a blame statement where the responsibility for my feeling bad is left with the other person. At this point, therapy and teaching merge because it is evident that Casey is ignorant about the difference and that he genuinely believes that he is expressing a feeling when he says "Nobody gives a shit about me."

70. Virginia: I want to say something, and Coby, I especially want you to hear it *(looking down and then at Casey)* and I'm taking a big risk at this moment. *(She concentrates silently.)* I feel, and I've been feeling this for about the last ten minutes, that I want to take you in my arms. Not because you're a baby, but because I think in your insides you've had all this longing to have something. *(Looking at Margie:)* And I want you on the other side. And I think for me . . . [it] is my reaching out into your insides for how hard you struggled, and feel that you haven't gotten what you hoped for, and I feel this strongly here.

70. The nature of the risk to which Virginia is referring is two-fold. First, at a personal level she is referring to a feeling that is not grounded in adult reality and is often irrational but that activates in us those same feelings we had in early infancy when the [inability to retrieve] love was synonymous to death and when our extreme dependency on others for our survival meant that we were completely vulnerable. This feeling can emerge in even the most mature person. The mature person overcomes the feeling, however, knowing that it does not fit present reality, whereas the less mature person will be submerged by it. One of the tasks of the therapist in the stage of chaos is to help people to take those kinds of risks. Specifically, in this interaction with Casey, Virginia is making herself vulnerable by being open to the possibility of a rejection. Second, at a therapeutic level, Virginia might have overestimated the trust level that has been established. Casey may not be ready for such demonstration of feelings, and he may close off.

71. Virginia *(Looking at Casey)***:** How do you feel about my saying that to you, Casey?

71. After taking what she considers a risky step, Virginia is checking the impact of her declaration. This is an extremely important follow-up, because if

Casey: Makes me feel good to hear somebody say something like that.

she sensed any negativity it would be extremely important to deal with it right away to avoid sabotaging the trust previously established.

Virginia again is taking the risk of a possible rejection. Only a secure and congruent therapist will knowingly allow himself to be put in a vulnerable position. Virginia is also modeling for family members the importance of checking the impact of their statements, even if it puts them in a vulnerable situation. Taking the risk of being hurt and experiencing pain is one of the conditions of real intimacy.

72. Virginia (*Addressing the whole family*)**:** And in a funny way I have a hunch that when people don't know how to say what they want, and don't know what to do to get it, fighting is the easiest way. See, I think if we don't know how to do what we really want and we do know how to fight, that does help us a little, but the pains are great in it. (*Looking down at Lisa:*) I want to find out something from you, Lisa.

72. By making a general statement on the meaning of fighting for people in general, Virginia is removing the stigma and blame attached to fighting in this specific family.

73. Is it all right with you if your mother feels sad, and she cries, will that be OK? And if you can say what you feel when that happens? Would you do that? (*Lisa nods.*) OK. I wonder if you could kind of sit over a little bit so you wouldn't be between you mother and daddy, because we have some things that need to be checked here.

73. Virginia is reconnecting with Lisa. In working with a family, Virginia attempts to have as many family members as possible connecting to the theme under focus. Lisa initiated the theme, and Virginia is now aiming at a closure with her, thus acknowledging her importance in the preceding interactions. She is also teaching the family not to get upset by feelings and to allow them to happen while also taking the freedom to comment on them.

(*Looking at Margie:*) I wonder what you felt when I said to Casey, "I want to take you in my arms."

74. Margie: Very warm.

74. It was important that Virginia also check with Margie about how she felt about the intimate statement that Virginia had made to Casey. Margie might have felt that Virginia was taking sides with Casey against her. She could also have felt some jealousy at Virginia's ability to express tenderness to Casey in a way that she was no longer able to do. Again, if Virginia had sensed any negativity in Margie's answer, she would probably have dealt with it at this point.

Virginia: And how did you feel when I said it about you?

Margie: Warm, and soft, and gentle.

Virginia: You see, I think all these parts are here, if you all know how to use them with each other. You started to say that what you wanted from Casey was that you could communicate with him better, and what I heard him say he wanted from you was to get out of the "bad guy" seat.

Margie: Which he has been. I have been taking over the authority. He just sits back.

This segment demonstrates Satir's spontaneous use of empathy but also includes a sophisticated way of working with the projective system. According to the commentary provided, Satir realizes that the feeling of being unwanted, originally revealed by one of the youngest members of the family, is indicative of a similar feeling between and within the parents. She creates understanding with the family, first by checking if her hunch is correct by asking various members, and then by revealing her own related feelings. She suggests and demonstrates that the feelings she experiences can be accessed by family members only if they express their vulnerability openly. Her empathy in this regard occurs because, unlike family members, she is able to detect their pain without their directly revealing it, and because she has not become part of their system to the extent that their angry projections can be used on her to make her feel unwanted.

Although her interventions are beautiful, what seems to be missing here is an explanation of the way the feelings of being unwanted are passed around from family member to family member. An opportunity for such an intervention using countertransference does occur, however, in the vulnerability she experienced when starting to reveal her own desire to soothe family members. Such an intervention might only require a few more words than Satir already uses. The therapist in this situation might state that she is feeling vulnerable and that she knows the other family members are feeling vulnerable, too, because it is so difficult for a person to admit her feelings when she expects to be yelled at or not supported in that vulnerable moment. The therapist could say:

"I've noticed myself feeling afraid to say something. I have a sense that what I have to say is unwanted. It seems like I might be in danger if I say something. I realize that, in a way, this feeling is caused by the sense that if I do say something like 'I want you to appreciate what I say,' that people in the family might not respond by appreciating me—maybe because they don't feel appreciated themselves. But the thing is, like we've just seen, you all are willing to appreciate each other and you do want my input, just like you love and want each other. I think it's really important that we all realize what acting angry does—how it makes our own unwanted feelings come out in others, and how all the anger stops us from receiving what we really want—which is to have others be there for us and love us. I think it's the anger in this family that makes me feel like I might be shot down or I might not get the appreciation I need. Bust as long as we are all afraid to say how we feel, no one will get their needs met or their fears soothed."

The simple addition of this stated understanding allows family members to know exactly how they create this "unwanted" feeling in each other. The family not only learns new behavior that helps them get what they want, but they also get an understanding of exactly how to avoid the continuation of bad feelings. Although this alternative intervention does not include any psychological theory, it is clearly evident in the kind of thinking that such an intervention would require, and the relational systems model is always kept in mind as a backdrop to interpersonal relations.

Carl Whitaker

Whitaker is well known for spontaneous activity that he believes creates salutary enactments within therapy. In this excerpt taken from his book with Napier (Napier and Whitaker 1978, p. 186), a classic Whitaker enactment takes place with a family that has both progressed and regressed within treatment.

When the Brices returned to therapy after a two-month absence, they had largely resolved the original crisis with Claudia, but they were now in the process of reorganizing their triangular conflict around Don. He was becoming the second scapegoat. When Carl saw the familiar pattern, he moved fast, chastising the parents forcefully for what they were doing to Don. The toughness in Carl's voice signaled the end of diplomacy. In response to the Brices' raising the stakes by returning to therapy, this time with the implicit goal of reorganizing the family structure, Carl also raised the intensity of his response. "Cut out the games," he said. "Grow up!" He was indignant, therapeutically indignant. Surely Carolyn didn't need to meddle in David's struggle with Don the way she did. Surely David could have done something to prevent Carolyn from invalidating and ignoring him. Why hadn't the couple turned to each other and argued out their obvious disagreement instead of putting Don in a bind? A thorough parental scolding, well deserved.

Something changed. Perhaps David and Carolyn felt genuinely ashamed. Don appeared at the next interview feeling liberated from the parental triangle, ready to fight. When Carl came to his defense, it gave his anger new license. First he attacked his mother, and she registered her week-long amazement at his ready irritability. Then, seemingly out of nowhere, he turned toward Carl, lashing out. Something unexpected happened in Carl, too, and he fought back. Before the astounded group the two of them tumbled into a physical fight.

The moment did not come out of nowhere. Don and Carl had irritated each other for some time. Don didn't like Carl's "sarcasm," and Carl often had to bite his tongue to keep from confronting Don's arrogant attitude. "It's really not my business if his parents let him talk to them like that," Carl said to himself. Inwardly, Don and Carl had scheduled a confrontation. When it came, the fight was part of everyone's need to raise the stakes of the therapy.

The authors go on to explain what happens when the therapist becomes part of the family or more deeply involved in the therapist–family system: "The therapist's contribution comes primarily out of his own person, not out of his professional skill. If the therapist is fighting with the family, it is because what is happening in that family has become very important to him. He is pushing for change" (p. 186).

The authors then discuss how Whitaker's behavior demonstrated alternate behaviors to the family and demonstrated for the son that the father is bigger than he is and cannot be pushed around. Whitaker's spontaneous action, well beyond what most therapists would try, would indeed challenge any family. Nevertheless, its effectiveness, no matter what the reason, need not be so ambiguous. This enactment within the therapy affords an especially good opportunity for an empathic and genuine discussion of how emotions were transferred in an intense moment, and how alternate behaviors helped to return the family to a healthier course. Another therapist might say,

"In working with you I was noticing myself getting irritated with the whole family, but often a lot of my irritation was directed at Don. Somehow my own immaturity got the best of me when I fought with Don—I just wasn't able to put into words anything I thought might get through to him—that he just had to stop being such an irritant. For a long time my irritation showed in my sarcasm, which is also immature, but right then I had just *had* it. I think, now, that the whole family was putting that irritation into Don by not recognizing him for his age-appropriate maturity, which means expecting him to respect you. You, Dad, never tell Don that he's out of line, which allows you to see yourself as the poor victim, but it's your immaturity that won't let you stand up to your own son appropriately—your immaturity and your irritation. You seem to try to do something, Mom, but you are really just as ineffectual as Mr. Brice, and I think that says something about your immaturity. But really, we're all immature to some extent, and I think that sometimes we just have to let that kind of behavior go—to free ourselves up from the confinement of maturity. I think, Mr. Brice, that if you'd just let yourself express your irritation, you'll show Don who's in charge. He will feel more comfortable with you clearly taking a stand and you'll slowly find yourself feeling less irritable. I suggest the same thing to you, Mrs. Brice. Let your son feel your strength as parents even if it sometimes means just letting your feelings out without thinking—or by wrestling a little bit. I know it will feel good to you—it felt very good for me just now."

By clearly explaining how feelings get transferred in the family, which requires some use of theory, but from the heart, the family learns from genuine empathy and action. Although Whitaker is known for stating that theory has no place within the process of therapy, when theory is well-integrated into one's understanding of human relationships it helps to connect understanding to genuine enactments, thus allowing new enactments of healthier behavior.

THE INTEGRATIONIST VIEW

The integrationist view holds the most potential for an approach similar to the relational systems perspective. However, most attempts at integration have difficulty with balanced, comprehensive, and consistent use of the specific theories they aim to integrate. Several examples of approaches which attempt to integrate analytic and systems theory were presented in Chapter 2. Vignettes from two therapists who have made such attempts are presented here.

Michael Nichols

The following example is taken from Nichols's 1987 book (pp. 130–132), and demonstrates his point of view on the importance of empathy. Throughout Nichols's presentation, analytic theory is invoked in explaining how intrapsychic understanding is necessary in making complete interventions. And Nichols is also specific about how countertransference can be used. Despite the use of countless examples within his text, however, Nichols never seems to demonstrate a use of countertransference in formulating interventions. A demonstration of the necessity for empathy would seem to be an especially good opportunity for discussing the merits of the use of countertransference, but within the following example no such use occurs.

Mrs. Polanski called about her son, Maxwell. "The problem, doctor, is masturbation." The boy was 15 years old and, according to his mother, "addicted to masturbation." She grumbled when I asked to see the whole family for a consultation, but grudgingly she agreed. Not, however, before giving me an earful of her version. Among the things I learned while I tried unsuccessfully to get off the phone were: The boy had been nothing but trouble since they adopted him as an infant; her husband was a lousy businessman and a lousy father; and they had consulted a psychiatrist last year, but "that fool told me not to worry about the masturbation, ease up on the boy—can you imagine!" (Forewarned is forearmed.)

I began the session by asking Mrs. Polanski to describe the problems she was having with her son. Her criticisms were interesting. She described him as willful, stubborn, interested in girls from an early age—at 14 he wrote graphic love letters to a girl he met at summer camp—and inconsiderate. She alluded to the masturbation, but apparently felt it was too embarrassing to speak about openly in front of the whole family. Aside from the obvious fact that she worried too much about too little, what was interesting in her complaints was that she was describing a strong, precocious, and mature young man. He was doing well in private school, was on the wrestling and soccer teams, and was extremely bright. And even though she was complaining, there was a touch of pride in her voice. Then she turned on her husband.

In response to my asking him what he thought, Mr. Polanski said that he agreed with his wife but didn't think the problems were so serious. At which she launched into a scathing diatribe. He was never a father, couldn't run the family business without her doing his jobs, and so on and on. At that point, my plan to use the father as an ally to support his son and challenge his wife seemed futile. His wife's angry disavowal provoked his withdrawal into silence and self-pity.

There was plenty of self-pity in this family. Each of them manifested it differently. The presenting complaint, the boy's masturbating while reading "men's" magazines in his room, could be seen as an adolescent expression of growing sexuality. (Leaving them where they could be discovered might be a way of engaging his mother in conflict.) But it was also his way of soothing himself, sexualized to be sure, but primarily a way of making himself feel good. Mrs. Polanski soothed herself with Valium and Mr. Polanski retreated by staying out late, drinking beer, and watching television.

Each of them had complaints which, like a baby's cry, were intended to call forth a soothing response. But it didn't happen. The lack of a sympathetic response set a process in motion where they disengaged from each other and tried to set up a new form of empathy, that of taking the self as its own soothing partner. All three of them were mired in self-pity, with an element of self-righteousness that was a protest against the other's failure to understand. The self-pitying responses had become a chronic, distorted way of trying to achieve a connection with the needed source of emotional support.

I offered an interpretation, tried to explain this to them, but my remark only felt like another attack. It just hurt. So I switched gears and tried to empathize at length with each of them in turn. Even this wasn't easy, because my listening sympathetically to one aggravated the others. I started with Mrs. Polanski, who obviously had the most to get off her chest. Only then did I try to speak to her husband, deliberately avoiding subjects that might put him at odds with his wife, concentrating instead on his own problems and his past history. He spoke without sentiment as though he were merely giving evidence. They were all so used to being attacked that they had trouble opening up. Even Mrs. Polanski had trouble talking about the hurt behind her anger. But I offered a model of acceptance that they were gradually able to emulate. I gave each one of them a chance to talk without interruption, to express his point of view, *and* to be heard by the others.

Did empathy solve this family's problems? No, that only happens in grade B movies. Empathy does not extinguish conflict. Even after they had a chance to talk and be heard, Mrs. Polanski still insisted on more control over her son than he could tolerate, and Mr. Polanski was still unwilling to stand up to his wife, leaving a vacant role for his son to fill. But the fact that they began to feel understood, at least a little, made them cooperative partners in trying to find a solution for these problems. And, more important, when therapy was concluded, they retained the ability to discuss their disagreements a little longer before retreating into defeatist self-pity.

Nichols's efforts to soothe this family's pain with empathy are admirable. But full integration of systems and object relations theory offers a more deeply felt and comprehensive systems-level empathy that includes the therapist within the family dialogue. The level of difficulty in this case is obvious, and so is Nichols's frustration. He describes the mother's speech as officious, "scathing," and suggests that the family is filled with "self-pity." These are not flattering remarks. The feelings engendered within him are clearly powerful and yet he apparently does not consider an intervention that could harness his countertransference on the way to describing the therapist–family system dynamic in a way that would provide understanding as well as holding for the family. An imagined relational systems intervention would bring the family dynamic into the room while allowing the family members to feel deeply understood. An opportunity for such an intervention presents itself most clearly at the point where Nichols perceives family complaints to be like a "baby's cry" aiming at evoking a soothing response. Such an alternative intervention might proceed in the following way, with various parts dispersed throughout the session and discussed for clarity:

"As I've been sitting here with you all, I've noticed myself feeling like I need to soothe you all, like somehow none of you are getting your needs met in this family. In a way I feel like I should try to soothe everyone, but when I try to soothe any one of you I find that someone else gets aggravated. I'm finding myself trying so hard not to hurt anyone, like I'm walking on eggshells. I've noticed that Maxwell tries very hard to be the best at everything, and I wonder if maybe that's his way of walking on eggshells. But because no one else is happy, he doesn't get any recognition, and in fact, he's often criticized for those few things he does that are perceived as less than perfect. Mr. Polanski, I feel as if you've just given up trying to get any love, and in the process you're not able to be there for anyone else. And Mrs. Polanski, I'm getting two pictures—in the one, you're desperate for love, but in the other, you're just trying to shake up the family. But then the shaking, which you do because you so badly need someone to soothe you, has the opposite effect, and everyone else feels your need for soothing when you criticize. I was feeling it, too. It was getting so difficult to speak with you, or even to give you my own opinion, that I felt stuck and dulled. I think I could easily listen to you, and maybe that would help, but I think it's important for you all to know the effect you have on me and on each other or you won't be able to start to change."

Such an intervention might be jarring to the reader. But families have a way of appreciating heartfelt language, especially when it seems to ring true with how they, themselves, are feeling. It is also important to recognize that, although the therapist has more education and knowledge, within the relational systems approach, he does not have a monopoly on understanding. Interventions must always be left open to change as the family experiences the situation differently. But the relational systems process moves toward openness in a different way than Nichols's procedure suggests. Because the therapist is open about his experience, the family, too, begins to realize that openness is possible. Nichols's response was both patient and prudent. A family would be likely to improve given his approach. But a more comprehensively integrated view allows for an intervention that demonstrates understanding of family interaction as experienced through the therapist–family dynamics; such interventions will not be incorrectly perceived because they are genuine and respectful of family disagreement.

Robin Skynner

What follows is a collection of brief vignettes from one therapy by Skynner (1981, pp. 61–71) that includes snippets from sessions one, two, three, four, and five, and the entire sixth session, with Skynner's own brief summary of the last three sessions (the complete case study is presented in Skynner's 1981 paper). These excerpts provide an essential understanding of the therapeutic process, but for the sake of brevity some imagination about the process occurring between the cuts is required, and I have provided some information in square brackets; Skynner offers his own thoughts in parentheses. The content of the therapy and of his thoughts during these sessions is indicative of a relational systems perspective. However, Skynner's approach, according to him, is not applicable to other methods, such as the strategic, structural, or narrative approaches, because he feels those methods do not allow the therapist to work from within the family. My view is that the therapist's part in the system with the family must always be recognized, and that this can lead to interventions that sensitively reflect the intrapsychic as well as interpersonal dynamics of the family regardless of whether those interventions take a directive form. The therapist's part in that process need only be recognized as part of the intervention.

Skynner discloses his feelings to the family as a way of mirroring their conflicts. He does not, however, suggest to family members how the emotions he experiences are caused by their behaviors. Thus the family cannot consciously make a connection between their own emotions and the behaviors they use to create unconsciously desired behaviors and emotions in other family members. Nevertheless, Skynner's approach is the most similar to the relational systems perspective of any family therapy model yet developed.

The family was middle-class and consisted of the parents, [and the children] Alan, aged 12, and Sacha, aged 8 . . . The mother did most of the talking.

Session One: I suggested that [Alan] had, in fact, lost a special relationship with his mother when the marriage improved, but somehow hadn't yet found a new relationship with his father as a replacement. This seemed to make some sense to them all.

(All this was rather intellectual, and I can recall no particular feelings during this session, but I was taking things slowly and concentrating on forming good relationships with them all in view of the boy's hostility to the previous therapy.)

Session Two: On enquiry, father said he had lost his own interest in food in childhood, and "liked to avoid eating between meals." This provoked the mother and developed into an argument between the parents, where mother asked him, "Why can't you bear people enjoying themselves?"

(*About 25 minutes of the hour had elapsed and I wrote in my notes during this discussion about food: "No feeling in me except frustration. Not clear at all whether I will be able to do anything with this session." I realized that I might have to rewrite the chapter for the* Handbook of Family Therapy, *admit I am a fraud and emigrate to a third-world country where there is no psychotherapy. Shortly after this I became aware that I was having, or rather having a conflict about, enjoyable sexual responses to the mother's vibrant sexuality. I was preventing my thought from proceeding towards the idea of what she would be like in bed, felt embarrassed at myself, struggled to keep my attention on the whole family and at first treated this distraction of my attention as personal and unrelated to the family problem, so that I did not report it or use it.*)

. . . I now reported these feelings frankly, saying, "I often find my own feelings during an interview tell me something about the family problem, as if I am tuning into it. At first I was concerned at feeling nothing, but *(to the mother)* I have just realized how aware I have been of what an attractive woman you are sexually and *(to the father, balancing things up and passing her back to him)* what a lucky man you are to have chosen her." I added that I had no idea what all this meant and that I had also felt very embarrassed at my sexual response, but wondered whether the parents were letting the children jealously interrupt their sexuality as well as their argument? I suggested that the sex was not "earthed" between the parents but was floating about and getting into the children, and into me.

. . . *(As the session ended I felt that no one seemed to like the ideas I was putting forward much. I felt I had made a mess of the session, gone too quickly and made them reject me).*

Fourth Session: (The next session occurred after a two-week interval. Since the last session I had described this case to illustrate a point at a seminar, ending by saying that Sacha was still a mystery to me. At this, a female student had said, with a teasing twinkle in her eye, "well, you called her a little sweetie!," as if suggesting that I was not recognizing some sexual attraction. I usually feel quite comfortable with such sexual feelings and, as the outline of my concepts indicates, believe that a right measure of sexual attraction between adults and children is beneficial. *But I found myself once again embarrassed as I had been over my feelings towards the mother. However, on reflection, I wondered if in some way I was "filling a vacuum" with Sacha as I had done with the mother, that is, having father's unfulfilled oedipal romance with Sacha, or feeling her need for it.*)

Fifth Session: As I met them, eight days later, *my attention was caught and held throughout the session by a very large and beautiful blue patterned tie the mother was wearing.*

The focus turned to father's feelings about Sacha. The sexual father/daughter aspect did indeed seem to be lacking; the relationship was clearly based more on father's vicarious infantile gratification. He said, "I enjoyed my early childhood when I was happy, when I was very small, and I may have tried to relive this through Sacha." Father also made a connection between his hostility to his father following this period and Alan's hostility to him.

Sacha's blinking was still increasing. *At this stage I was feeling increasingly isolated and rejected by the family for the views I was expressing about the desirability of sexual feelings between father and daughter, and the fact that I had felt attraction of this kind myself.* Mother clearly understood and agreed, but I felt her basic loyalty had to be to the family denial.

My attention was still caught by mother's prominent tie and I felt impelled to mention it.

Mother grinned and said, "You mean I am the man in the family?" (Father had on a black polo-neck sweater.) Mother suggested another possible sexual link we had not explored—that between the males. This was avoided by them, but the relevance seemed confirmed when it was next revealed that Alan did up mother's tie for her. Alan looked uncomfortable and, suddenly, in a breakthrough, the mother said she had realized vividly how the sexual pattern between herself and her husband was always dictated by the children: "We like to make love on Saturday and Sunday but they barge in whenever they feel like it. There is always some excuse to disturb us and we are fools; we pretend we are doing something quite different altogether when they enter the room. The one thing I am longing to get away on holiday for is so we can make love as often as we like, without worrying about the children at all." Father nodded agreement, but though mother and the children seemed quite at ease during this discussion, father appeared much more embarrassed. He said, "Do you want us to have a notice on the door saying 'vacant' or 'engaged,' to tell you what we are doing? Why can't you knock?" I suggested that it was genuinely difficult for everybody if there were not some clear indication, such as a locked door, and Alan said to the parents, "Why don't you tell us? What's the problem about telling us, so we know when to stay away?"

. . . Time was up. As they left I found myself chatting with father in a man-to-man way about the business trip on which he would shortly be taking his wife. I felt as if I was offering the supportive "homosexual" relationship he had lacked with his father.

I was left feeling that all was now well between the parents, or well enough for them to develop the relationship, but that I still needed to help the children to cope with this change.

Sixth Session: I began the session two weeks later still feeling I had to do something to help the children to cope with the loss of their parents, who were closer to each other sexually. Sacha's unusual liveliness, animation and confidence were striking. After we were seated, I asked if anyone wished to change places, and mother said she would like to change with father. He reluctantly complied. . . .

Mother began by saying that Sacha would probably do all the talking, as she had been very lively, woken up first and got the rest of the family up. Mother continued by saying that since moving her chair she had realized she wanted to put more space between herself and Sacha, that she resented Sacha's attachment and dependency. (Alan said that was mother's fault, implying the dependency was mutual.) Mother expressed increasing anger at Sacha's dependence, and said she wished Sacha would fight back instead of denying her hostility. Sacha was blinking steadily with a hostile stare, which I described as "stopping the daggers from flying out of her eyes." Soon we were again like spectators watching a tennis match, but now between mother and Sacha.

I found myself thinking Sacha could not grow away from mother because father would not accept her oedipal attachment, and I expressed this in simple language. Father complained again that both children stayed up late and interfered with his relationship with his wife.

I felt again that I had enabled the parents to be comfortable about their sexuality and to be closer, but that somehow the children were stranded. Reporting this, I confessed that I did not yet see how to help the children cope with the new situation, and particularly with their own sexuality.

Sacha responded to my mention of "the children's sexuality" by complaining that Alan's anger and teasing prevented a good relationship between them, as if the aggressiveness were a defense against enjoyable sexual feeling.

Still feeling blocked by the father's reluctance to acknowledge his side of the oedipal romance with Sacha, I mentioned that I had a beautiful daughter who obviously enjoyed her sexual feelings to me as much as I did mine towards her. I mentioned also how skillful she was at playing my wife and I [sic] off against each other, and commented that Sacha seemed unable to do this. Mother confirmed this, saying of Sacha, "She always failed to pull her father on her side against me" and of father, "he was never really ready to be her white knight on a charger."

The family next discussed an incident where Sacha had gone home to seek father's support when a rough boy had pushed her off a swing. Father had gone with her to the playground, but had spoken to the boy mildly, disappointing Sacha, who had screamed repeatedly that father was "a coward." As the story unfolded, it was Sacha who disclosed that, returning home to seek father's protection, she had become aware that her parents were "upstairs making love." Despite her feeling that she should not interrupt them, she had intruded and father had got up and gone with her, leaving mother. As the discussion continued, it became obvious that the motives for Sacha's interruption were mixed, and that neither female was pleased with the way father dealt with the situation!

(At this point I experienced a strong feeling that these children, and children in general, must find it difficult to lose the bodily intimacy of babyhood and also accept exclusion from their parents' intimate sexuality, unless they could find a substitute in their own sexuality.)

Reporting this, I acknowledged I still could not understand it well enough to help them. *I was also strongly feeling the lack of some normal sexual attraction and enjoyment between Alan and Sacha.*

I did not report this, but the relevance of my feelings was verified when mother immediately continued, "There is a terrific sexual tension between the children when they are left alone, but *(teasingly)* they are too afraid to have a good time like mum and dad."

Following this the parents continued to talk in terms of adult sexuality, while the children responded appropriately to each statement, but as if translating into another language where nonsexual games and play substituted for sex. Sacha said, "The difference is that when they like each other men and women can say they want to be with each other, but children can't." I suggested that she was speaking about intercourse, and this led to a relaxed discussion of what it meant. Alan confirmed his knowledge about it, but Sacha blocked as if she knew but was denying her knowledge. I explained the details, and said it was exciting and enjoyable. The children said they did not wish to do anything like that yet.

The theme changed to complaints about father's inhibitions over being aggressive, forceful and potent. Sacha, in particular, angrily protested to father, "You never even shout at me, let alone hit me," as if greatly deprived.

Father repeatedly avoided this confrontation, but Sacha pursued the subject, shouting angrily, "I am asking for you to hit me and you keep trying to change the subject!" Father finally acknowledged that he was realizing he did not want to feel "sexual overtones coming towards him from Sacha." Mother said teasingly to her, "Oh, she is faithful to Daddy only, and to prove it she doesn't show interest in any other boy, but Daddy doesn't care and she is angry with him for it!" Mother went on to describe her awareness in childhood of her own father's strong sexual feelings for her, and his jealousy of any other males, "It made me feel good, but it was really very bad for me. I felt that somehow I could get my father though really I couldn't."

I was struck by the father's fear of violent, animal feelings, including sexuality and aggression. Drawing attention to this, I pointed out that father could have "been a beast" and enjoyed himself three times over in the incident described earlier; he could have finished making love to his wife, smacked Sacha for interrupting, and shouted at the boy who bullied her. Everyone found this hugely amusing.

They continued on the theme of the desire of all other members that father should be the strongest in the family. Mother described how the children wanted him to win when they all played games together and how upset they got when he once suggested that in the future he would let mother win. Mother continued, "When the father is the strongest in the family, everything comes back to peace and quiet; there is order, harmony, no wars. But in reality I am the strongest." An argument developed between the children and mother about who was the strongest, and Alan said to father, "If you didn't have a son, you'd have no one to bully," as if he had to "put himself down" to keep his father above him.

(Throughout the interview I had been preoccupied with a family therapy session carried out by a colleague at the Institute of Family Therapy, which was part of a program our Institute was making for BBC television. The family concerned also contained a dominant mother, withdrawn father and a stealing boy whose rivalry was not being adequately contested. The staff at the Institute, which had watched the film, had seemed to me as inhibited about discussing the sexual, oedipal problems as the therapist had been with the family. I had found this intensely frustrating and had almost exploded. At the same time, I had admired the fact that this colleague paid real attention to the children's needs, and realized that I tended to neglect this aspect.

I recognized for the first time that this was connected with the fact that while I had become relaxed and comfortable at talking about parental sexuality in front of children, I was much more embarrassed about talking about children's sexuality in front of adults. Although more in a "parental" role in the Institute, as its "founder" and first Chairman, I suddenly found myself identifying with the children in the family being watched, and taking a "child" role in relation to the Institute "family" as if it were my own. I had reported this to my colleagues, saying that watching the film had made me identify with the children and have the fantasy that "I shall masturbate as much as I like, any time I like, and no one will stop me." I had not understood the significance of this at the time, but felt sure it was the key to the television family interview.)

I reported all this to the family I was treating, saying it kept coming to my mind as if it had some connection. I then realized, and reported, that the fathers in both families were like my own father, fearful of their own potency, and that perhaps as a child I had also been frightened of my own developing sexual potency, and embarrassed over masturbation because of a need to be weaker than my father and keep him strong, and out of fear that my parents would allow me to inhibit their sexuality if mine was too strongly experienced.

As I was reporting this, I had a profound feeling that many things I had not previously understood, in my personal life, my family of origin, my theoretical conceptions and my professional work, had fallen into place and become connected together. I said to the family that I had perhaps brought myself in more personally than usual because I had been learning something important about my own family of origin and myself. They left looking quiet and thoughtful. There was no time for further discussion but I felt a deep assurance that I had given the children what they needed, and that the main work was done.

Final Three Sessions: A six-week interval followed, since a visit by the parents abroad—the first without the children—overlapped with my teaching visit to the U.S. As the deadline of delivery for this chapter had arrived, I took it with me, including the report as summarized so far. I did not realize until my return the extent to which "the chips were down," since my firm prediction, now in the editor's hands, was still to be tested.

The family came for three more sessions at intervals of two weeks. The seating remained unchanged except that mother and father changed places with each other twice. At the first of these (session 7), father took an authoritative position for the first time, criticizing Alan for lack of effort at school. Alan said the school was too permissive and that he wanted to change to another with more discipline and educational "stretching," which I personally also thought he needed. The females "sat this one out," looking relaxed, but when mother tried once to dominate, father told her to "keep out of it . . . you take too much territory." *I still felt some lack of connection between Alan and father, and found myself thinking repeatedly that the father's father had failed in his relationship with the father in some way, and that the males in the family were uncomfortable with their homo-erotic feelings.* I said this and while father showed discomfort, mother and Sacha agreed, saying the females, by contrast, were getting along famously. *I felt myself to be occupying paternal grandfather's role, giving the males permission for a more comfortable attitude to their homosexual feelings.*

At the next (8th) session, the father looked much more manly, showing a new quiet firmness, as well as an obviously sexual enjoyment of his wife, moving his chair close and leaning towards her. Both expressed feelings of increasing differentiation, mother saying she "had her own universe instead of seeing the family as an extension of herself," the father agreeing. The children, rather bored, asked why they were still coming for therapy.

The final (9th) session began with the parents saying that on the way to the interview they had both found themselves having the same thought—that this would be the last visit. Sadness at parting was expressed, together with pleasure at the changes. Mother reported that Alan had "changed drastically," was a "pleasure to be with" and could "express his pain instead of keeping it inside him." The changes in Alan and the family were confirmed by other members.

In addition, there were three further sessions, six months later, for the parental couple without the children, to help them deal with a long-standing problem presented by the father's elder brother who had regularly intruded into, and tried to disrupt, their marriage. As the final draft of this chapter had been dispatched, it was no longer necessary to keep the technique "pure" for the sake of clarity; the approach at this family of origin level could therefore be eclectic and so more swift—enabling the entanglement of the brother in this marital system to be dealt with in one final session where an essentially psychoanalytic understanding (that he had displaced into his brother's marriage the oedipal conflict which had never been resolved in relation to his parents) was presented in systemic, paradoxical form (namely, that his attempt to disrupt his parents' marriage, and now that of his brother, had the positive purpose of stimulating father and brother towards greater potency, and so strengthening the marital bonds in each case by provoking and "testing" them; further, as the effect was clearly most beneficial, he should continue to intrude between them as much as possible, even though it was recognized that this required a generous sacrifice of his own life and freedom). A spate of international phone calls and letters from this brother, both to the couple and to myself—sometimes several within an hour and each canceling the one before—indicated that the medicine had been internalized and was operating effectively. The couple confirmed that they now felt able to exclude him from the marital relationship.

This excerpt is fascinating in many ways. It demonstrates Skynner's view that becoming part of the projective system of the family is highly effective. But beyond that, the particular projective system discussed is clearly oedipal. Thus countertransference is used with relatively highly functioning family members. It is also interesting that despite Skynner's feeling that strategic models do not fit with his perspective, he reveals the use of a strategic intervention when circumstances do not require a "pure" approach. And that intervention is analytic in origin. Perhaps the most refreshing aspect of Skynner's work is the level of genuine self-disclosure he advocates. Yet the self-disclosure of countertransference he advocates does not include any formulation of how his countertransference feelings were evoked. His ability to say to the family that he does not understand why his feelings were evoked is appropriate at times. It would seem consistent with his type of analysis, however, especially given the importance he attributes to the projective system, to describe for the family how his own sexual feelings might have become evoked. Such an intervention might take the following form:

I have been telling you how I've been feeling many times within these sessions. And I've shared with you my belief that the therapist often gets caught up in important emotions within the family. Now I'm thinking that it would be helpful to explore how that happens, because often the therapist gets caught up in those emotions in the same way that family members do. The strongest thing I feel most consistently is sort of a sexual power which, it seems, is transferred from you, Mother. The way you wear your clothing seems designed to attract even if you don't know you are doing it, and I have the sensation of it filling me with manliness. The way you seem so impressed with the things I say and listen to me so intently, even leaning toward me at times—I think that's what does it. It feels good. And when I think of it, it seems like there's an unconscious agreement between you two parents that this will happen. You don't seem comfortable, Dad, with having that sexual power, which is rightly yours, so you allow it to be given to me. I think something similar happens with Alan. Sometimes he does get the power but then he feels bad because it seems to him that he might be chosen over Daddy by Mommy, which is, of course, very dangerous for him. When it seemed as if I were being chosen over you, Dad, I felt that danger even while Mother was filling me with sexual power. I wonder, too, if you stop your spontaneity with Sacha because you're scared that she'll become more desirable to you than your wife? But even so she feels your unconscious desire and so she enacts it more strongly. I mean she can sense in you the desire for her, but since you won't let yourself notice it, she's left expressing it without any overt reaction from you, which frustrates her. Meanwhile Mom continues to teach her to be the way she is—feminine and attractive, and she teaches Alan to be like her ideal little man, when all Sacha wants from Mom is acceptance to be a young girl and all Alan wants is to have a spontaneous friendship with his Dad. But Dad, you don't need to be afraid of your own power. The whole family clearly would like you to have it, even if it sometimes seems like they don't want you to have it. When they don't seem to be respecting your authority, you might even recognize that as their way of testing you and expressing their desire for you to pass that test. It is possible that you have this fear because you, yourself were afraid as a child that showing too much prowess would make you win your mother's affection over your father. Mom takes that power so easily because she almost succeeded in stealing her father's affection away from her mother, and continues to feel good when she thinks she could have had her father's affection—now she attempts to feel good by attracting the attention of men she sees as powerful. But Dad, if you follow your desires without too much fear, you are bound to have an admiring relationship with your son, your daughter will feel recognized by you and her mother for her femininity as well as her eight-year-old self without needing to wonder about her appropriate place, and your wife will only desire to put that feeling of power into you because she will like that you demand it.

Such an intervention goes one step further than the process suggested by Skynner. The family learns what behaviors they use to ward off uncomfortable feelings. They also learn why they might be having these feelings and that they don't need to fend them off. The relational systems perspective allows the therapist to share his experience of the intrapsychic and interpersonal systems with the family and retain the knowledge of how such systems work while describing that experience. Thus emotional experience is connected to behavior at the systemic level and the family is able to change those behaviors while understanding how the same needs that were met by the behaviors can continue to be met in more satisfactory ways within the family.

THE FLEXIBILITY OF THE RELATIONAL SYSTEMS PERSPECTIVE

In this chapter I have detailed the relational systems perspective for family therapy and demonstrated how it can be used with analytic, integrationist, experiential, systems, and solution-oriented effectiveness. In areas where other models cannot make full use of countertransference, the relational systems perspective does so by focusing on the connection of intrapsychic to interpersonal within all members of the system, including the therapist. The relational systems perspective views the therapist as within the therapist–family system, and thus does not deny the effect of the prereflective use of countertransference as do current analytic family therapy models. The relational systems model is a full integration of interpersonal and intrapsychic systems, and interventions are formulated with the theory in mind so that the absence of theoretically consistent interventions characteristic of integrationist models is avoided. The fact that theory is ever-present within the relational systems model allows for access to interventions that are typically not used by experiential therapists, who do not subscribe to the use of theory. Finally, because therapists using the relational systems model attempt to be aware of their countertransference reactions, they are able to make use of those reactions in formulating systems and solution-oriented interventions. Interventions that have strategic, structural, or solution-oriented effects are developed without a hidden agenda. The relational systems perspective is able to accommodate all therapeutic strategies by bridging the gap between systems and psychoanalytic models. Being human is something we all have in common. The relational systems model merely aims to describe the intrapsychic and interpersonal human process.

Conclusion

Countertransference is always involved in therapy, and I have described it as integral within all the major family therapy approaches. An important aspect of this study is that it shows that what some therapists say they do allows the actual process involved to remain mysterious primarily for the purpose of clearly presenting an approach. In contrast, the relational systems perspective explains what occurs in therapy that makes it curative, whether the approach is analytic, systems oriented, or involves any other model. Human systems function in a manner that can be understood in a cohesive way. The relational systems perspective integrates analytic and systems viewpoints, which in spite of their similarities have often been considered incompatible, in the effort to present a cohesive understanding of human systems.

The use of countertransference offers a potentially powerful tool, one that so far has not been well-understood or utilized. It is a tool that can potentially be employed to bridge many approaches to family therapy and be used in attaining many very different therapeutic goals. However, when ideas are integrated in a new way there is always likely to be resistance. In fact, such resistance has already led to the two factors that have limited the use of countertransference. First, therapists have not viewed themselves as part of the therapist–family system despite the wide use of systems theory that would indicate such inclusion. Second, although many approaches to psychotherapy attempt a complete explanation of human behavior, no theory of communication that addresses both intrapsychic and interpersonal phenomena has been adequately applied to the full range of events that occurs within psychotherapy. Many other issues are related to these two areas, such as the prereflective use of countertransference, the definition of projective identification, and—perhaps the stickiest issue of all—the mental health of the therapist. What is significantly different about the relational systems perspective, however, is the application of a comprehensive theoretical model that applies to both therapist and family equally, with all their history and context considered. The only essential difference between therapist and family within the relational systems perspective is the self-reflectiveness of the therapist as he or she attempts to be therapeutic.

Finally, it seems all therapies bear remarkable similarities due to the simple fact that clients and therapists are "more human than otherwise" (to quote Sullivan). By demonstrating some of those similarities it becomes clear that the use of countertransference can be valuable to all therapists. The relational systems perspective shows that countertransference is always a part of therapy. Although therapists will always have the choice of either using countertransference self-reflectively or simply accepting the fact that they are using it prereflectively, its intentional use has been shown to be a vital technique. Using countertransference provides limitless opportunities for therapeutic intervention because it refers to the therapist's sensitivity to emotional interaction, and our emotions are always involved in our work. The possibilities are endless in the same way that openness to experience leads to endless possibilities in a world of relationships among all things.

References

Ackerman, N. W. (1959). Transference and countertransference. *Psychoanalysis and Psychoanalytic Review* 46:17–28.

———. (1966). *Treating the Troubled Family*. New York: Basic Books.

Ackerman, N. W., and Sobel, R. (1950). Family diagnosis: an approach to the preschool child. *American Journal of Orthopsychiatry* 20:744–753.

Adler, A. (1917). *The Neurotic Constitution*. New York: Mofatt Yard.

Aponte, H. J., and VanDeusen, J. M. (1981). Structural family therapy. In *Handbook of Family Therapy* ed. A. S. Gurman and D. P. Kniskern, pp. 310–360. New York: Brunner/Mazel.

Aponte, H. J., and Winter, J. E. (1987). The person and practice of the therapist: treatment and training. *Journal of Psychotherapy and the Family* 3:85–111.

Arlow, J. A. (1985). Some technical problems of countertransference. *Psychoanalytic Quarterly* 54:164–174.

Aron, L. (1992). Interpretation as expression of the analyst's subjectivity. *Psychoanalytic Dialogues* 2:475–508.

Ashbach, C., and Schermer, V. L. (1987). *Object Relations, the Self, and the Group: A Conceptual Paradigm*. New York: Routledge & Kegan Paul.

Atwood, G. E., and Stolorow, R. D. (1984). *Structures of Subjectivity: Explorations in Psychoanalytic Phenomenology*. Hillsdale, NJ: Analytic Press.

Balint, A., and Balint, M. (1939). On transference and counter-transference. *International Journal of Psycho-analysis* 20:223–230.

Bateson, G. (1958). *Naven*, rev. ed. Stanford, CA: Stanford University Press.

———. (1962). A note on the double bind. *Family Process* 2:154–161.

————. (1972). *Steps to an Ecology of Mind*. New York: Ballantine.

————. (1977). The birth of a matrix or double bind and epistemology. In *Beyond the Double Bind*, ed. M Berger. New York: Brunner/Mazel.

————. (1979). *Mind and Nature: A Necessary Unity*. New York: Dutton.

Bateson, G., Jackson, D. D., Haley, J., and Weakland, J. H. (1956). Toward a theory of schizophrenia. In *Family Therapy: The Major Contributions*, ed. R. J. Green and J. L. Framo, pp. 41–68. Madison, CT: International Universities Press, 1981.

Berman, L. (1949). Countertransferences and attitudes of the analyst in the therapeutic process. *Psychiatry* 12:159–166.

Bion, W. R. (1959a). Attacks on linking. *International Journal of Psycho-analysis* 40:308–315.

————. (1959b). *Experiences in Groups*. New York: Basic Books.

————. (1967). Notes on memory and desire. *Psychoanalytic Forum* 2: 217–280.

————. (1970). *Attention and Interpretation*. London: Tavistock.

Bollas, C. (1983). Expressive uses of the countertransference: notes to the patient from oneself. *Contemporary Psychoanalysis* 19(1):1–34.

————. (1987). *The Shadow of the Object: Psychoanalysis of the Unthought Known*. New York: Columbia University Press.

Boszormenyi-Nagy, I. (1966). From family therapy to a psychology of relationships: fictions of the individual and fictions of the family. *Comparative Psychiatry* 7:408–423.

Boszormenyi-Nagy, I., and Framo, J. L. (1987). Hospital organization and family-oriented psychotherapy of schizophrenia. In *Foundations of Contextual Therapy: Collected Papers of Ivan Boszormenyi-Nagy, M.D.*, ed. I. Boszormenyi-Nagy, pp. 8–19. New York: Brunner/Mazel.

Boszormenyi-Nagy, I., and Krasner, B. R. (1986). *Between Give and Take: A Clinical Guide to Contextual Therapy*. New York: Brunner/Mazel.

————. (1987). Trust based therapy: a contextual approach. In *Foundations of Contextual Therapy: Collected Papers of Ivan Boszormenyi-Nagy, M.D.*, ed. I. Boszormenyi-Nagy, pp. 213–237. New York: Brunner/Mazel.

Bowen, M. (1965). Family psychotherapy with schizophrenia in the hospital and in private practice. In *Intensive Family Therapy*, ed. I. Boszormenyi-Nagy, pp. 213–243. New York: Harper & Row.

————. (1972). Toward a differentiation of a self in one's own family. In *Family Interaction*, ed. J. L. Framo, pp. 111–173. New York: Springer.

————. (1978). *Family Therapy in Clinical Practice*. New York: Jason Aronson.

Bowlby, F. (1969). *Attachment*. New York: Basic Books.

————. (1973). *Separation: Anxiety and Anger*. New York: Basic Books.

————. (1975). *Loss: Sadness and Depression.* New York: Basic Books.

Box, S., Copley, B., Magagna, J., and Moustaki, E., eds. (1981). *Psychotherapy with Families: An Analytic Approach.* London: Routledge and Kegan Paul.

Boyer, L. B. (1983). *The Regressed Patient.* New York: Jason Aronson.

Brenner, C. (1985). Countertransference as compromise formation. *Psychoanalytic Quarterly* 54:155–163.

Burke, W. F. (1992). Countertransference disclosure and the asymmetry/mutuality dilemma. *Psychoanalytic Dialogues* 2(2):241–271.

Burke, W. F., and Tansey, M. J. (1991). Countertransference disclosure and models of therapeutic action. *Contemporary Psychoanalysis* 27(2): 351–384.

Carr, A. (1989). Countertransference to families where child abuse has occurred. *Journal of Family Therapy* 11: 87–97.

Chused, J. F. (1992). The patient's perception of the analyst: the hidden transference. *Psychoanalytic Quarterly* 61:161–184.

deShazer, S. (1985). *Keys to Solution in Brief Therapy.* New York: Norton.

Dickerson, V. C., and Zimmerman, J. L. (1993). A narrative approach to families with adolescents. In *The New Language of Change: Constructive Collaboration in Therapy*, ed. S. Friedman, pp. 226–250. New York: Guilford.

Dicks, H. V. (1967). *Marital Tensions: Clinical Studies towards a Psychological Theory of Interaction.* New York: Basic Books.

Durkin, H. E. (1972). Analytic group therapy and general systems theory. In *Progress in Group and Family Therapy*, ed. C. J. Sager and H. S. Kaplan, pp. 9–17. New York: Brunner/Mazel.

Edelson, M. (1970). *Sociotherapy and Psychotherapy.* Chicago: University of Chicago Press.

Ehrenberg, D. B. (1992). *The Intimate Edge.* New York: Norton.

English, O. S., and Pearson, H. J. (1937). *Common Neuroses of Children and Adults.* New York: Norton.

Erickson, M. H., and Rossi, E. (1983). *Healing in Hypnosis.* New York: Irvington.

Erikson, E. H. (1956). The problem of ego identity. *Journal of the American Psychoanalytic Association* 4:56–121.

Fairbairn, W. R. D. (1941). A revised psychopathology of the psychoses and psychoneuroses. *International Journal of Psycho-Analysis* 22:250–279.

————. (1943). The repression and the return of bad objects (with special reference to the 'war neuroses'). *British Journal of Medical Psychology* 19:327–341.

————. (1946). Object-relationships and dynamic structures. *International Journal of Psycho-Analysis* 27:30–37.

Federn, P. (1952). *Ego Psychology and the Psychoses*, ed. E. Weiss. New York: Basic Books.

Ferenczi, S. (1909). Introjection and transference. In *Sex in Psychoanalysis*, ed. S. Ferenczi, pp. 35–93. New York: Basic Books, 1950.

———. (1988). *The Clinical Diary of Sandor Ferenczi*, ed. J. Dupont. Cambridge: Harvard University Press.

Ferenczi, S., and Rank, O. (1923). *The Development of Psychoanalysis*. New York and Washington: Nervous & Mental Disease Publishing Company, 1925.

Ferreira, A. (1963). Family myths and homeostasis. *Archives of General Psychiatry* 9:457–463.

Fliess, R. (1942). The metapsychology of the analyst. *Psychoanalytic Quarterly* 11:211–227.

———. (1953). Countertransference and counteridentification. *Journal of the American Psychoanalytic Association* 1:268–284.

Framo, J. L. (1965). Rationale and techniques of intensive family therapy. In *Intensive Family Therapy: Theoretical and Practical Applications*, ed. I. Boszormenyi-Nagy and J. Framo, pp. 143–212. New York: Brunner/Mazel.

———. (1968). My families, my family. *Voices: Art and Science of Psychotherapy* 4:18–27.

Franklin, G. (1990). The multiple meanings of neutrality. *Journal of the American Psychoanalytic Association* 38:195–220.

Freud, A. (1936). *The Ego and the Mechanisms of Defence*. New York: International Universities Press, 1946.

———. (1965). *Normality and Pathology in Childhood*. New York: International Universities Press.

Freud S. (1905). Fragment of an analysis of a case of hysteria. *Standard Edition* 7:3–122.

———. (1910). The future prospects of psychoanalytic psychotherapy. *Standard Edition* 11:139–151.

———. (1912a). The dynamics of the transference. *Standard Edition* 12:97–108.

———. (1912b). Recommendations to physicians on the psychoanalytic method of treatment. *Standard Edition* 12:109–121.

———. (1914a). Observations on transference-love. *Standard Edition* 12:157–171.

———. (1914b). Remembering, repeating, and working through. *Standard Edition* 12:145–156.

———. (1920). Beyond the pleasure principle. *Standard Edition* 18:3–64.

———. (1921). Group psychology and the analysis of the ego. *Standard Edition* 18:67–143.

Fromm-Reichmann, F. (1948). Notes on the development of treatment of schizophrenics by psychoanalytical psychotherapy. *Psychiatry* 11:263–273.

Ganzarain, R. (1977). General systems and object-relations theories: their usefulness in group psychotherapy. *International Journal of Group Psychotherapy* 27:441–456.

———. (1989). *Object Relations Group Psychotherapy: The Group as an Object, a Tool, and a Training Base.* Madison, CT: International Universities Press.

———. (1992). Introduction to object relations group psychotherapy. *International Journal of Group Psychotherapy* 42:205–223.

Giovacchini, P. L. (1975a). *Psychoanalysis of Character Disorders.* New York: Jason Aronson.

———. (1975b). *Tactics and Techniques in Psychoanalytic Therapy, vol. 2: Countertransference.* New York: Jason Aronson.

———. (1979). *Treatment of Primitive Mental States.* New York: Jason Aronson.

———. (1989). *Countertransference Triumphs and Catastrophes.* Northvale, NJ: Jason Aronson.

Greenberg, J. R. (1986). Theoretical models and the analyst's neutrality. *Contemporary Psychoanalysis* 22:87–106.

———. (1991). *Oedipus and Beyond.* Cambridge, MA: Harvard University Press.

———. (1995). Self-disclosure: Is it psychoanalytic? *Contemporary Psychoanalysis* 31 (2): 193–205.

Greenberg, J., and Mitchell, S. (1983). *Object Relations in Psychoanalytic Theory.* Cambridge, MA: Harvard University Press.

Greenson, R. (1960). Empathy and its vicissitudes. *International Journal of Psycho-Analysis* 41:418–424.

———. (1967). *The Technique and Practice of Psychoanalysis. Vol. 1.* New York: International Universities Press.

Grinberg, L. (1962). On a specific aspect of countertransference due to the patient's projective identification. *International Journal of Psycho-Analysis* 43:436–440.

———. (1968). On acting out and its role in the psychoanalytic process. *International Journal of Psycho-Analysis* 49:171–178.

———. (1979). Countertransference and projective counteridentification. *Contemporary Psychoanalysis* 15:226–247.

Grotstein, J. S. (1981). *Splitting and Projective Identification.* New York: Jason Aronson.

Guntrip, H. (1969). *Schizoid Phenomena, Object Relations and the Self.* New York: International Universities Press.

Gurman, A. S. (1981). *Questions and Answers in the Practice of Family Therapy.* New York: Brunner/Mazel.

———. (1987). The effective family therapist: some old data and some new directions. *Journal of Psychotherapy and the Family* 3:113–125.

Gurman, A. S. and Kniskern, D. P. (1981). *Handbook of Family Therapy*. New York: Brunner/Mazel.

Haley, J. (1971). Family therapy: a radical change. In *Changing Families: A Family Therapy Reader*, ed. J. Haley, pp. 272–284. New York: Norton.

———. (1976). *Problem Solving Therapy*. San Francisco: Jossey-Bass.

———. (1977). Toward a theory of pathological systems. In *The Interaction View*, ed. P. Watzlawick and J. Weakland. New York: Norton.

Hall, A., and Fagan, B. (1956). Definition of system. *General Systems Yearbook* 1:18.

Halperin, S. M. (1991). Countertransference and the developing family therapist: treatment and supervision issues. *Contemporary Family Therapy* 13:127–141.

Hartmann, H. (1964). *Essays on Ego Psychology*. New York: International Universities Press.

Heimann, P. (1950). On countertransference. *International Journal of Psycho-Analysis* 31:81–84.

———. (1956). Dynamics of transference interpretations. *International Journal of Psycho-Analysis* 37:303–310.

Hoffman, I. Z. (1991). Toward a social-constructivist view of the psychoanalytic situation: Discussion of papers by L. Aron, A. Modell, and J. Greenberg. *Psychoanalytic Dialogues* 1:74–105.

———. (1992a). Expressive participation and psychoanalytic discipline. *Contemporary Psychoanalysis* 28(1):1–15.

———. (1992b). Some practical implications of a social-constructivist view of the psychoanalytic situation. *Psychoanalytic Dialogues* 2(3):287–304.

Hoffman, L. (1981). *Foundations of Family Therapy*. New York: Basic Books.

Horney, K. (1937). *The Neurotic Personality of Our Time*. New York: Norton.

Horwitz, L. (1983). Projective identification in dyads and groups. *International Journal of Group Psychotherapy* 33:259–279.

Jackson, D. D. (1956). Countertransference and psychotherapy. In *Progress in Psychotherapy*, ed. F. Fromm-Reichmann and J. C. Moreno, pp. 234–238. New York: Grune & Stratton.

———. (1957). The question of family homeostasis. *Psychiatric Quarterly* (Suppl.) 31:79–90.

Jackson, D. D., and Haley, J. (1963). Transference revisited. In *Therapy, Communication and Change: Human Communication, volume II*, ed. D. Jackson, pp. 115–128. Palo Alto: Science and Behavior Books, 1968.

Jackson, D. D., and Weakland, J. H. (1961). Conjoint family therapy: some considerations on theory, technique, and results. In *Changing Families: A Family Therapy Reader*, ed. J. Haley, pp. 13–35. New York: Grune & Stratton, 1971.

Jacobs, T. J. (1991). *The Use of the Self: Countertransference and Communication in the Analytic Situation.* Madison, CT: International Universities Press.

Jacobson, E. (1964). *The Self and the Object World.* New York: International Universities Press.

Jung, C. G. (1927). *The Psychology of the Unconscious.* New York: Dodd, Mead.

Keith, D. V. (1987). The self in family therapy: a field guide. *Journal of Psychotherapy and the Family* 3:61–70.

Kempler, W. (1965). Experiential family therapy. *International Journal of Group Psychotherapy* 15:57–71.

———. (1968). Experiential psychotherapy with families. *Family Process* 7:88–99.

Kernberg, O. F. (1965). Notes on countertransference. *Journal of the American Psychoanalytic Association* 13:38–56.

———. (1975). *Borderline Conditions and Pathological Narcissism.* New York: Jason Aronson.

———. (1976). *Object Relations Theory and Clinical Psychoanalysis.* New York: Jason Aronson.

———. (1984). *Severe Personality Disorders: Psychotherapeutic Strategies.* New Haven: Yale University Press.

———. (1989). *Psychodynamic Psychotherapy of Borderline Patients.* New York: Basic Books.

Kleckner, T., Frank, L., Bland, C., et al. (1992). The myth of the unfeeling strategic therapist. *Journal of Marital and Family Therapy* 18:41–51.

Klein, M. (1935). A contribution to the psychogenesis of manic-depressive states. *International Journal of Psycho-Analysis* 16:145–174.

———. (1940). Mourning and its relation to manic-depressive states. In *Love, Guilt and Reparation, 1921–1945,* pp. 344–369. New York: Free Press, 1975.

———. (1946). Notes on some schizoid mechanisms. *International Journal of Psycho-Analysis* 27:99–110.

———. (1948a). On the theory of anxiety and guilt. In *Envy and Gratitude 1946–1963,* pp. 25–42. New York: Dell, 1975.

———. (1948b). *The Psychoanalysis of Children.* London: Hogarth.

———. (1957). Envy and gratitude. In *Envy and Gratitude 1946–1963,* pp. 176–235. New York: Dell, 1975.

Kohut, H. (1959). Introspection, empathy, and psychoanalysis: an examination of the relationship between mode of observation and theory. *Journal of the American Psychoanalytic Association* 7:459–483.

———. (1971). *The Analysis of the Self.* New York: International Universities Press.

———. (1977). *The Restoration of the Self.* New York: International Universities Press.

———. (1984). *How Does Analysis Cure?* Chicago: University of Chicago Press.

Landis, B. (1970). Ego boundaries. *Psychological Issues Monograph* 24(6). New York: International Universities Press.

Langs, R. (1973). *The Technique of Psychoanalytic Psychotherapy: Volume I.* New York: Jason Aronson.

———. (1976a). *The Bipersonal Field.* New York: Jason Aronson.

———. (1976b). *The Therapeutic Interaction.* New York: Jason Aronson.

———. (1978). *Technique in Transition.* New York: Jason Aronson.

———. (1983). The interactional dimension of countertransference. In *Countertransference: The Therapist's Contribution to the Therapeutic Situation*, ed. L. J. Epstein and A. Feiner, pp. 71–103. New York: Jason Aronson.

Lichtenberg, J. (1983). *Psychoanalysis and Infant Research.* Hillsdale, NJ: Analytic Press.

Lidz, T. (1973). *The Origin and Treatment of Schizophrenic Disorders.* New York: Basic Books.

Little, M. (1951). Countertransference and the patient's response to it. *International Journal of Psycho-Analysis* 32:32–40.

Loewald, H. (1960). On the therapeutic action of psychoanalysis. *International Journal of Psycho-Analysis* 41:16–33.

Luepnitz, D. A. (1988). *The Family Interpreted: Feminist Theory in Clinical Practice.* New York: Basic Books.

Luthman, S. G. (1974). *The Dynamic Family.* Palo Alto: Science and Behavior Books.

Madanes, C., and Haley, J. (1977). Dimensions of family therapy. *Journal of Nervous and Mental Disease* 165:88–98.

Mahler, M., Pine, F., and Bergman, A. (1975). *The Psychological Birth of the Human Infant.* New York: Basic Books.

Malin, A., and Grotstein, J. S. (1966). Projective identification in the therapeutic process. *International Journal of Psycho-Analysis* 47:26–31.

Maruyama, M. (1963). The second cybernetics: deviation-amplifying mutual causal processes. *American Scientist* 51:164–179.

Masler, E. G. (1969). The interpretation of projective identification in group psychotherapy. *International Journal of Group Psychotherapy* 19:441–447.

Masterson, J. F. (1981). *The Narcissistic and Borderline Disorders.* New York: Brunner/Mazel.

———. (1983). *Countertransference and Psychotherapeutic Technique: Teach-*

ing Seminars on Psychotherapy of the Borderline Adult. New York: Brunner/ Mazel.

Maturana, H. (1978). Biology of language: the epistemology of reality. In *Psychology and Biology of Language and Thought*, ed. G. A. Miller and E. Lenneberg. New York: Academic Press.

————. (1980). Autopoiesis and evolution. In *Autopoiesis, Dissipitive Structures, and Spontaneous Social Orders*, ed. M. Zaleny. Boulder, CO: Westview.

McElroy, L. P., and McElroy R. A. (1991). Countertransference issues in the treatment of incest families. *Psychotherapy* 28:48–54.

Miller, E. J., and Rice, A. K. (1963). *Systems of Organization*. London: Tavistock.

Millon, T, and Davis, R. D. (1996). *Disorders of Personality: DSM-IV and Beyond, Second Edition*. New York: Wiley.

Minuchin, S. (1974). *Families and Family Therapy*. Cambridge: Harvard University Press.

Minuchin, S., and Fishman, C. H. (1982). *Family Therapy Techniques*. Cambridge: Harvard University Press.

Mitchell, S. (1988). *Relational Concepts in Psychoanalysis*. Cambridge, MA: Harvard University Press.

Moustaki, E. (1981). Glossary: a discussion and application of terms. In *Psychotherapy with Families: An Analytic Approach*, ed. S. Box, B. Copley, J. Magagna, and E. Moustaki, pp. 160–172. London: Routledge & Kegan Paul.

Napier, A. Y., and Whitaker, C. A. (1978). *The Family Crucible*. New York: Harper & Row.

Neill, J. R., and Kniskern, D. P. (1982). *From Psyche to System: The Evolving Therapy of Carl Whitaker*. New York: Guilford.

Nichols, M. P. (1984). *Family Therapy: Concepts and Methods*. New York: Gardner.

————. (1987). *The Self in the System: Expanding the Limits of Family Therapy*. New York: Brunner/Mazel.

Nichols, M. P., and Schwartz, R. C. (1991). *Family Therapy: Concepts and Methods*, 2nd ed. Boston: Allyn and Bacon.

Ogden, T. H. (1979). On projective identification. *International Journal of Psycho-Analysis* 60:357–373.

————. (1989). *The Primitive edge of Experience*. Northvale, NJ: Jason Aronson.

————. (1994a). The analytic third: working with intersubjective clinical facts. *International Journal of Psycho-Analysis* 75:3–19.

————. (1994b). *Subjects of Analysis*. Northvale, NJ: Jason Aronson.

O'Hanlon, W. H., and Weiner-Davis, M. (1989). *In Search of Solutions: A New Direction in Psychotherapy*. New York: Norton.

Orr, D. (1954). Transference and countertransference: a historical survey. *Journal of the American Psychoanalytic Association* 2:647–662.

Palazzoli, M. S., Boscolo, L., Cecchin, G., and Prata, G. (1978). *Paradox and Counterparadox.* New York: Jason Aronson.

Piaget, J. (1954). *The Construction of Reality in the Child.* New York: Basic Books.

———. (1974). *The Place of the Sciences of Man in the System of Sciences.* New York: Harper & Row.

Pittman, F. S. (1985). Children of the rich. *Family Process* 24:461–472.

Poland, W. S. (1981). On the analyst's neutrality. *Journal of the American Psychoanalytic Association* 32:283–299.

Pollak, J., and Levy, S. (1989). Countertransference and failure to report child abuse and neglect. *Child Abuse and Neglect* 13:515–522.

Prigogine, I. (1976). Order through fluctuation: self-organization and social system. In *Evolution and Consciousness: Human Systems in Transition,* ed. E. Jantsch and C. H. Waddinton. Reading, MA: Addison-Wesley.

Racker, H. (1953). A contribution to the problem of countertransference. *International Journal of Psycho-Analysis* 34:313–324.

———. (1957). The meanings and uses of countertransference. *Psychoanalytic Quarterly* 26:303–357.

Reich, A. (1951). On countertransference. *International Journal of Psycho-Analysis* 32:25–31.

Reich, W. (1949). *Character Analysis,* 3rd ed. New York: Orgone Institute.

Reik, T. (1964). *Listening with the Third Ear.* New York: Pyramid.

Renik, O. (1995). The ideal of the anonymous analyst and the problem of self-disclosure. *Psychoanalytic Quarterly* 64:466–495.

Reynolds, M. P., and Levitan, S. (1990). Countertransference issues in the in-home treatment of child sexual abuse. *Child Welfare* 69:53–61.

Rice, A. K. (1967). *Learning for Leadership: Interpersonal and Intergroup Relations.* London: Tavistock.

———. (1969). Individual, group and intergroup processes. *Human Relations* 22:565–584.

Sandler, J. (1976). Countertransference and role-responsiveness. *International Review of Psycho-Analysis* 3:43–47.

Sandler, J., Dare, C., and Holder, A. (1973). *The Patient and the Analyst: The Basis of the Psychoanalytic Process.* London: Allen & Unwin.

Sass, L. A. (1988). Humanism, hermeneutics, and the concept of the human subject. In *Hermeneutics and Psychological Theory,* ed. S. B. Messer, L. A. Sass, and R. L. Woolfolk, pp. 222–271. New Brunswick, NJ: Rutgers University Press.

Satir, V. (1964). *Conjoint Family Therapy*. Palo Alto: Science and Behavior Books.

———. (1987). The therapist story. *Journal of Psychotherapy and the Family* 3:17–25.

Satir, V., and Baldwin, M. (1983). *Satir Step by Step*. Palo Alto: Science and Behavior Books.

Schafer, R. (1959). Generative empathy in the treatment situation. *Psychoanalytic Quarterly* 28:347–373.

———. (1968). *Aspects of Internalization*. New York: International Universities Press.

———. (1978). *Language and Insight*. New Haven: Yale University Press.

———. (1983). *The Analytic Attitude*. New York: Basic Books.

Schaffer, L., Wynne, L. C., Day, J., et al. (1962). On the nature and sources of the psychiatrist's experience with the family of the schizophrenic. *Psychiatry* 5:32–45.

Scharff, D. E. (1991). Transference, countertransference, and technique in object relations family therapy. In *Foundations of Object Relations Family Therapy*, ed. J. S. Scharff, pp. 421–446. Northvale, NJ: Jason Aronson.

Scharff, D. E., and Scharff, J. S. (1987). *Object Relations Family Therapy*. Northvale, NJ: Jason Aronson.

Scharff, J. S. (1989). *Foundations of Object Relations Family Therapy*. Northvale, NJ: Jason Aronson.

———. (1992). *Projective and Introjective Identification and the Use of the Therapist's Self*. Northvale, NJ: Jason Aronson.

Scheflen, A. E. (1968). Human communication: behavioral programs and their integration in interaction. *Behavioral Science* 13:86–102.

Schwaber, E. (1979). On the "self" within the matrix of analytic theory—some clinical reflections and reconsiderations. *International Journal of Psycho-Analysis* 60:467–479.

Searles, H. F. (1958). The schizophrenic's vulnerability to the therapist's unconscious processes. In *Collected Papers on Schizophrenia and Related Subjects*, ed. H. F. Searles. New York: International Universities Press, 1965.

———. (1959a). The effort to drive the other person crazy—an element in the aetiology and psychotherapy of schizophrenia. In *Collected Papers on Schizophrenia and Related Subjects*, ed. H. F. Searles. New York: International Universities Press, 1965.

———. (1959b). Oedipal love in the countertransference. In *Collected Papers on Schizophrenia and Related Subjects*, ed. H. F. Searles. New York: International Universities Press, 1965.

————. (1963). Transference psychosis in the psychotherapy of chronic schizo-phrenia. In *Collected Papers on Schizophrenia and Related Subjects*, ed. H. F. Searles, pp. 654–716. New York: International Universities Press, 1965.

————. (1964). The contributions of family treatment to the psychotherapy of schizophrenia. In *Intensive Family Therapy: Theoretical and Practical Applications*, ed. I. Boszormenyi-Nagy. New York: Brunner/Mazel, 1965.

————. (1965). *Collected Papers on Schizophrenia and Related Subjects*. New York: International Universities Press.

————. (1975). Countertransference and theoretical model. In *Psychotherapy of Schizophrenia*, ed, J. G. Gunderson and L. R. Mosher. New York: Jason Aronson.

Segal, H. (1973). *Introduction to the Work of Melanie Klein,* new, enlarged edition. London: Hogarth.

Shapiro, E. R., Shapiro, R. L., Zinner, J., and Berkowitz, D. A. (1977). The borderline ego and the working alliance: indications for family and individual treatment in adolescence. *International Journal of Psycho-Analysis* 58:77–87.

Shapiro, R. L. (1979). Family dynamics and object relations theory: an analytic, group interpretive approach to family therapy. In *Foundations of Object Relations Family Therapy*, ed. J. S. Scharff, pp. 225–246. Northvale, NJ: Jason Aronson, 1991.

Shapiro, R. L. (1981). Countertransference reactions in family therapy. In *Questions and Answers in the Practice of Family Therapy*, ed. A. S. Gurman, pp. 195–200. New York: Brunner/Mazel.

Shapiro, R. L., and Zinner, J. (1979). The adolescent, the family, and the group: boundary considerations. In *Foundations of Object Relations Family Therapy*, ed. J. S. Scharff, pp. 203–224. Northvale, NJ: Jason Aronson, 1991.

Shapiro, T. (1984). On neutrality. *Journal of the American Psychoanalytic Association* 32:269–282.

Sharpe, E. F. (1947). The psycho-analyst. *International Journal of Psycho-Analysis* 28:1–6.

Shay, J. J. (1992). Countertransference in the family therapy of survivors of sexual abuse. *Child Abuse and Neglect* 16:585–593.

Skynner, A. C. R. (1976). *Systems of Family and Marital Psychotherapy*. New York: Brunner/Mazel.

————. (1981). An open-systems, group analytic approach to family therapy. In *Handbook of Family Therapy*, ed. A. S. Gurman and D. P. Kniskern, pp. 39–84. New York: Brunner/Mazel.

Slipp, S. (1980). Interactions between the interpersonal in families and individual intrapsychic dynamics. In *Family Therapy: Combining Psychodynamic and Family Systems Approaches*, ed. J. K. Pearce and L. J. Friedman. New York: Grune & Stratton.

———. (1984). *Object Relations: A Dynamic Bridge Between Individual and Family Treatment*. New York: Jason Aronson.

———. (1988). *The Technique and Practice of Object Relations Family Therapy*. Northvale, NJ: Jason Aronson.

Spotnitz, H. (1969). *Modern Psychoanalysis of the Schizophrenic Patient*. New York: Grune & Stratton.

Springer, C. (1991). Clinical work with adolescents and their parents during family transitions: transference and countertransference issues. *Clinical Social Work Journal* 19:405–415.

Sterba, R. (1960). Dynamics of the dissolution of the transference resistance. *Psychoanalytic Quarterly* 9:363–379.

Stern, A. (1924). On the counter-transference in psychoanalysis. *Psychoanalytic Review* 11:166–174.

Stern, D. (1985). *The Interpersonal World of the Infant*. New York: Basic Books.

Stierlin, H. (1977). Countertransference in family therapy with adolescents. In *Psychoanalysis and Family Therapy*, ed. H. Stierlin, pp. 301–322. New York: Jason Aronson.

Stolorow, R., and Atwood, G. (1979). *Faces in a Cloud: Intersubjectivity in Personality Theory*. New York: Jason Aronson.

Stolorow, R. D., Atwood, G. E, and Brandchaft, B. (1994). *The Intersubjective Perspective*. Northvale, NJ: Jason Aronson.

Sullivan, H. S. (1953a). *The Collected Works of Harry Stack Sullivan*. New York: Norton.

———. (1953b). *The Interpersonal Theory of Psychiatry*. New York: Norton.

———. (1954). *The Psychiatric Interview*. New York: Norton.

———. (1962). *Schizophrenia as a Human Process*. New York: Norton.

Summers, F. (1994). *Object Relations Theories and Psychopathology: A Comprehensive Text*. Hillsdale, NJ: Analytic Press.

Tansey, M. J., and Burke, W. F. (1985). Projective identification and the empathic process. *Contemporary Psychoanalysis* 21:42–69.

———. (1989). *Understanding Countertransference: From Projective Identification to Empathy*. Hillsdale, NJ: Analytic Press.

Vogel, E. F., and Bell, N. W. (1960). The emotionally disturbed child as the family scapegoat. In *A Modern Introduction to the Family*, ed. N. W. Bell and E. F. Vogel, pp. 412–427. New York: The Free Press.

von Bertalanffy, L. (1968). *General Systems Theory*. New York: George Braziller.

———. (1974). General system theory and psychiatry. In *American Handbook of Psychiatry*, 2nd ed., ed. S. Arieti. New York: Basic Books.

Wachtel, E. F., and Wachtel, P. L. (1986). *Family Dynamics in Individual Psychotherapy*. New York: Guilford.

Wachtel, P. L. (1986). On the limits of therapeutic neutrality. *Contemporary Psychoanalysis* 22(1):60–70.

———. (1987). *Action and Insight*. New York: Guilford.

———. (1997). *Psychoanalysis, Behavior Therapy, and the Relational World*. Washington, DC: American Psychological Association.

Wallerstein, J. S. (1990). Transference and countertransference in clinical intervention with divorcing families. *American Journal of Orthopsychiatry* 60:337–345.

Wangh, M. (1962). The evocation of a proxy: a psychological manoeuvre, its use as a defence, its purposes and genesis. *Psychoanalytic Study of the Child* 17:451–469. New York: International Universities Press.

Watzlawick, P., Beavin, J. H., and Jackson, D. D. (1967). *Pragmatics of Human Communication*. New York: Norton.

Weiner, N. (1954). *The Human Use of Human Beings: Cybernetics and Society*. New York: Doubleday.

Whitaker, C.A. (1946). Ormsby Village: an experiment with forced psychotherapy in the rehabilitation of the delinquent adolescent. *Psychiatry* 9 (3): 239–250.

———. (1947). Induced regressive behavior as therapy for adults. American Orthopsychiatric Association, unpublished with movie.

———. (1958). Psychotherapy with couples. *American Journal of Psychotherapy* 12 (1): 18–23.

Whitaker, C. A., Felder, R. E., and Warkentin, J. (1965). Countertransference in the family treatment of schizophrenia. In *Intensive Family Therapy*, ed. I. Boszormenyi-Nagy and J. L. Framo. New York: Brunner/Mazel.

Whitaker, C. A., and Keith, D. V. (1981). Symbolic-experiential family therapy. In *Handbook of Family Therapy*, ed. A. S. Gurman and D. P. Kniskern, pp. 187–225. New York: Brunner/Mazel.

Whitaker, C. A., Warkentin, J., and Malone, T. P. (1959). The involvement of the professional therapist. In *Case Studies in Counseling and Psychotherapy*. Englewood Cliffs, NJ: Prentice Hall.

White, M. (1991). Deconstruction and therapy. *Dulwich Centre Newsletter* 3:21–40.

White, M., and Epston, D. (1990). *Narrative Means to Therapeutic Ends*. New York: Norton.

White, R. (1963). Ego and reality in psychoanalytic theory. *Psychological Issues, Monograph 11* 3(3). New York: International Universities Press.

Whitehead, A. N., and Russell, B. (1910). *Principia Mathematica*. Cambridge, England: Cambridge University Press.

Wilkinson, M. (1992). How do we understand empathy systemically? *Journal of Family Therapy* 14:193–205.

Winnicott, D. W. (1949). Hate in the countertransference. *International Journal of Psycho-Analysis* 30:69–74.

———. (1952). Psychoses and child care. In *Through Paediatrics to Psycho-Analysis*, pp. 219–228. New York: Basic Books, 1975.

———. (1960). The theory of the parent-infant relationship. *International Journal of Psycho-Analysis* 41:585–595.

———. (1963a). From dependence toward independence in the development of the individual. In *The Maturational Processes and the Facilitating Environment*, pp. 83–92. New York: International Universities Press, 1965.

———. (1963b). The development of the capacity for concern. In *The Maturational Processes and the Facilitating Environment*, pp. 73–82. New York: International Universities Press, 1965.

———. (1965a). Ego distortion in terms of true and false self. In *The Maturational Processes and the Facilitating Environment*, pp. 140–152. London: Hogarth.

———. (1965b). *The Maturational Processes and the Facilitating Environment*. London: Hogarth.

———. (1969). The use of an object and relating through identifications. In *Playing and Reality*, ed. D. W. Winnicott. New York: Basic Books, 1971.

Wolf, E. (1966). Learning theory and psychoanalysis. *British Journal of Medical Psychology* 39:1–10.

———. (1988). *Treating the Self: Elements of Clinical Self Psychology*. New York: Guilford.

Wynne, L. C. (1965). Some indications and contraindications for exploratory family therapy. In *Intensive Family Therapy: Theoretical and Practical Applications*, ed. I. Boszormenyi-Nagy and J. L. Framo, pp. 289–322. New York: Brunner/Mazel.

Wynne, L. C., Ryckoff, I. R., Day, J., and Hirsch, S. I. (1958). Pseudo-mutuality in the family relations of schizophrenics. *Psychiatry* 21:205–220.

Zinner, J., and Shapiro, R. L. (1972). Projective identification as a mode of perception and behavior in families of adolescents. In *Foundations of Object Relations Family Therapy*, ed. J. S. Scharff, pp. 109–126. Northvale, NJ: Jason Aronson, 1991.

———. (1974). The family group as a single psychic entity: implications for acting out in adolescence. In *Foundations of Object Relations Family Therapy*, ed. J. S. Scharff, pp. 187–202. Northvale, NJ: Jason Aronson, 1991.

CREDITS

Index

ABOUT THE AUTHOR

Daniel A. Bochner, Ph.D., is currently practicing in the United States Navy where he is the department head of the Mental Health Unit at Parris Island in South Carolina. As a naval psychologist, in addition to providing individual, couple, family, and group treatment, he is responsible for providing clinical supervision, critical incident stress debriefing, stress management seminars, and divorce mediation. As a member of the adjunct faculty at the Savannah Campus of the Georgia School of Professional Psychology, he teaches counseling theory and leads a clinical seminar. Dr. Bochner has been working with families since 1987 in community mental health centers, psychiatric facilities, and in the Navy. He studied under Stephen J. Schultz, Ph.D. (author of the book *Family Systems Thinking*) at the California School of Professional Psychology, Berkeley/Alameda, where his primary focus was on the application of psychoanalytic theories to family treatment. Dr. Bochner currently resides in Savannah, Georgia.